1 MONTH OF
FREE
READING

at
www.ForgottenBooks.com

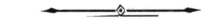

By purchasing this book you are eligible for one month membership to ForgottenBooks.com, giving you unlimited access to our entire collection of over 1,000,000 titles via our web site and mobile apps.

To claim your free month visit:
www.forgottenbooks.com/free157043

ISBN 978-0-483-14163-6
PIBN 10157043

PRINCIPLES AND PRACTICE

OF

MODERN OTOLOGY

BY

JOHN F. BARNHILL, M. D.

PROFESSOR OF OTOLOGY, LARYNGOLOGY, AND RHINOLOGY, INDIANA UNIVERSITY
SCHOOL OF MEDICINE; OTOLOGIST AND LARYNGOLOGIST TO
DEACONESS AND STATE COLLEGE HOSPITALS, ETC.

AND

ERNEST deWOLFE WALES, B. S., M. D.

ASSOCIATE PROFESSOR OF OTOLOGY, LARYNGOLOGY, AND RHINOLOGY, INDIANA UNIVERSITY
SCHOOL OF MEDICINE; FORMER ASSISTANT IN OTOLOGY, HARVARD MEDICAL
SCHOOL; FORMER ASSISTANT AURAL SURGEON, MASSACHUSETTS
CHARITABLE EYE AND EAR INFIRMARY, ETC.

WITH 305 ORIGINAL ILLUSTRATIONS, MANY IN COLORS

PHILADELPHIA AND LONDON

W. B. SAUNDERS COMPANY

1907

PRESS OF
W. B. SAUNDERS COMPANY

ENGLISH SPEAKING STUDENTS AND PRACTITIONERS OF

INE THIS VOLUME IS DEDICATED BY THE AUTHORS

PREFACE

In the preparation of this work, which is intended for the use of students and practitioners of general medicine, among others the following objects have been kept in view:

1. To modernize the subject.

The methods of practice in otology have changed so rapidly that much concerning the subject which was only recently accepted as a standard of guidance is now almost entirely obsolete. This statement is especially true of the suppurative affections of the temporal bone, the treatment of which is now based upon a more thorough knowledge of the anatomy of this bone and its environs, upon more accurate diagnostic methods, and upon more nearly correct medical and surgical principles.

The text has been written from the valued personal instruction received from such eminent teachers as J. E. Sheppard of New York, Dundas Grant and Percy Jakins of London, Jansen of Berlin, and Alt of Vienna; from the authors' personal experience as practitioners and teachers; from the opinions of contemporaries gained by active participation in the several American societies devoted to otology; and, lastly, from recent American and European literature. Of the literature, however, no attempt has been made to give a complete digest.

2. To correct certain traditional beliefs.

Several factors have greatly limited the progress of otology in the past. Chief among these are the strangely persistent beliefs that children will outgrow their aural ailments, and that a discharging ear is nothing more than an annoyance, or is even beneficial to the individual. Since neither belief has any basis in fact, and since abundant clinical and postmortem evidence proves the absurdity of both, the effort has been made to point out the far-reaching and harmful results of these traditions, and in their stead—

3. To advocate the earliest possible prophylaxis or treatment.

While much, but not too much, attention has recently been given to the surgical aspect of otology, certainly too little has been paid to the prevention of aural affections. Throughout this entire work, therefore, on all proper occasions, the fact is stated that prevention of aural diseases is usually easy in early childhood, whereas benefit or cure as a result of treatment in later life is often impossible.

4. To emphasize the importance of a thorough examination and a definite diagnosis as a basis for rational treatment.

Empiricism in both diagnosis and treatment have heretofore played too large a part in the practice of otology. Since success in the practice of this branch of medicine depends almost wholly upon correct diagnosis, the methods of investigation into the nature of aural diseases are given in detail, and their practice is insisted upon in every case, however simple it may appear.

5. To thoroughly illustrate the text.

The preparation of the illustrations has been given the greatest care. A large number of the drawings have been made by Mr. H. F. Aitken,—some directly from the anatomic specimen and others from the actual patient during the progress of an examination, treatment, or surgical operation,—a few are schematic, and only a very few have been copied. The instruments shown are those in daily use by the authors. Therefore, some are bent and apparently misshapen,—a form necessary in actual practice to meet the requirements of some individual case. While, therefore, they do not have that stiff and precise shape of the mechanical drawings usually shown in works on otology, it is believed that the illustrations of tools that have been taken directly from active service are better suited to a practical work of this kind.

Thanks are due to Mr. H. F. Aitken for his faithful and painstaking work in illustration; to Harvard University for the loan of the several most excellent specimens showing the ravages of suppurative necrosis of the temporal bone, and to Mr. Willard C. Greene who faithfully photographed the same; to Mr. John Nicholson and the Stafford Engraving Company, who executed the photography and art work in the representation of many subjects and instruments; to Dr. Paul B. Coble, who has read the proof; and, lastly, to the publishers upon whom devolved the final task of producing a masterpiece in bookmaking.

The first three chapters and the pathology have been prepared by Dr. Wales; the balance of the work by Dr. Barnhill.

INDIANAPOLIS, *October,* 1907.

CONTENTS

CHAPTER VI

CHAPTER VII

CHAPTER VIII

CHAPTER IX

CHAPTER X

CHAPTER XI

CHAPTER XVIII

The Watch Test, The Voice Test, Politzer's Acumeter, Tuning-fork, The Schwabach Test, Weber's Test, Rinné's Test.
Summary of the Various Tuning-fork Tests and of the Interpretation of the Results Obtained from Each, or from All Used Collectively.

CHAPTER XIX

Adenoids—Diagnosis, Treatment.

Preliminary Remarks.

CHAPTER XX

Acute Myringitis—Symptoms, Diagnosis, Treatment.
Chronic Myringitis—Symptoms, Treatment.
Injuries to the Membrana Tympani—Symptoms, Treatment.

CHAPTER XXI

Causation, Pathology, Symptoms, Diagnosis, Prognosis, Treatment.

CHAPTER XXII

Causation, Symptoms, Prognosis, Treatment.

CHAPTER XXIII

Causation, Pathology, Symptoms, Prognosis, Treatment.
Differential Diagnosis of Acute Tubotympanic Catarrh, Acute Catarrhal Otitis Media, and Acute Suppurative Otitis Media.

CHAPTER XXIV

Causation.
Diagnosis—The Physical Condition of the Patient, the External Manifestations over the Mastoid Region, Changes at Inner End of Auditory Canal, Membrana Tympani, and in the Middle Ear.
Prognosis, Treatment.

CHAPTER XXV

CHAPTER XXVI

CHAPTER XXVII

CHAPTER XXVIII

CHAPTER XXIX

CHAPTER XXX

CHAPTER XXXI

CHAPTER XXXII

CHAPTER XXXIII

CHAPTER XXXIV

CHAPTER XXXV

CHAPTER XXXVI

CHAPTER XXXVII

CHAPTER XXXVIII

CHAPTER XXXIX

CHAPTER XLVII

CHAPTER XLVIII

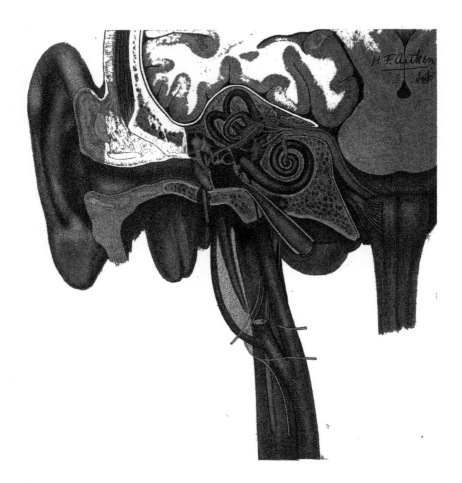

Fig. 1.— Diagram to Show Relations of Organ of Hearing to Brain, Blood-vessels, and Nerves.
(Wales)

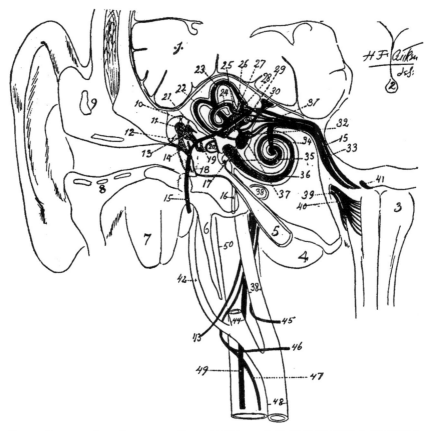

Fig. 1.—Diagram to Show Relations of Organ of Hearing to Brain, Blood-vessels, and Nerves.
(Wales.)

1, Cerebrum; 2, third ventricle; 3, medulla oblongata; 4, condyle; 5, Eustachian tube; 6, styloid process; 7, mastoid process; 8, fissura Santorini; 9, cut cartilage of auricle; 10, superior ligament of malleus; 11, head of malleus; 12, external ligament; 13, body of incus; 14, chorda tympani nerve; 15, facial nerve; 16, aqueductus cochleæ; 17, saccule; 18, drum membrane; 19, stapedius nerve; 20, stapes in vestibular window; 21, superior ligament of incus; 22, cerebral semicircular canal; 23, cerebellar semicircular canal; 24, tympanomastoid semicircular canal; 25, ampullary branch of vestibular nerve to 24 ampulla; 26, utricle; 27, ampullary branch of vestibular nerve to 22 ampulla; 28, ampullary branch of vestibular nerve to 23 ampulla; 29, utricular branch; 30, saccus endolymphaticus; 31, vestibular nerve; 32, saccular branch; 33, auditory nerve; 34, cochlear nerve; 35, membrane of cochlear window; 36, ductus cochlearis; 37, ductus utriculosaccularis; 38, internal carotid artery; 39, hypoglossal nerve; 40, glossopharyngeal nerve; 41, abducens nerve; 42, occipital artery; 43, spinal accessory nerve; 44, external carotid artery; 45, glossopharyngeal nerve; 46, hypoglossal nerve; 47, descending branch of the hypoglossal nerve; 48, common carotid artery; 49, pneumogastric nerve; 50, internal jugular vein.

THE PRINCIPLES AND PRACTICE

OF

OTOLOGY

CHAPTER I

ANATOMY OF THE TEMPORAL BONE

Introduction.—The temporal bone is one of the most important and most interesting bones in the human skull. Imbedded within its substance are the endings of the eighth nerve, which spread out, forming the complex labyrinth, the cochlear portion of this nerve passing to the organ of hearing and the vestibular portion passing to the organ of equilibration. The temporal bone contains a portion of the carotid artery. Along its intracranial surfaces and borders courses the sigmoid portion of the lateral sinus, ending at the jugular bulb, which forms the jugular fossa; also the petrosal sinuses, and at its apex the cavernous sinus. The Gasserian ganglion of the fifth nerve rests in a hollow near the apex. Descending with the jugular vein are the glossopharyngeal, the vagus, and the spinal accessory nerves. Roughly speaking, its whole inner surface is in contact with the dura, covering a portion of the cerebrum and cerebellum, while its outer surface is covered with muscles; the temporal bone gives origin to eleven muscles and insertion to three (Macalister), according to Gray, fifteen muscles. The temporal bone is in relation to the capsule of the jaw and to the parotid gland.

The first gill cleft (tubotympanal sinus) projects from the pharynx and forms the middle ear; the middle ear includes the Eustachian tube, the tympanic cavity, and the antrum with its mastoid cells; these structures, with the exception of the fibrocartilaginous portion of the Eustachian tube, all lie within the temporal bone. The tympanic portion of the middle ear contains the ossicles with their muscles and ligaments, forming the accommodative apparatus of the organ of hearing and connecting the internal ear with the external ear. The tympanic space lies between the petrous portion and the squamotympanic portion of the temporal bone.

The endings of the eighth nerve are incased within very hard, dense bone. External to the internal ear is the middle-ear space, which is well protected from injury by the squamotympanic portion of the temporal bone with its covering of muscles and fasciæ. Even the auricle acts as a protective pad. Holding the lower half of the skull before a strong light, certain parts will appear translucent and other parts opaque (Fig. 2). The petrous portion of the temporal bone acts as a column of support. This denser section of bone passes from the dense bone around the foramen magnum to the plane of the mastoid process, and helps protect the base of the brain, with its vessels, from injury.

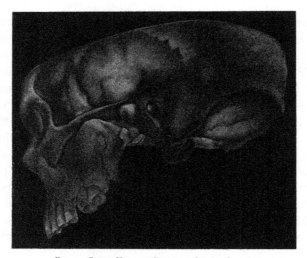

FIG. 2.—SKULL HELD UP BEFORE A STRONG LIGHT.

Note the thin (lighter) portions of the central portion of the squamous portion of the temporal bone, the glenoid fossa, the tegmen tympani, and the occipital bone covering the posterior brain fossa below the lateral sinus.

From the fact that the temporal bone contains and is surrounded by these important structures, the otologist must have a practical knowledge of its anatomy; primarily to save life and secondarily to preserve the hearing. To obtain this practical knowledge it is well to own several infant and adult bones for study and reference. With a jeweler's saw make seven to ten horizontal sections of an adult temporal bone (Figs. 3 and 4); then make vertical sections of another. The student should then study the structure of the different sections, noting the relations of its cavities with neighboring dura, sinus, nerves, or blood-vessels; note the difference between cortical bone and bone in contact with the dura; also note carefully the great differences between the adult bone and the infant temporal bone. Under instruction perform the different mastoid operations on wet specimens of both the adult and infant temporal bones. For anatomic detail the student is referred to the works of Schwalbe and Siebenmann, Zuckerkandl, Testut, Söndermann, Katz, Preysing, Shambaugh, and Körner.

Position of the Temporal Bone in the Skull.—The temporal bone occupies the lower middle third of the side of the skull and articulates with five cranial bones. The temporal bone in the infant consists

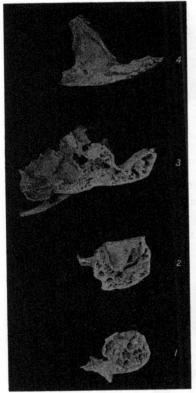 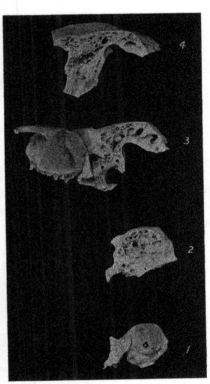

FIG. 3.—HORIZONTAL SECTIONS THROUGH ADULT TEMPORAL BONE, VIEWED FROM ABOVE.

FIG. 4.—HORIZONTAL SECTIONS THROUGH ADULT TEMPORAL BONE, VIEWED FROM BELOW.

Figs. 3 and 4 are views of the same temporal bone.

of three parts, which may be separated several months after birth. These are the squamous, the tympanic, and the petrous portions. These parts are united by fibrous tissue at birth. This fibrous tissue ossifies toward the end of the first year of life, sometimes later. The squamous and tympanic portions are produced from fibrocartilage, the petrous and styloid portions from cartilage. The temporal bone is weakened by the middle-ear cavities, the carotid canal, and by the external and internal auditory canals. Fractures of the skull are apt to follow these natural passages, transversely through the external and internal auditory meati, or longitudinally through the middle ear, depending on the direction of the blow, whether on the side or the back of the head.[1]

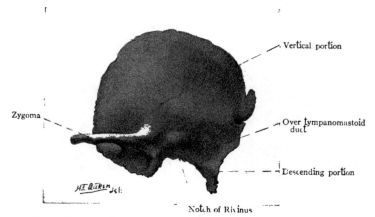

FIG. 5.—EXTERNAL SURFACE OF THE LEFT SQUAMOUS BONE OF INFANT.

The Squamous Portion of the Temporal Bone.—The squamous portion forms a part of the cranial box and articulates with the parietal, a small portion of the frontal, and the great wing of the sphenoid bone. Anteriorly its zygomatic process articulates with the malar bone. The

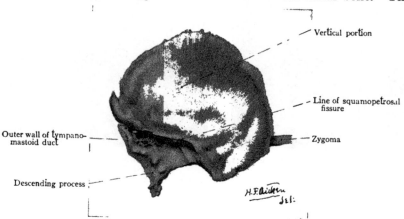

FIG. 6.—INNER VIEW OF THE LEFT SQUAMOUS BONE OF INFANT.

squamous portion is like an inverted letter T on coronal section, the elliptic part forming the stem. The elliptic, or vertical portion (Figs. 5 and 6), is thinner in its central portion than toward the periphery. Its

[1] Read Dr. A. Passow's book on "Die Verletzungen der Gehörorganes."

outer surface is greater than the inner surface, since its inner surface is beveled and overlaps the parietal bone. The inner surface forms a part of the outer boundary of the middle cranial fossa. The middle meningeal artery deeply grooves this inner surface. The basal horizontal part of the squamous bone is broader anteriorly and vanishes to the thin vertical portion posteriorly, like a wedge (Fig. 7). Its inner horizontal basal portion extends inwardly to join the external or tegmental border of the petrous bone and thus forms the squamopetrosal fissure. This fissure is important at birth, since it contains the squamopetrous sinus, which rarely persists; here, too, the dura with blood-vessels dips into the fissure and communicates with the mucous membrane of the middle ear. The inner horizontal portion of the squamous bone helps in the formation of the outer part of the tegmen over the middle ear. Beneath the anterior part of the horizontal portion or base of the inverted T is the glenoid fossa for the condyle of the lower jaw. The bone in the depth of this fossa is often as thin as paper. Posterior to the glenoid

Tip of descending portion of squama   Notch of Rivinus   Glenoid fossa

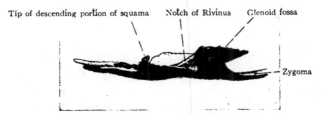

Zygoma

FIG. 7.—LEFT SQUAMOUS PORTION OF TEMPORAL BONE OF INFANT, VIEWED FROM BELOW.

fossa is the posterior articular tubercle. This tubercle varies greatly in its development. Sometimes it is so strongly developed that it forms a barrier against which the jaw would fracture; again it is so weakly developed that a blow on the jaw would fracture the skull.[1]

Posterior to the glenoid fossa is that part of the squamous bone which forms the roof of the external auditory meatus. The distance between the inner horizontal plate and the roof of the external auditory meatus varies from 2 to 14 mm. (see Fig. 263). When the lamellæ are close together the brain lies close to the roof of the external auditory meatus, whereas when pneumatic cells develop between the lamellæ the thickness may reach 14 mm. The higher the attic of the tympanic cavity the thicker the bone between the brain and the roof of the external auditory meatus. Posterior to the meatal portion is the descending plate of the squamous bone, which in the infant forms the lid, covering the external wall of the antrum (tympanomastoid duct).[2] As the pneumatic cells which lie

[1] "Die Verletzungen der Gehörorganes," von Dr. A. Passow, S. 36.
[2] In this book mastoid antrum, antrum, and tympanomastoid duct are synonymous.

on the inner surface of the descending plate develop along with the development of the bony external auditory meatus, the antrum lies deeper from the cortex, so that in the adult the antrum lies from 15 to 30 mm. from the cortical surface instead of 1 or 2 mm., as in the infant at birth. The posterior part of the outer horizontal portion of the squamous bone begins at the posterior part of the vertical portion of the squamous bone near the angle of the incisura parietalis, and widens as it extends anteriorly over the external auditory meatus, forming the linea temporalis or supramastoid crest (Fig. 8). This crest broadens ante-

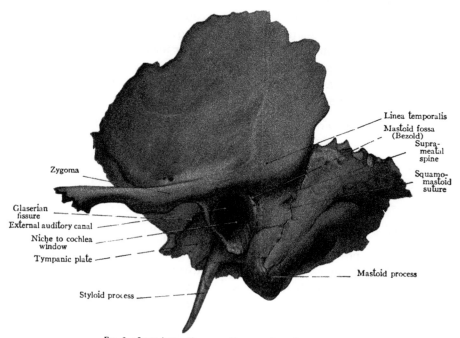

FIG. 8.—LEFT ADULT TEMPORAL BONE, TO SHOW LANDMARKS.

riorly into a process called the zygoma. Beneath the linea temporalis at the upper posterior part of the external auditory meatus is the spine of the suprameatus or spine of Henle. This spine is often wanting. The mastoid fossa is triangular in shape, about the size of the ball of the thumb. The mastoid fossa is bounded above by the linea temporalis, anteriorly by the posterior upper wall of the meatus, and posteriorly, in the infant, by the squamomastoid fissure. This fissure closes in the adult, as a rule, but is present in 37 per cent. of adult temporal bones, according to Sato. The linea temporalis usually lies somewhat deeper than the floor of the middle fossa. A hole drilled from the center of the mastoid fossa parallel to the upper posterior wall of the external auditory canal is the most direct route to the mastoid antrum (tympano-mastoid duct).   A line drawn from the incisura parietalis to the tip of

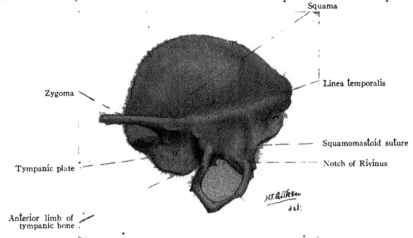

FIG. 9.—SQUAMOTYMPANIC PORTION OF LEFT TEMPORAL BONE OF INFANT, EXTERNAL VIEW.

the mastoid is called Macewen's line, and in the adult it passes through the anterior border, the middle, or the posterior border of the sigmoid sinus.   This line in the infant is far anterior to the sigmoid sinus.

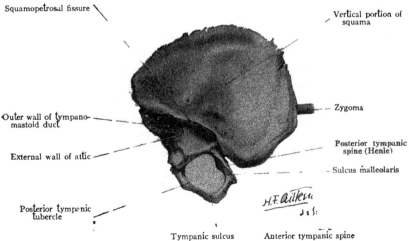

FIG. 10.—INNER VIEW OF SQUAMOTYMPANIC PORTION OF LEFT TEMPORAL BONE OF INFANT.

The Tympanic Bone (Fig. 9).—The tympanic portion of the temporal bone in the infant is shaped like a ring open above and anteriorly. The inner part of the ring, or annulus tympanicus, is grooved and called the tympanic sulcus, which gives attachment to the drum membrane (Figs. 10 and 11).   Anteriorly it is separated from the squamous bone by the Glaserian fissure.   Posteriorly it is separated from the mastoid portion of the petrous bone by the tympanomastoid fissure. The styloid process is directed downward and forward from the most prominent part of the vaginal process of the tympanic bone (see Fig. 8).   In operating upon the bulb the styloid process is an important landmark.   Immediately internal to the styloid process is the jugular bulb.

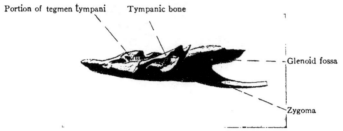

Portion of tegmen tympani   Tympanic bone

Glenoid fossa

Zygoma

FIG. 11.—LEFT SQUAMOTYMPANIC PORTION OF TEMPORAL BONE OF INFANT, VIEWED FROM BELOW.

The Petrous Bone.—The petrous portion is the most important part of the temporal bone.   It is an irregular four-sided pyramid with its oblique base projecting backward, so that it is much larger than the base of a quadrilateral pyramid.   The base forms a small portion of the external surface of the skull and is called the mastoid region (see Fig. 8). The projecting intracranial part of the base is grooved by the sigmoid sinus.   The groove is generally deeper and wider on the right side of the skull than on the left.   At birth there is no mastoid process, nothing but a small tubercle (Fig. 12), which slowly develops until about the third year it assumes the adult type.   The apex of the quadrilateral pyramid is directed forward and inward to the anterior lacerated foramen.   The pyramid has an upper, a lower, an inner, and an outer border.   Two of its surfaces are intracranial and two are extracranial. The intracranial surfaces face upward, the extracranial surfaces face downward.   The intracranial surfaces are called the anterior upper or cerebral surface, and the posterior upper or cerebellar surface. The extracranial surfaces are called the anterior lower or tympanic surface, and the posterior lower or jugular surface.   The base or mastoid region is five sided in shape and projects beyond the base of the pyramid, forming an intracranial surface.   The base is rough externally. It is bounded above by the parietomastoid suture; anteriorly by the squamomastoid suture and tympanomastoid fissure; a lower border to which the digastric muscle is attached and a posterior border bounded by the occipitomastoid suture. The mastoid process varies greatly in size and shape. Its tip is usually directed forward and downward. Into its outer rough surface the sternocleidomastoid, the splenius capitis, and the trachelomastoid muscles are attached. Internal to the mastoid tip is the digastric fossa, to which the digastric muscle is attached; behind this is a ridge which is sometimes so greatly developed that it resembles a second mastoid tip. Internal to this ridge is the groove for the occipital artery. The stylomastoid foramen lies at the anterior end of the digastric groove behind the styloid process. Near the occipitomastoid suture, and sometimes within it, are from one to five holes—as a rule only one or two—called the mastoid foramina.

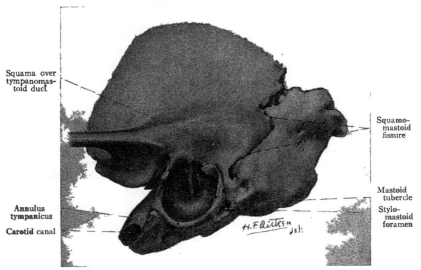

Squama over tympanomastoid duct

Annulus tympanicus

Carotid canal

Squamomastoid fissure

Mastoid tubercle

Stylomastoid foramen

H.F.Aitken Del:

FIG. 12.—LEFT TEMPORAL BONE OF INFANT.

That part of the base which is intracranial is concave and forms the anterolateral portion of the posterior fossa.

Mastoid Process.—The mastoid process makes up the base of the petrous portion and forms the posterior and the lower part, while the squamous portion forms the anterior and upper part (Fig. 13). The anterior border is thick and rounded and generally vertical. The infant at birth has no mastoid process. At the age of three years the mastoid process assumes the adult type and continues to grow till it attains the full development of the adult mastoid (see Fig. 36). Above and anterior to the squamomastoid suture in the infant at birth is the cavity of the antrum (tympanomastoid duct of Söndermann), and this is the important landmark in opening the infant antrum. Posterior and below this suture is the cartilaginous bone of the petrous bone containing the semicircular canals. Below and apparently about the middle of the posterior arm of the tympanic ring appears the exit of the facial nerve (see Fig. 12). In the adult the squamomastoid suture loses its surgical importance, and in those cases where it persists extends from the parietal notch obliquely across the mastoid in the direction of the tip. By the development of the mastoid cells from the floor of the antrum (petrous portion) and the development of the cells forming the external cover of the antrum (squamous portion) this suture moves downward and

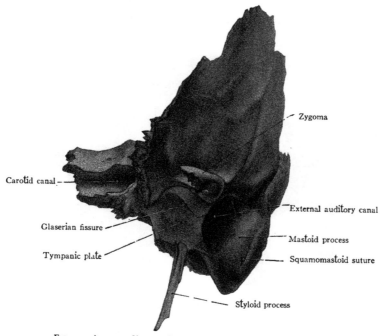

FIG. 13.—ANTERIOR VIEW OF LEFT ADULT TEMPORAL BONE.

backward. The periosteum is often closely adherent and dips into this suture.

The mastoid cells may be pneumatic (36.8 per cent.), diploetic (20 per cent.), or a combination of pneumatic and diploetic (43 per cent.). By pathologic changes the bone may become compact and hard like ivory. The size of the adult mastoid process is variable, depending on the size and the position of the sigmoid sinus in its relation to the external auditory canal (see Fig. 18). The depth is also variable. The depth of the antrum varies from 2 to 30 mm. from the mastoid fossa. To find the antrum, enter the mastoid fossa below the linea temporalis and chisel in a direction parallel to the upper posterior wall of the external auditory canal. Operate in every case as if the most dangerous condition existed; that is, as if the sinus came close to the external auditory canal. The cortex of the mastoid may be thin as paper or it may be very thick and hard (6 mm.).

PNEUMATIC CELLS IN THE TEMPORAL BONE OF THE INFANT

In the infant the cellular construction is not so extensively developed as in the adult. · The bony cells extend from the floor of the tympanic

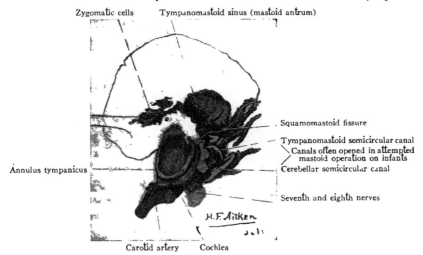

Fig. 14.—View of Tympanic or Anterior Inferior Surface of Infant Left Temporal Bone from a Corrosion. (Prepared by Wales.)

cavity along the tegmen, around the Eustachian tube, and around the antrum (tympanomastoid duct). This development is well shown in

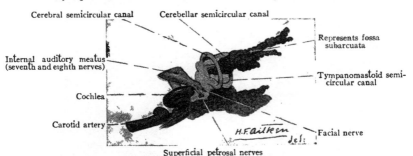

Fig. 15.—View of Cerebral or Anterior Superior Surface of Infant Left Temporal Bone from a Corrosion. (Prepared by Wales.)

corrosions of the infant temporal bone (Figs. 14 to 17). In the adult the growth of pneumatic cells invades the whole substance of the tem-

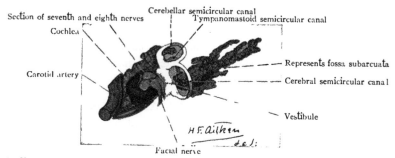

FIG. 16.—VIEW OF CEREBELLAR OR POSTERIOR SUPERIOR SURFACE OF INFANT LEFT TEMPORAL BONE FROM A CORROSION. (Prepared by Wales.)

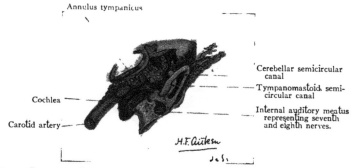

FIG. 17.—VIEW OF JUGULAR OR POSTERIOR INFERIOR SURFACE OF INFANT LEFT TEMPORAL BONE FROM A CORROSION. (Prepared by Wales.)

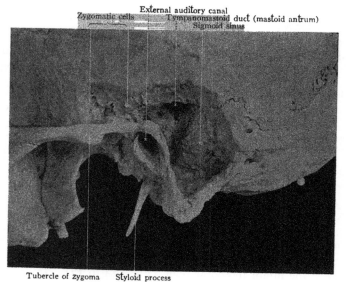

FIG. 18.—SKULL SHOWING GREAT DEVELOPMENT OF ZYGOMATIC CELLS. (Wales.)

poral bone except over the cerebral and tympanomastoid semicircular canals, the promontory, and around the internal and external auditory meatus. The mastoid cells vary in size in the adult. A large cell at the mastoid tip is common. The cells sometimes invade the zygoma and the squamous part of the temporal bone (Fig. 18). The cells may also extend around the Eustachian tube and the carotid canal. Another group of cells extends between the sigmoid sinus and the facial canal to the bulb of the jugular; the cells extend backward toward the occiput; they often extend downward to join the cells of the occipital bone and communicate with the sphenoid sinus and nasopharynx. These cells are lined by mucous membrane, which in turn may divide the bony mastoid cells.

THE PETROUS BONE

The *cerebral,* or *superior anterior surface of the petrous bone,* forms the posterior part of the floor of the middle fossa (Fig. 19). Near its apex is the hollow for the Gasserian ganglion of the fifth nerve. The

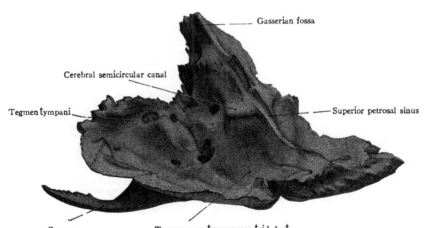

FIG. 19.—THE SUPERIOR ANTERIOR OR CEREBRAL SURFACE OF THE ADULT PETROUS BONE.

greater superficial petrosal nerve passes forward from the hiatus Fallopii in a small groove to the anterior lacerated foramen (Fig. 20); a smaller hole, external to the hiatus Fallopii, gives exit to the lesser petrosal nerve, a continuation of the tympanic nerve. This nerve runs parallel to the great superficial petrosal nerve. The eminentia arcuata is the outcropping of the superior cerebral semicircular canal. External to this eminence is the tegmen tympani and antri. This part of the cerebral surface may be thin as paper or may be entirely lacking in parts (dehiscences).   These dehiscences are filled in with fibrous tissue and hence may become pus channels connecting the cerebral fossa with the middle

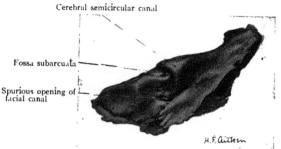

FIG. 20.—SUPERIOR ANTERIOR OF CEREBRAL SURFACE OF LEFT PETROUS PORTION OF INFANT TEMPORAL BONE.

ear.   External to the tegmen is the petrosquamous suture.   In the infant the suture is like a fissure, filled in with fibrous tissue and pierced by blood-vessels.

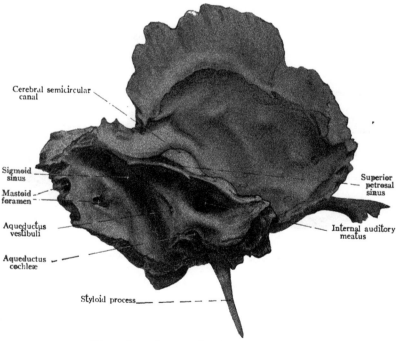

FIG. 21.—INNER ASPECT OF LEFT ADULT TEMPORAL BONE.
Showing landmarks of the posterior superior or cerebellar surface of petrous portion of temporal bone.

The Cerebellar Surface of the Petrous Bone.—The cerebellar, or posterior superior surface, is in relation to the cerebellum and forms the anterolateral wall of the cerebellar fossa (Fig. 21). Nearer the superior border than the inferior border and about midway between the apex and the anterior border of the sigmoid sulcus is the internal auditory meatus, which is surrounded by dense bone. Its axis is nearly in a line with that of the external auditory meatus. In the depth of the internal auditory meatus there is a transverse ridge, called crista transversa, dividing the fundus into an upper and lower half (Fig. 22). In the anterior upper half there is a foramen for the passage of the facial nerve; posterior to this is the area vestibularis superior, with several fine openings in which the upper-end branches of the vestibular nerve are conducted to the macula cribrosa superior of the vestibule. The lower half contains a grooved area called the area cochleæ, which contains a broad spiral groove with numerous openings for the branches of the cochlearis nerve, called the tractus spiralis foraminosus. In the posterior part of

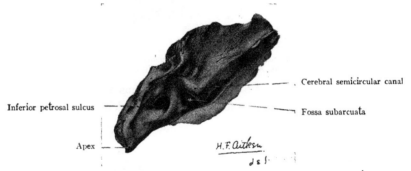

Inferior petrosal sulcus

Apex

Cerebral semicircular canal

Fossa subarcuata

H.F. Aitken

FIG. 22.—SUPERIOR POSTERIOR OR CEREBELLAR SURFACE OF LEFT PETROUS BONE OF INFANT.

the lower half, near the crista transversa, is a field with small openings, called the area vestibularis inferior, containing fine openings of canals which carry bundles of the vestibular nerve to the macula cribrosa media of the vestibule. Somewhat medially and posterior from this area is a single large hole, called the foramen singulare, which conducts the nerve ampullaris posterior to the macula cribrosa inferior.

The Facial or Fallopian Canal.—The facial canal begins at the internal auditory canal and ends at the stylomastoid foramen and has an opening on the cerebral surface of the petrous bone called the spurious opening (Fig. 23). Since the facial canal is not straight between the entrance and exit, but forms two knee-like bends, it may be divided into three parts (see Fig. 1). The first and shortest section begins at the upper anterior part of the fundus of the internal auditory canal and passes laterally to the spurious opening; here the canal bends posteriorly the inner wall of the tympanic cavity and passes above the vestibular window (at this point a dehiscence is common) till it reaches the eminentia pyramidalis posteriorly; above the canal lies the prominence of the tympanomastoid lateral semicircular canal.   The length of the middle

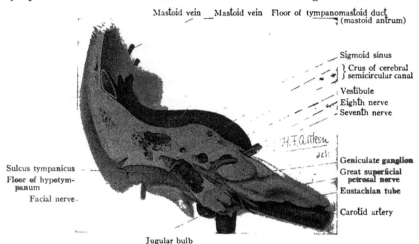

Mastoid vein __ Mastoid vein Floor of tympanomastoid duct (mastoid antrum)

Sigmoid sinus
Crus of cerebral semicircular canal
Vestibule
Eighth nerve
Seventh nerve

H.F.Aitken del:

Geniculate ganglion
Great superficial petrosal nerve
Eustachian tube
Carotid artery

Sulcus tympanicus
Floor of hypotympanum
Facial nerve

Jugular bulb

FIG. 23.—TRANSVERSE SECTION THROUGH RIGHT TEMPORAL BONE, FROM ABOVE.
Berlin Anatomical Institute.   (Wales.)

section of the canal is about 6 mm.   The canal has a medial portion in relation to the labyrinth wall and a lateral wall which projects into the

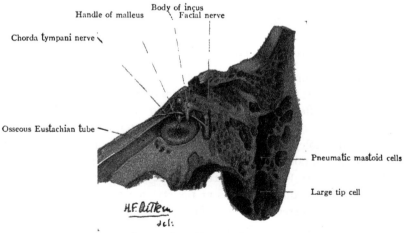

Body of incus
Handle of malleus   \ Facial nerve

Chorda tympani nerve \

Osseous Eustachian tube —

Pneumatic mastoid cells

Large tip cell

H.F.Aitken
del:

FIG. 24.—RIGHT TEMPORAL BONE.
Vertical section through middle ear, viewed from within.

tympanic cavity and is often so thin that the nerve shines through it. This wall is penetrated by a hole through which the stapedial artery, a branch of the stylomastoid artery, passes, and is important on account of disease processes of the middle ear making their way to the facial canal. The third and last section lies between the eminentia pyramidalis and the stylomastoid foramen (Fig. 24). Above the stylomastoid foramen the canal for the chorda tympani nerve is given off, which ends at an opening on the posterior wall of the tympanic cavity behind the sulcus of the membrana tympani.

The size of the spurious opening varies greatly; sometimes it is so wide that on detaching the dura mater the geniculate ganglion is visible, while in other cases it is so small that it is hard to find.

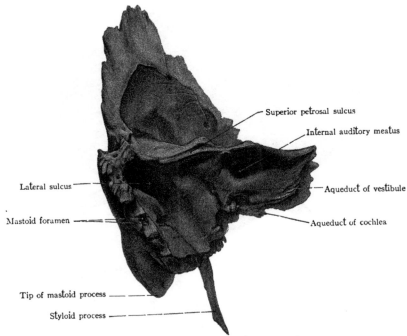

Superior petrosal sulcus

Internal auditory meatus

Lateral sulcus

Aqueduct of vestibule

Mastoid foramen

Aqueduct of cochlea

Tip of mastoid process

Styloid process

FIG. 25.—ADULT LEFT TEMPORAL BONE, VIEWED FROM BEHIND.

Below the internal auditory meatus is the three-sided aqueductus cochleæ (Fig. 25). The cerebellar surface is shorter than the other two sides and so presents a sulcus. The depth of the aqueductus cochleæ is seen best from the jugular surface of the petrous bone. The aqueductus cochleæ is about 10 mm. long and begins at the floor of the scala tympani in the neighborhood of the cochleæ window. From the jugular surface of the petrous bone the aqueductus cochleæ looks like a bayonet or specula. This canal forms a communication between the perilymphatic fluid of the internal ear and the arachnoid space of the posterior brain fossa. The vena aqueductus cochleæ is relatively of

3

large size and runs in a canal of its own, the canalis accessorius aqueductus cochleæ, and takes the venous blood from all the cochleæ canals, as well as part of the vestibule, and empties into the bulb of the jugular vein.

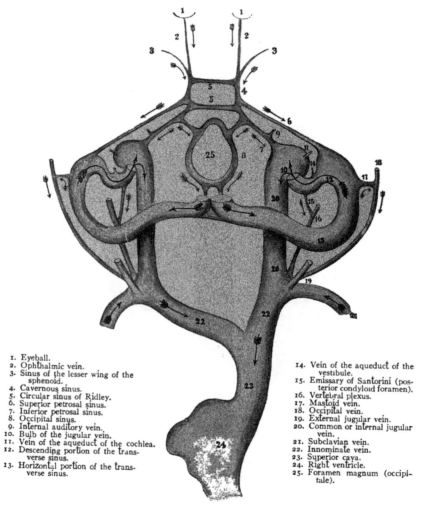

1. Eyeball.
2. Ophthalmic vein.
3. Sinus of the lesser wing of the sphenoid.
4. Cavernous sinus.
5. Circular sinus of Ridley.
6. Superior petrosal sinus.
7. Inferior petrosal sinus.
8. Occipital sinus.
9. Internal auditory vein.
10. Bulb of the jugular vein.
11. Vein of the aqueduct of the cochlea.
12. Descending portion of the transverse sinus.
13. Horizontal portion of the transverse sinus.

14. Vein of the aqueduct of the vestibule.
15. Emissary of Santorini (posterior condyloid foramen).
16. Vertebral plexus.
17. Mastoid vein.
18. Occipital vein.
19. External jugular vein.
20. Common or internal jugular vein.
21. Subclavian vein.
22. Innominate vein.
23. Superior cava.
24. Right ventricle.
25. Foramen magnum (occipitale).

FIG. 26.—DIAGRAM OF THE VENOUS SYSTEM THAT CARRIES OFF THE BLOOD FROM THE INTERIOR OF THE CRANIUM.
Base of the skull, viewed from above and behind. (Bruhl and Politzer.)

Between the internal auditory meatus and the cerebral surface along the superior border of the petrous bone runs the superior petrosal sinus, from the sigmoid sinus to the cavernous sinus. Below this sinus and behind the internal auditory meatus is the fossa subarcuatus, very

large in the infant, tunneling under the cerebral semicircular canals
(see Fig. 22). In the adult bone the fossa subarcuatus is often wanting,
often marked by a small foramen. Behind and below the fossa subarcuatus is the slit-like opening of the aqueductus vestibuli, covered by a
thin plate of bone. The aqueductus vestibuli begins with two thin forked
tubes, one leading from the utricle and the other from the saccule.
These tubes join and form a common tube which is 5 to 6 mm. long,
ending at the hiatus aqueductus vestibuli, where it spreads out toward
the sigmoid sinus into a blind sac about 15 mm. long in the dura mater,
called the saccus endolymphaticus (see Fig. 1). The base of the cerebellar surface ends at the anterior border of the sigmoid sinus; its
borders are nearly surrounded by venous sinuses (Fig. 26).

The Jugular Surface or Inferior Posterior Surface.—This surface is the most irregular of the surfaces of the petrous bone (Fig. 27).

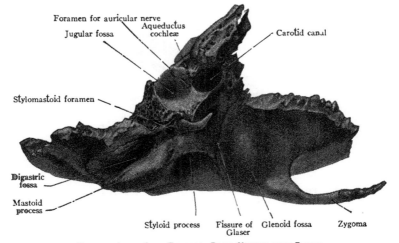

FIG. 27.—ADULT LEFT TEMPORAL BONE, VIEWED FROM BELOW.

The apex is rough and covered by the cartilage of the occipitopetrosal
synchondrosis. About midway between the apex and the base is the oval
opening of the carotid canal. The carotid canal ascends along the anterior wall of the tympanic cavity to the bony wall of the Eustachian tube
and then bends in a horizontal direction, ending at the apex of the petrous
bone. The lateral and upper walls are formed by a thin plate which is
often defective; frequently in detaching the dura from the middle fossa a
long strip of the horizontal portion of the carotid canal is exposed. The
medial wall of the perpendicular ascending portion of the canal forms
the anterior wall of the tympanic cavity. This wall is thin and perforated

by small holes which carry vessels and nerves. This wall is sometimes wanting. If the defect is great the internal carotid artery may project into the tympanic cavity. The horizontal part of this canal is in relation to the cochleæ and is tangent to the first turn of the cochlea. Between the internal carotid artery and its canal there is a network of veins. External to the carotid opening is the vaginal process of the tympanic plate. Just behind the opening is a sharp ridge called the carotid ridge, which separates the carotid and jugular fossæ. The jugular fossa at birth scarcely shows any depression for the bulb of the jugular vein (Fig. 28). The size and extent of this fossa, as well as the thickness of its walls, seems to depend on the size of the jugular. According to Zuckerkandl the fossa is larger on the right side in 54 per cent. of cases than on the left, and of equal size in 14 per cent. If the jugular fossa is deep the cellar of the tympanic cavity is shallow and the floor is often

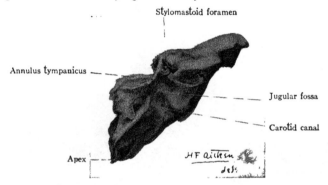

Stylomastoid foramen

Annulus tympanicus

Jugular fossa

Carotid canal

Apex

FIG. 28.—PETROUS PORTION OF LEFT INFANT TEMPORAL BONE.
Showing inferior posterior or jugular surface of petrous bone.

thin as paper. The jugular bulb may project into the tympanic cavity (Fig. 29). Dehiscences sometimes occur, but the danger of cutting the jugular bulb in incising the drum membrane is, according to C. Grunert, as dangerous as the possibility of a falling star striking one's head. By extension of its inner half and by dehiscences the vestibule and the internal auditory canal may be opened, and the jugular bulb is then in relation to the structures of these spaces. If the fossa jugularis is shallow the floor of the tympanic cavity may be from 5 to 6 mm. thick. Most temporal bones appear translucent on holding them up before a light (see Fig. 2). The floor of the tympanic cavity appears light on looking through the external auditory meatus. In the carotid ridge is a minute opening for the tympanic branch of the glossopharyngeal nerve. Behind the vaginal process of the tympanic plate is the styloid process, and behind the styloid process and at the anterior end of the digastic fossa is the Fallopian canal, where the facial nerve leaves the petrous bone. When the jugular fossa is small and insignificant on the jugular surface of the petrous bone the jugular bulb may make

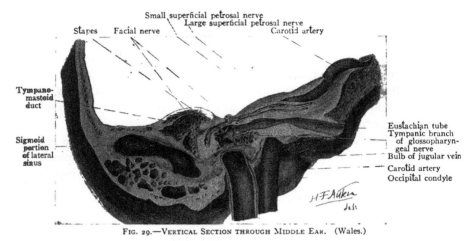

FIG. 29.—VERTICAL SECTION THROUGH MIDDLE EAR. (Wales.)

compensatory room in the occipital bone, thus the size of the jugular fossa does not necessarily indicate the size of the jugular vein.

The Tympanomastoid or Anterior Inferior Surface of the Petrous Bone (Fig. 30).—This wall is the most interesting and important to the

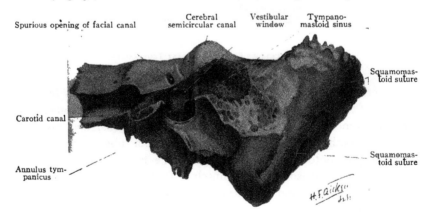

FIG. 30.—ADULT LEFT TEMPORAL BONE.
Squamous portion of temporal bone has been broken off, leaving petrous and tympanic portions.

otologist because it is the operative gateway to the petrous bone and the limiting wall of mastoid and middle-ear operations. On the inner wall of the antrum or tympanomastoid duct is the hard white bone of the tympanomastoid horizontal semicircular canal. This is an important landmark in operations on the mastoid and vestibule. Beneath the semicircular canal is the horizontal portion of the facial canal, and beneath the smooth, thin bony wall containing the facial nerve is the fossa which contains the vestibular window in which the foot-plate of the stapes is attached by fibrous tissue, called the annular ligament. Immediately below and slightly posterior is the tympanic sinus. Projecting over this sinus in its posterior part is the pyramid through which the ligament of the stapedius muscle passes to the head of the stapes. And at the lowest anterior part of this sinus is the niche leading to the cochlea window. The sinus varies in size and sometimes undermines the cerebellar posterior semicircular canal (Fig. 31).

Anterior to the fossa is the promontory, which is formed by the first turn of the cochlea. On the promontory are grooves for the plexus tympanicus. Posterior and inferior to the promontory is the jugular

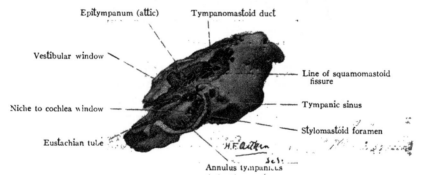

FIG. 31.—LEFT PETROUS PORTION OF INFANT TEMPORAL BONE.
Showing inferior anterior or tympanic surface of petrous bone.

wall covering the jugular bulb. The bulb may mount up as high as the niche of the cochlea window. Immediately beneath the promontory, there are some pneumatic cells, called tympanic cells, and anterior there is a smooth surface leading to the Eustachian tube. Immediately above the promontory and projecting into the tympanic cavity is the bony canal for the tensor tympani muscle. Its termination immediately anterior to the stapes and on a level with the facial canal is called the processus cochleariformis. This bony canal (canalis musculotubarius) lies near the tegmen and runs along the roof to the Eustachian tube. Internal to the opening of the Eustachian tube is a thin bony wall covering the carotid canal (Fig. 32).

The Infant Temporal Bone.—Some of the differences between the adult bone and the infant temporal bone are as follows:

·· In the infant there is no osseous external auditory canal. The mastoid process does not exist. It is indicated by a small tubercle without pneumatic cells. The antrum lies superficially. The fissures petrososquamosa and squamosomastoidea are present. The internal auditory canal is wide and shallow and the landmarks at the fundus of the canal are easily discerned. The contour of the cerebral and cerebellar semicircular canals are more prominent than in the adult. The fossa subarcuata is large. The fossa jugularis is flat. The swollen fetal mucous membrane fills up the tympanic cavity and is slowly absorbed. This process of absorption takes place most slowly on the roof of the tympanic cavity and in the mastoid antrum. The Eustachian

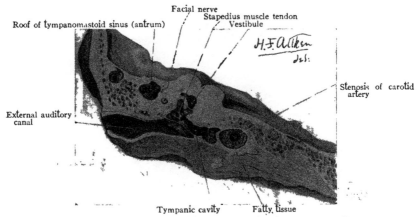

FIG. 32—TRANSVERSE SECTION THROUGH THE LEFT TEMPORAL BONE, FROM BELOW. From a section obtained from the Berlin Anatomical Institute. (Wales.)

tube is relatively wide and short and on a level with the hard palate. Its upper and lower walls lie on each other in the median section. This narrow cleft is filled with loosened and macerated epidermis. The drum membrane is thicker, especially the epidermal layer, and therefore appears cloudy and lustreless.

THE AURICLE

The auricle projects from the side of the head and in man is probably of little use. The auricle is made up of an irregular framework of yellow elastic fibrocartilage covered with perichondrium and skin. The cartilage does not extend into the lobule. Generally concave externally with its upper and posterior edges rolled in, forming the helix. Every concavity is represented on the other side by a convexity and *vice versa*. The skin over the outer part is firmly adherent to the perichondrium by elastic fibers, while on the internal side the skin is loose with considerable fatty tissue beneath the epidermis.

The posterior line of insertion is along the squamomastoid suture, and thus the inferior part of the insertion approaches the inferior wall of the external auditory meatus. The linea temporalis is about on a level with the upper border of the concha, which is formed by the lower arm of the forked portion of the anthelix. In operations on the infant temporal bone the insertion of the auricle and its fibrocartilaginous canal serve as important landmarks in making the first incision and in locating the tympanomastoid duct (antrum). At birth the exit of the facial from its bony canal is close beneath the lower part of the insertion of the auricle.

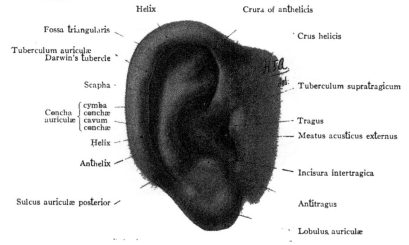

FIG. 33.—RIGHT AURICLE. (Nomenclature after Spalteholz.)

For the names of the different ridges, concavities, and incisures the student is referred to the illustration of the auricle (Fig. 33). These parts are important only in locating exactly the position of a wen or other pathologic process. The cartilage of the auricle extends into the external auditory meatus to help form its fibrocartilaginous canal. Near the concha the cartilage is lacking on the upper wall and on the upper part of the posterior wall of the auditory canal; the cartilage then tapers down to a flat piece attached to the inferior wall of the osseous canal. In the anterior wall of this cartilage are two slits called the incisures of Santorini (see Fig. 1). Through these slits pus may make its way from the external auditory canal or from infections of the parotid gland to the auditory canal. The fascia covering the parotid gland is wanting in this region, as well as a small area in relation to the tonsils, which gives a possible route of infection from the external auditory canal to the throat.

THE EXTERNAL OSSEOUS CANAL

The external osseous canal is developed after birth (Fig. 34). The anterior wall, the inferior wall, and the lower portion of the posterior wall are developed from the tympanic ring (Fig. 35). The upper portion of the posterior wall and the superior wall or roof are developed from the squamous portion of the temporal bone. At the age of three years the development is so much advanced that the canal resembles the adult type (Fig. 36). A small dehiscence is found in the anterior wall, commonly up to the sixth year of life. Sometimes through lack of development the dehiscence persists and becomes a

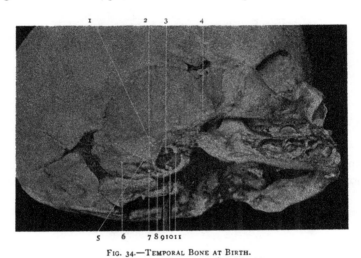

FIG. 34.—TEMPORAL BONE AT BIRTH.
(Warren Museum, Harvard Medical School.)
1, Line of linea temporalis; 2, lid over tympanomastoid duct; 3, notch of Rivinus; 4, zygoma; 5, line of squamopetrosal fissure; 6, petrous bone; 7, mastoid tubercle; 8, stylomastoid foramen; 9, annulus tympanicus; 10, posterior tubercle; 11, anterior tubercle.

possible pus channel for infection to pass from the auditory canal to the articulation of the jaw (Fig. 37). The superior wall is the shortest of the four walls. Above, the superior wall is made up of smooth cortical bone, then comes a thin or thick layer of diploë, and then the harder inner layer lining the middle fossa. In the adult the thickness of the bone between the upper wall of the osseous canal and the middle fossa of the brain varies between 2 and 14 mm. in thickness. The space between these two bony layers may be taken up by pneumatic cells which communicate with the zygoma and the attic of the tympanic cavity. The thicker this wall separating the osseous canal from the brain cavity, the higher the attic becomes, so that in the case of a chronic suppurative otitis media with loss of ossicles the

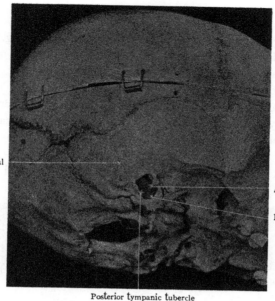

Squamopetrosal suture

Anterior tympanic tubercle

Dehiscence

Posterior tympanic tubercle

FIG. 35.—DEVELOPMENT OF OSSEOUS CANAL.
Child eighteen months old. (Warren Museum, Harvard Medical School.)

thickness of this wall may be judged by the aural probe.   The inner
portion of the upper wall sometimes shuts off a direct view of the vestib-

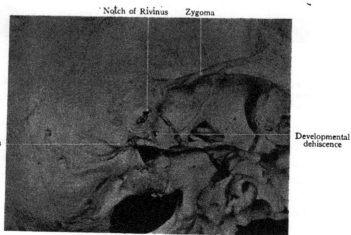

Notch of Rivinus   Zygoma

Mastoid process

Developmental dehiscence

FIG. 36.—DEVELOPMENT OF OSSEOUS CANAL.
Child four years old.   (Warren Museum, Harvard Medical School.)

ular window.   Above this inner portion is the epitympanum or attic,
containing the head of the malleus, articulating with the body of the
incus (see Fig. 1).

The posterior wall of the external auditory canal is in relation to the mastoid cells. This wall may be paper thin to 5 mm. in thickness. The descending portion of the facial canal is in relation to the inner part of the posterior wall and has been named by the surgeon the facial ridge. Rarely the sigmoid sinus comes very close to this wall. The antrum or tympanomastoid duct lies above and posterior to the inner part of the external auditory osseous meatus. Small canaliculi containing blood-vessels make their way from the tympanomastoid duct to the upper posterior part of the osseous meatus, close to the drum membrane, and it is due to these vessels that inflammation is carried from the

Tubercle   External auditory osseous canal

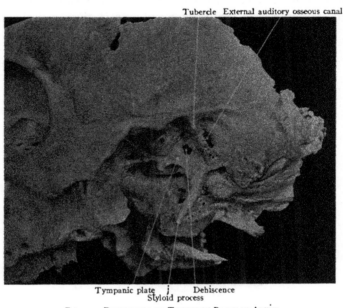

Tympanic plate   Dehiscence
Styloid process
FIG. 37.—DEHISCENCE OF TYMPANUM PLATE IN ADULT.
Pus channel to articulation of jaw and parotid gland.

antrum to the upper posterior part of the canal and manifests itself by redness and bulging in any acute disease of the tympanomastoid duct.

The inferior wall is generally composed of compact bone, rarely containing pneumatic cells. This wall is rarely in relation to the jugular bulb in that portion nearest the drum. The descending portion of the facial canal is at a depth equal to about half the length of this inferior wall. The parotid gland is in relation to the under surface of this inferior wall.

The anterior wall is behind the condyle of the lower jaw and is in relation to the parotid gland. This wall may be paper thin or, through lack of development, it may be perforated.

A sharp instrument or probe carried along the junction of the anterior and superior walls of the auditory canal in a direction parallel to the bone would pierce the drum membrane and tegmen tympani posterior to the horizontal portion of the carotid artery and above the opening of the Eustachian tube, into the middle cranial fossa.

THE DRUM MEMBRANE

The drum membrane lies at the end of the osseous auditory canal and forms the external wall of the tympanic cavity. Since the anterior wall of the external auditory canal is longer and extends further inward than the posterior wall the drum membrane is given a declination of

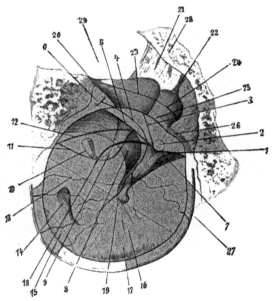

FIG. 38.—THE DRUM-HEAD AND TYMPANIC OSSICLES (Schematic.)

1, Anterior boundary fold; 2, short process of malleus; 3, superior fold; 4, arteria manubrium mallei; 5, posterior boundary fold; 6, branch of deep auricular artery; 7, anterior pouch of tympanic membrane; 8, posterior pouch of tympanic membrane; 9, long process of incus; 10, stapes; 11, tendon of stapedius muscle; 12, chorda tympani; 13, anastomosis of arteria manubrii mallei with peripheral system of blood-vessels; 14, fenestra cochleæ; 15, bulb of jugular vein; 16, cone of light; 17, tympanic cells; 18, posterior fold; 19, umbo; 20, posterior ligament of incus; 21, superior ligament of incus; 22, superior ligament of malleus; 23, lateral fold of incus; 24, lateral fold of malleus; 25, external ligament of malleus; 26, anterior ligament of malleus; 27, peripheral system of blood-vessels; 28, tegmen tympani; 29, threshold of antrum. (Brühl and Politzer.)

50 degrees. Since the inferior wall is longer than the superior wall, the inferior pole lies further inward and the drum membrane is given an inclination of about 45 degrees. Between the lower pole and the inferior wall of the external auditory meatus is the external auditory sinus, where small foreign bodies often lodge and where water gives

the sensation of a bubble in the ear. The drum is not a plane surface, but indrawn like a funnel, the umbo forming the apex. The drum membrane is inserted in a small groove called the annulus tympanicus, except at the upper part of the membrane, where the drum is attached to the squama in the incisura Rivini. The size of the drum membrane varies; it is about 8 mm. wide and 9 mm. high, and normally about $\frac{1}{10}$ mm. thick. In the upper anterior part there is a yellowish-white protuberance, the short process of the malleus, and from this protuberance running downward and slightly backward is the handle of the malleus ending in a spatula-like end, called the umbo. For convenience of description the drum membrane is divided into quadrants. The

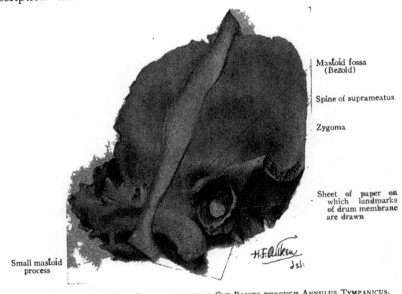

FIG. 39.—ADULT TEMPORAL BONE SECTIONED SO THAT CUT PASSES THROUGH ANNULUS TYMPANICUS.
Cut shows piece of bond paper interposed. Phantom used to teach student to incise drum membrane (Wales).
(See *Transactions of American Otological Society*, 1906.)

anatomic quadrants vary greatly from the pathologic quadrants.[1] A line drawn through the short process and umbo and another straight line at right angles to this passing through the umbo divides the drum membrane into four parts—an anterior upper, an anterior lower, a posterior upper, and a posterior lower quadrant (Fig. 38). The anterior lower quadrant is the smallest anatomic quadrant, the posterior upper quadrant is the largest anatomic quadrant. Behind the anterior upper quadrant lies the opening into the Eustachian tube, the canal for the tensor tympani, and the anterior mucous pouch of the drum. Behind

[1] Passow, "Transactions of the German Otological Society," 1906, p. 203.

the anterior lower quadrant lies the carotid canal. Behind the posterior upper quadrant is the long process of the incus, the stapes in the vestibular window, the pyramid containing the stapedius muscle, the chorda tympani nerve, and the posterior mucous pocket of the drum membrane. Behind the posterior lower quadrant is the niche to the cochlea window and the bulb of the jugular vein. Beneath Shrapnell's membrane is the neck of the malleus and Prussak's space.

The membrana tympani consists of three layers, an outer cutaneous, a middle fibrinous, and an inner mucous layer. The membrana flaccida or Shrapnell's membrane consists of two layers, an outer cutaneous and an inner mucous layer.

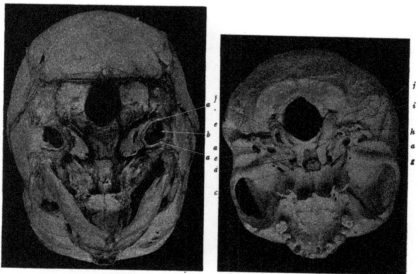

FIG. 39 (a).—INFANT SKULL.   FIG. 39 (b).—ADULT SKULL.

Note position of annulus tympanicus in Fig. 39 (a) and compare with adult in Fig. 39 (b): a, Annulus tympanicus; b, upper border, notch of Rivinus; c, sphenoid sinus; d, probe in basilar process of occipital bone; e, probe; f, condyle fenestrated; g, carotid canal; h, facial canal; i, sigmoid sinus; j, jugular fossa. (Warren Museum, Harvard Medical School.)

The epithelial layer of the drum membrane is made up of layers of flat epithelium with cylindric cells in the deepest layers. The epithelial layer contains blood-vessels and nerves. The fibrous layer consists of an outer radiating layer and an inner circular layer poor in elastic tissue-fibers. The mucous layer consists of simple cuboidal epithelium. This layer as it passes from the drum to the tympanic cavity becomes higher and on the floor of the tympanic cavity the cells are ciliated. The drum membrane of the infant has the same relative position as in the adult and is not more horizontal. This can be seen by comparison (Randall) in Fig. 39 (a) and Fig. 39 (b).

THE OSSICLES

There are three ossicles—the malleus, the incus, and the stapes. The stapes lies in the vestibular window, the malleus lies on the drum membrane; between the stapes and the malleus is the incus. The malleus presents a head lying behind the membrana flaccida and a handle which lies in the drum membrane. Behind the head of the

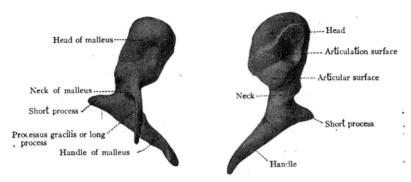

Head of malleus

Neck of malleus

Short process

Processus gracilis or long process

Handle of malleus

Head

Articulation surface

Articular surface

Neck

Short process

Handle

FIG. 40.—THE RIGHT MALLEUS. (Spalteholz.)

malleus there is a figure-of-eight articulation of the incus. The malleus (Fig. 40) has a tooth-like process which locks with the incus when the drum is pushed inward and unlocks when the drum is pushed outward. Anteriorly the neck of the malleus presents a long process, the remains of Meckel's cartilage. Outwardly the short process at the beginning of

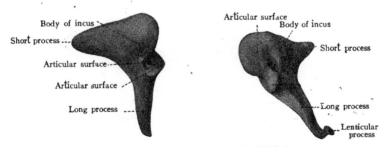

Body of incus

Short process

Articular surface

Articular surface

Long process

Articular surface

Body of incus

Short process

Long process

Lenticular process

FIG. 41.—THE RIGHT INCUS. (Spalteholz.)

the handle projects prominently. Opposite and on the inner aspect of the malleus there is a rough spot for the attachment of the tendon of the tensor tympani muscle.

The incus has somewhat the appearance of a tooth; its head articulates with the head of the malleus (Fig. 41). A short process rests in the fossa incudis, attached by a ligament. Its long process articulates with the stapes. This process is nearly parallel to the handle of the malleus and is often seen through the normal or atrophied drum membrane.

The stapes (Fig. 42) or stirrup consists of a foot-plate which is attached by an annular ligament into the vestibular window (Fig. 43).

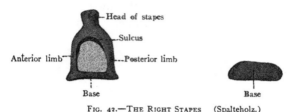

FIG. 42.—THE RIGHT STAPES (Spalteholz.)

From the foot-plate two arms or cruræ arise and join (Fig. 44), forming a neck which slightly swells to form a head. The stapedius muscle, lying in the pyramid, takes origin along the ascending part of the facial canal (Fig. 45). The muscle is about 5 mm. long and is attached to the neck of the stapes by a small ligament. The tensor tympani is

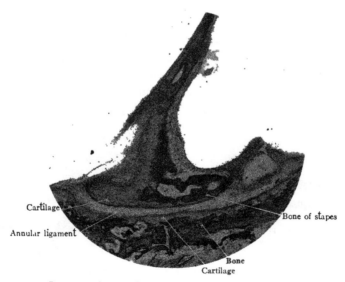

FIG. 43.—PORTION OF ANNULAR LIGAMENT. OSTEOPOROSIS. (Prepared by Wales.)

the antagonist to the stapedius muscle and is four times as long as that muscle, lying in the canalis musculotubarius.

Supporting the ossicles in the tympanic cavity there are five ligaments (see Fig. 1):

Anterior ligament of malleus, superior ligament of malleus, and the

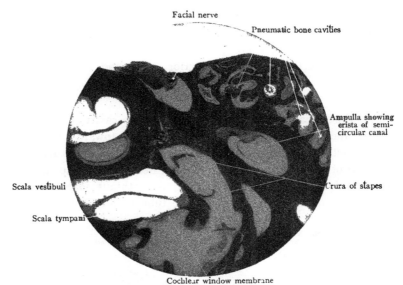

Facial nerve

Pneumatic bone cavities

Ampulla showing crista of semi-circular canal

Scala vestibuli

Crura of stapes

Scala tympani

Cochlear window membrane

FIG. 44.—VERTICAL SECTION THROUGH LEFT TEMPORAL BONE. (Prepared by Wales.)

lateral ligament of the malleus, which passes to the upper edge of the incisura Rivini. The superior ligament of the incus, passing to the

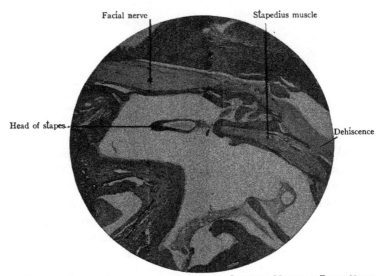

Facial nerve

Stapedius muscle

Head of stapes

Dehiscence

FIG. 45.—VERTICAL SECTION SHOWING RELATION OF STAPEDIUS MUSCLE TO FACIAL NERVE.

tegmen tympani, and the ligament of the short process of the incus, passing to the fossa incudis on the floor of the antrum. Folds of mucous membrane are thrown around the ossicles, their muscles, ligaments,

4

and the chorda tympani nerve forming pockets which are the means of guiding pus to certain parts of the drum membrane (see Fig. 38). Three of these pouches are in contact with the drum membrane, namely, the anterior pouch, the posterior pouch, and Prussak's space.

THE EUSTACHIAN TUBE

The Eustachian tube connects the tympanic cavity with the naso-pharynx and is about 36 mm. long. Its lumen toward the tympanic end is about 4 mm. high and toward the pharyngeal end about 5 mm. One-third of the tube is osseous, that part nearest the tympanic cavity, and two-thirds cartilaginomembranous; the isthmus joins both these parts and is about 2 mm. broad. The tube runs downward, inward,

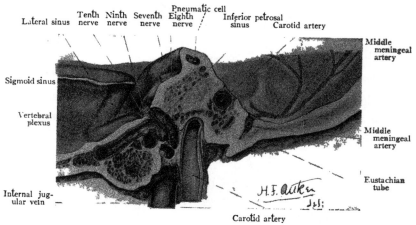

Fig. 46 —Vertical Section to show Relation of Eustachian Tube to Carotid Artery and Middle Meningeal Artery.
Berlin Anatomical Institute. (Specimen of Wales.)

and forward and its ostium pharyngeum lies 25 mm. deeper than the ostium tympani tubæ. Note the relation of the tube to the internal carotid artery and the middle meningeal artery (Fig. 46).

The membranocartilaginous portion consists of a medial carti-laginous part and an outer part made up of connective tissue. The tube passes between the palatine muscles and the tensor palati externus in front, while the levator palati muscle is internal and behind.

The levator palati muscle arises from the lower and outer part of the Eustachian cartilage and from the rough, under side of the apex of the petrous bone in front of the carotid canal. It descends inward and slightly forward to be attached to the soft palate. This muscle is supplied by a branch of the facial nerve, conveyed to the muscle through the great superficial petrosal, Meckel's ganglion, and the posterior palatine nerves.

The tensor palati lies anterior and external, separated from the levator palati muscle by the pharyngeal aponeurosis. It arises from the linear outer margin of the scaphoid fossa, from the spine of the sphenoid, and from the outer surface and lower border of the Eustachian cartilage. As it descends its fibers converge to unite in a tendon which winds round the hamular process, from without inward, passing thence horizontally to be inserted into the transverse ridge on the posterior surface of the palate plate and into the palatine aponeurosis. Beneath the tendon there is a small bursa over the hamular process. The tensor palati muscle is supplied by the inferior maxillary division of the fifth nerve.

The walls of the tube normally are in contact except during swallowing and in some pathologic conditions. The mucous membrane of the Eustachian tube consists of three layers: first, the ciliated epithelium; second, the adenoid layer; third, the glandular layer. All these layers are separated from one another by elastic fiber layers. The cartilage of the tube is elastic cartilage and contains clefts and holes.

THE OSSEOUS LABYRINTH

The three semicircular canals with their ampullæ form a part of the labyrinth. The osseous semicircular canals surround a thin-walled membranous structure called the membranous semicircular canals. The osseous canal consists of compact bone. Its lumen is from $1\frac{1}{2}$ to 2 mm. and on cross-section has an elliptic form. The position of the semicircular canals in the petrous portion of the temporal bone to the rest of the labyrinth is posterior and lateral, while the anterior part forms the cochlea, which is mostly medial. Each of the three semicircular canals originates with an elliptic enlargement, the so-called osseous ampullæ, from the walls of the vestibule, and after making nearly a whole circular turn they re-enter the vestibule. These three semicircular canals unite with the vestibule by five openings, since the cerebral and cerebellar canals join and enter by a canal in common. The planes of the semicircular canals are nearly perpendicular to each other. They are called the cerebral or superior vertical (frontal) semicircular canal, the cerebellar or posterior vertical (sagittal), and the tympanomastoid or external lateral (horizontal) semicircular canal (Fig. 47).

The cerebral canal is perpendicular to the superior border of the petrous bone and the hard bony wall of its convexity comes to the surface of the cerebral face of the petrous bone, forming the eminentia arcuata. The cerebellar canal lies deeper than the cerebral canal and its convexity is directed backward. Its plane lies nearly parallel to the cerebellar face of the petrous bone. The tympanomastoid canal is also directed backward and its outer arm forms a prominence on the tympano-antral face of the petrous bone and lies somewhat parallel, upward and backward from the facial canal. The prominence of this canal is seen on opening the mastoid antrum and is an important guide to the facial nerve. Here, too, is the most common point of caries in disease of the vestibule, and inspection under a strong artificial light is essential. The length of the loops of the semicircular canals varies. The cerebellar is the longest, the tympanomastoid is the shortest. The

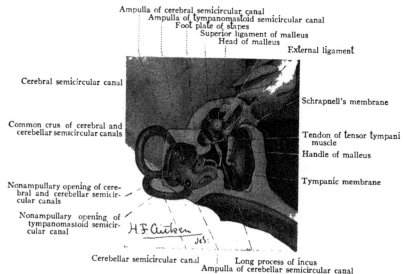

Ampulla of cerebral semicircular canal
Ampulla of tympanomastoid semicircular canal
Foot plate of stapes
Superior ligament of malleus
Head of malleus
External ligament

Cerebral semicircular canal

Common crus of cerebral and cerebellar semicircular canals

Nonampullary opening of cerebral and cerebellar semicircular canals

Nonampullary opening of tympanomastoid semicircular canal

Schrapnell's membrane

Tendon of tensor tympani muscle

Handle of malleus

Tympanic membrane

Cerebellar semicircular canal
Long process of incus
Ampulla of cerebellar semicircular canal

FIG. 47.—SCHEMATIC VIEW OF VESTIBULE AND TYMPANIC PORTION OF MIDDLE EAR.

inner surface of the osseous semicircular canal is covered with a periosteal lining or endosteum. The space between the membranous semicircular canal and the endosteum is called the perilymphatic space. This space communicates with the labyrinth and to the posterior cerebellar fossa by means of the aqueductus cochlea to the subarachnoid space.

The delicate membranous semicircular canal is filled with endolymph. The shape and position of the three membranous semicircular canals with their ampullæ corresponds to the osseous semicircular canal. The average diameter of the membranous semicircular canal is about one-third the diameter of the osseous semicircular canal (Fig. 48). The membranous semicircular canal is attached to the outer peripheral wall of the osseous semicircular canal. From the free circumference bordering on the perilymphatic space are numerous connective-tissue bands or ligaments which are attached to the endosteum of the osseous semicircular canal. The membranous ampullæ are from 2 to $2\frac{1}{2}$ mm.

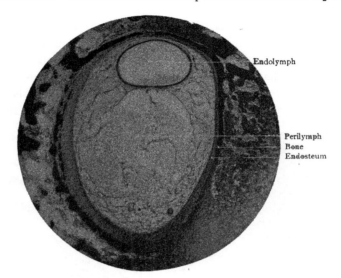

Endolymph

Perilymph
Bone
Endosteum

FIG. 48.—RELATIVE SIZE OF MEMBRANOUS SEMICIRCULAR CANAL TO OSSEOUS SEMICIRCULAR CANAL.
(Prepared by Wales.)

in diameter in the direction of the semicircular canal and about $1\frac{1}{2}$ mm. perpendicular to that direction. In a small groove on the floor of the ampullæ, called the sulcus transversus, the ampullæ nerve enters the crista acustica.

THE VESTIBULE

The vestibule lies between the cochlea and the semicircular canals, the cochlea anterior and the semicircular canals posterior. The vestibule may be compared to a cube. It has six surfaces nearly perpendicular to each other, but not of equal area. The upper side or roof has a smaller surface than the base or any of the four sides. One of the four sides is in about the same plane as the cerebral (anterior vertical) semicircular canal. It is, therefore, at right angles to the superior border of the petrous bone. This surface looks forward and inward and Söndermann calls it the sellar wall of the vestibule because it looks toward the sella turcica. The wall running parallel to this in the direction of the mastoid is called the mastoid wall. Perpendicular to these two surfaces, in the long direction of the pyramid, looking internal and posterior, is the posterior, medial wall. The other wall, looking external and anterior, is called the anterolateral surface or wall.

The sellar wall separates the internal auditory meatus from the vestibule. The recessus sphericus lies below and posterior medially from the recessus ellipticus, and also lies somewhat deeper in the bone in the direction of the sella turcica toward the apex of the pyramid. The recessus sphericus is separated from the recessus ellipticus by the crista vestibuli which projects into the vestibule from the middle of the sellar surface, having a horizontal direction. The anterolateral end of the crista thickens and forms a swelling like a pyramid, called pyramis cristæ. The posteromedial end is forked, surrounding the fossula

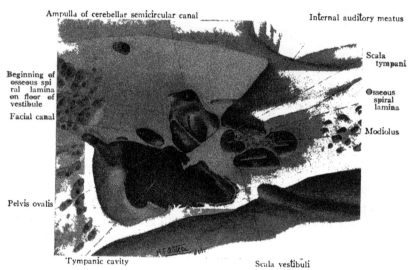

Fig. 49.—Horizontal Section showing Floor of Vestibule and Relation of Cochlea to Internal Auditory Meatus.

sulciformis. This fossula closes the vestibular end of the aqueductus vestibuli, a definite canal taken up by the ductus endolymphaticus communis. The fossula sinks deeper into the sellar wall to the corner where the sellar, the posteromedial, and the upper wall or roof of the vestibule meet. From there the aqueductus vestibuli is directed up and posterior in the substance of the pyramid crossing the posteromedial arm of the cerebellar semicircular canal and ending in the apertura aqueductus vestibuli on the cerebellar surface of the pyramid. There the ductus endolymphaticus swells out into the saccus endolymphaticus.

The floor or lower wall of the vestibule corresponds to the medial wall of the tympanic cavity and lies more horizontal than vertical; in other words, the tympanic cavity undermines the floor of the vestibule (Fig. 49). In the floor is the vestibular window. This window extends the whole length of the floor from the sellar to the mastoid wall. Toward the sellar wall it is nearer the anterolateral wall than the posteromedial wall, below the place where the recessus sphericus and ellipticus come together. Toward the mastoid end the vestibular window is in the floor midway between the two openings of the external lateral semicircular canal. Its greatest extent is, therefore, somewhat oblique to the long axis of the pyramid in the floor of the vestibule. Toward the sellar wall is the beginning of the scala vestibuli, called by Söndermann canalis vestibuli cochlearis. The lower edge of the recessus sphericus is undermined by the scala vestibuli.

The posteromedial wall of the vestibule contains the ampulla end of the cerebellar semicircular canal.

The upper wall or roof of the vestibule contains the entrance of the crus commune near its posteromedial edge.

The anterolateral wall contains the ampulla end of the cerebral semicircular canal.

The mastoid wall is perpendicular to the long axis of the pyramid and contains the ampulla and non-ampulla ends of the external lateral semicircular canal.

THE COCHLEA

The cochlea is cone shaped and surrounded by hard bone. Its axis is nearly horizontal. Its base lies against the anterior part of the fundus of the internal auditory meatus. Its lower anterior wall is in relation to the first knee of the internal carotid artery and its rounded apex is directed toward the canal for the tensor tympani muscle (Fig. 50). In the adult the apex is 4 to $4\frac{1}{2}$ mm. anterior to the anterior border of the vestibular window. The modiolus of the cochlea extends from the base to the apex, it is cone shaped and made up of spongy bone, around which the spiral cone makes two and three-quarter turns (Fig. 51). From the modiolus a plate of bone projects (spiral osseous lamina) into the spiral canal, a distance of little more than one-half its diameter, dividing the space into two compartments. The modiolus is filled with small canals which run parallel to the axis; these canals are arranged at the base of the modiolus in a spiral manner and end at the base of the osseous spiral lamina, where they open into the spiral canal of the modiolus (canal of Rosenthal) for the spiral ganglia.

The secondary osseous spiral lamina begins near the mastoid end of the vestibular window in a broad bony plate above the cochlea window and runs along, gradually growing smaller, till it vanishes, ending at a

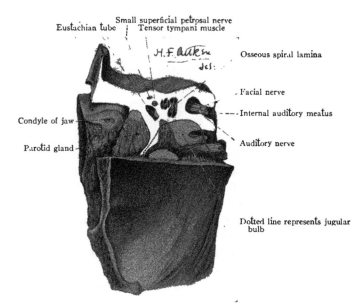

FIG. 50.—VERTICAL SECTION SHOWING RELATION OF APEX OF MODIOLUS TO TENSOR TYMPANI MUSCLE.
Berlin Anatomical Institute. (Prepared by Wales.)

point about one-half the length of the first turn of the cochlea.   The
osseous spiral lamina begins on the floor of the vestibule near the

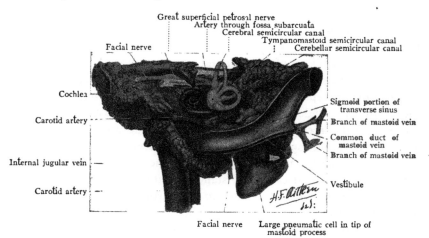

FIG. 51.—CORROSION OF ADULT RIGHT TEMPORAL BONE.
Medial view. (Prepared by Wales.)

recessus cochlearis, starting in a direction parallel to the axis of the
modiolus, turning while in the vestibule to become perpendicular to the
axis of the modiolus, and ends at the hamulus.   Between the concave

edge of the hamulus and the lamina modioli the end of the cochlea duct forms a round opening, called the heliotrema, where the scala vestibuli and scala tympani join, having been separated the whole length of the bony spiral lamina by the cochlea duct. The cleft between the osseous spiral lamina and the secondary spiral lamina in the vestibule gradually broadens as the secondary osseous spiral lamina grows smaller.

MEMBRANOUS LABYRINTH

The membranous labyrinth is formed by a system of hollow spaces containing a fluid poor in albumin, called endolymph; these hollow spaces are lined with epithelium and contain the nerve-endings of the

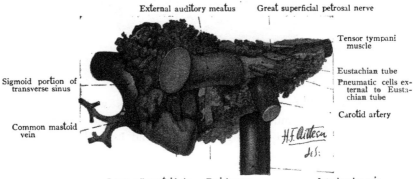

FIG. 52.—CORROSION OF ADULT RIGHT TEMPORAL BONE (LATERAL VIEW). (Prepared by Wales.)

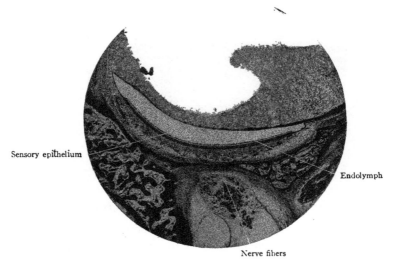

FIG. 53.—HUMAN MACULA ACUSTICA. (Wales.)

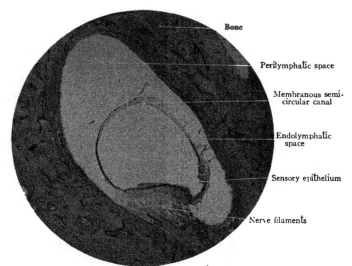

Fig. 54.—Crista Acustica of Adult. (Ampulla.)
Boston City Hospital. (Wales.)

eighth nerve. The membranous labyrinth lies within the bony labyrinth, appearing much smaller in cross-section, and attached here and there by connective-tissue strands. Around its delicate structure

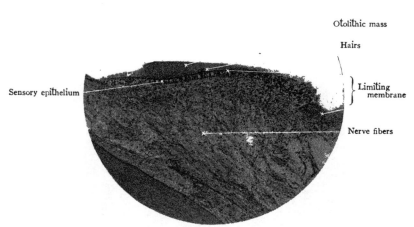

Fig. 55.—Human Crista Acustica.
Higher magnification of sensory epithelium of Fig. 54. (Prepared by Wales.)

there is a space filled with a fluid also poor in albumin, called perilymph. This space is lined with endothelium. In the bony vestibule there are two vestibular sacs, the utricle and the saccule. The utricle lies in the recessus ellipticus of the vestibule, where it is held to the bone by connective tissue, and the utriculus nerve enters the macula cribrosa superior. The fibers of the utriculus nerve end in the macula acustica utriculi (Fig. 53). The membranous semicircular canals end in five openings. They lie on the convex side of the bony canals and are about one-third the size of the bony canals. Through the sulcus ampullaris in the ampullæ the ampullaris nerve ends in the crista ampullaris (Figs. 54 and 55). The sacculus is smaller than the utriculus, lies in the recessus sphericus of the vestibule, and is fastened to the bone by connective tissue and fibers of the saccularis nerve coming through the macula cribrosa media. Its lower end narrows to the

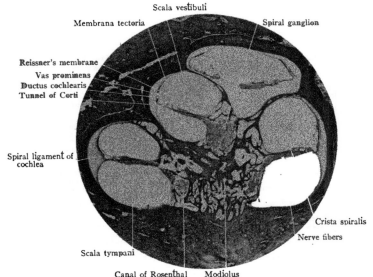

Scala vestibuli

Membrana tectoria   Spiral ganglion

Reissner's membrane
Vas prominens
Ductus cochlearis
Tunnel of Corti

Spiral ligament of
cochlea

Crista spiralis
Nerve fibers

Scala tympani

Canal of Rosenthal   Modiolus

FIG. 56.—COCHLEA OF ADULT. (Prepared by Wales.)

ductus reuniens, which joins the ductus cochlearis. The saccularis nerve ends in the macula acustica sacculi. The utricle is joined to the saccule through the forked end of the ductus endolymphaticus.

The membranous labyrinth is formed by the ductus cochlearis, which begins in the recessus cochlearis of the vestibule, the cæcum vestibulare, and ends blindly in the cupula, to help form the helicotrema. On cross-section it is for the most part triangular, its outer wall uniting with the thickened periosteum of the inner surface of the osseous cochlear canal. Its base connects with the osseous spiral lamina and the free edge of the spiral ligament on the outer wall; it consists of a fibrous connective tissue, the lamina basilaris, which supports the organ of Corti (Fig. 56).

ANATOMY

Vascular and Nervous Supply of the Organ of Hearing, Copied from Brühl-Politzer's *Atlas and Epitome of Otology*:

Part supplied.		Vessel.	Course.
Auricle..........	Helix, tragus, lobe.	Anterior auricular artery (superficial temporal).	In front of the ear.
	Greater part of the auricle.	Posterior auricular artery (external carotid), perforating branches. Veins empty into the superficial temporal and external jugular veins.	Posterior auricular fossa and through the cartilage.
External auditory canal	Cartilaginous. Anterior wall.	Anterior auricular artery.	Entrance through junction of the cartilaginous and bony auditory canal.
	Posterior wall.	Posterior auricular artery.	
	Bony.	Deep auricular artery (internal maxillary).	
Drum-head	Stratum cutaneum.	Anteria manubrii mallei (deep auricular).	Annulus tendineus and stratum cutaneum behind manubrium mallei. Radial anastomosis.
	Stratum mucosum.	Anterior tympanic (internal maxillary) perforating branches (anastomosis between stratum cutaneum and stratum mucosum).	Through Glaserian fissure and stratum cutaneum behind manubrium mallei.
Eustachian tube ..	Roof.	Branches of the middle meningeal artery (internal maxillary).	Radial anastomosis.
	Floor.	Basilar branch of ascending pharyngeal artery (external carotid) and vidian artery (superior palatine).	Petrosquamous fissure.
Mastoid process ...	Mastoid cells.	Mastoid branches (stylomastoid artery).	From the Fallopian canal.
	Attic and antrum.	Branches of the middle meningeal artery. Veins empty into the posterior auricular vein and transverse sinus.	Petrosquamous fissure.
Tympanic cavity...	Anterior portion.	Caroticotympanic branch of external carotid artery.	Caroticotympanic canaliculi.
Tympanic cavity..	Anterior ligament of malleus.	Anterior tympanic artery (internal maxillary artery).	Glaserian fissure.
	Posterior portion.	Posterior tympanic artery (stylomastoid).	Canal for chorda tympani.
	Stapedius muscle.	Stapedic (stylomastoid artery).	Pyramidal eminence.
	Stapes.	Branch to the stapes (stylomastoid artery). Anastomosis of stylomastoid artery with superficial petrosal branch.	From the Fallopian canal.
Tympanic cavity ...	Tensor tympani muscle.	Branch to tensor tympani (middle meningeal artery).	Spurious hiatus.
	Upper portion.	Superior tympanic artery (middle meningeal). Superficial petrosal branch (middle meningeal).	Roof of tubes.
	Lower portion.	Inferior tympanic artery (ascending pharyngeal).	Apertura superius canaliculi tympanici.
	Wall of promontory and endosteum of labyrinth.	Branches that communicate with branches of the internal auditory artery. Veins empty into middle meningeal and deep auricular veins.	Vascular perforations in promontorial wall (Politzer).
Labyrinth	Osseous semicircular canal capsule.	Arteria subarcuata. Internal auditory artery (basilar).	Fossa subarcuata. Porus acusticus internum.
	Membranous semicircular canals, utricle, and saccule, especially the cristæ and maculæ acusticæ.	Vestibular artery (internal auditory).	With vestibular nerve.
	Cochlea, nerve, spiral ganglia osseous spiral lamina, scala vestibuli, periosteum of walls of scalæ, spiral ligament.	Cochlear artery (internal auditory).	With cochlear nerve. Venous blood flows off in scala tympani (vas spirale).
	Utricle and saccule, cochlea.	Internal auditory vein.	Into inferior petrosal sinus.
	Semicircular canals, utricle.	Vena aqueductus vestibuli.	Into transverse sinus.
	Cochlea.	Vena aqueductus cochleæ.	Into bulb of jugular vein.

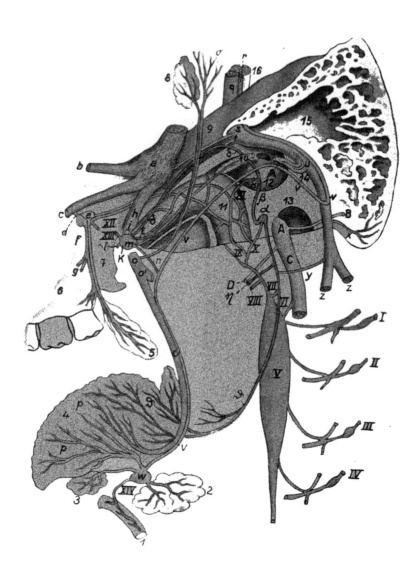

FIG. 57.—FOR DESCRIPTION, SEE PAGES 61 AND 62.

PART DRAINED	LYMPH-GLAND.	LYMPH-VESSEL.
Lymph channels. Cavum conchæ, external auditory canal.	Lymph-gland in front of tragus.	Lower anterior lymphatic vessel.
Triangular fossa, anterior surface of helix.	Highest mastoid gland.	Upper anterior lymphatic vessel.
Helix, antihelix, posterior surface.	Mastoid and cervical glands.	Posterior lymphatic vessel.
Lobe, auditory canal.	Parotid glands.	Posterior lymphatic vessel.
Drum-head, tympanic cavity.	Mastoid glands on sternocleidomastoid.	
Labyrinth.		Aquæductus cochleæ in subarachnoid.

NERVE SUPPLY.	MOTOR.	SENSORY.
Extrinsic muscles of the ear.	Posterior auricular nerve (facial nerve).	Muscle of the ear. Auricular canal. Cartilaginous.
	Anterior auricular nerve (right temporal nerve—seventh).	Auricularis magnus nerve (third cervical nerve).
Stapedius muscle.	Stapedius nerve (seventh nerve).	Auriculotemporal nerve (fifth nerve).
Tensor tympani muscle.	Tensor tympanic nerve (otic ganglion and fifth nerve).	Bony posterior wall. Drum-head. Tympanic cavity. Eustachian tube.
	Seventh nerve through great superficial petrosal nerve (from geniculate ganglion through spurious hiatus, anterior lacerated foramen, vidian canal to the nasal ganglion, pterygopalatine nerves).	Nerve of the external auditory meatus (auriculotemporal nerve). Auricular nerve, vagus nerve (tympanomastoid fissure). Nervi membranæ tympani (nerve of the external auditory meatus). Plexus tympanicus.
		(a) Caroticotympanic branch (lesser deep petrosal nerve). Internal carotid plexus of sympathetic.
Tensor veli muscle.	Otic ganglion, fifth nerve.	
Retrahens tubæ.	Pharyngeal plexus, vagus nerve.	(b) Tympanic (Jacobson's) nerve from petrous ganglion.
Vaso constrictors of the entire ear.	Sympathetic nerve.	Ninth nerve through inferior aperture and superior tympanic canal to small superficial petrosal nerve. Anastomosis with eighth nerve through the anterior lacerated foramen to the otic ganglion of the fifth nerve and parotid.
Secretory. **Taste of anterior half of tongue; salivary secretion of submaxillary and sublingual glands.**	Chorda tympani (seventh nerve); fibers of the chorda tympani are joined to the seventh nerve by the intermediate portion of the ninth and extend through the apertura canaliculi chorda between folds of drum-head; through the Glaserian fissure to the lingual nerve (fifth nerve).	

FIG. 57.—SCHEMATIC VIEW OF THE UNION OF THE NERVES OF THE MIDDLE EAR WITH THE SURROUNDING NERVES (BRÜHL AND POLITZER, AFTER LANDUS).

1. External maxillary artery.
2. Submaxillary gland.
3. Sublingual gland.
4. Tongue.
5. Uvula.
6. Upper jaw.
7. Pterygoid promontory.
8. Parotid gland.
9. Cerebral surface of the pyramid.
10. Tensor tympani muscle.
11. Carotid.
12. Promontory.
13. Bulb of jugular vein.
14. Stapedius muscle.
15. Tympanomastoid duct (antrum).
16. Eighth nerve.

Green—Fifth nerve.

(a) Gasserian ganglion.
(b) Ophthalmic branch (sensory).
(c) Maxillary branch (sensory and motor). Major superficial petrosal nerve yellow.
(d) Root to.
(e) Sphenopalatine ganglion.
(f) Sphenopalatine nerve (sensory).
(g) Postinferior nasal nerve (sensory).
(h) Mandibular branch (sensory and motor).
(i) Root to.
(j) Otic ganglion.
(k) Branch from the otic ganglion to the tensor veli palatine muscle (motor).
(l) Branch of the otic ganglion to the tensor tympani muscle (motor).
(m) Mastoid branch to the chorda tympani.
(n) Auriculotemporal nerve (secretory).
(o) Lingual nerve.
(p) Lingual branches (sensory).

Yellow—Seventh nerve (solely motor).

(q) Seventh nerve in the porus acusticus internus.
(r) Intermediary nerve (glossopharyngeal nerve).
(s) Geniculate ganglion and great superficial petrosal to the sphenopalatine ganglion (e) and the postpalatine to the muscles of the palate (5) motor.
(t) Anastomosis to the lesser superficial petrosal nerve.
(u) Stapedius nerve.
(v) Chorda tympani, continuation of the intermediary nerve to the lingual nerve and submaxillary gland (2) to the
(w) Sublingual ganglion and os, the lingual running to the tongue (p) (anterior half) and sublingual gland (3).
(x) Posterior auricular nerve.
(y) Anastomosis with the ninth nerve.
(z) End branch (per anserinus major).

White—Tenth nerve.

A. Jugular ganglion.
B. Auricular nerve to the tenth (sensory).   Anastomosis with the seventh, where the two cross each other.
C. Ganglion nodosum.
D. Pharyngeal rami (motor).

Red—Ninth nerve.

(α) Petrosal ganglion.
(β) Tympanic nerve (Jacobson's nerve).
(γ) Caroticotympanic nerve (deep lesser petrosal).
(δ) Superficial lesser petrosal nerve (continuation of the tympanic nerve), to the ganglion (*k*) and a branch.
(ε) For the auriculotemporal nerve (parotid).
(η) Pharyngeal branch (sensory).
(ϑ) Lingual branch (taste posterior half of tongue).

Blue—Sympathetic nerve.

I., II., III., IV. Four cervical nerves (cer plexus).
V. Superior cervical ganglion.
VI. Anastomosis to the tenth nerve.
VII. Anastomosis to the ninth nerve.
VIII. Pharyngeal branches.
IX. Internal carotid nerve (plexum).
X. Anastomosis with the petrosal ganglion.
XI. Lesser deep petrosal nerve (to the tym nerve).
XII. Great deep petrosal nerve (Vidian nerve). the sphenopalatine ganglion (*e*), and here to the nose (glands).
XIII. Union of the otic ganglion to the meningeal pl
XIV. Union of the sublingual ganglion to the maxi plexus.

CHAPTER II

PHYSIOLOGY OF THE ORGAN OF HEARING

VERY little is actually known about the function of hearing. The physiology of the internal ear is wholly theoretic, and theory is but another term for ignorance. To understand these theories it is essential to have a knowledge of the physics of sound and also of the minute anatomy of the brain and temporal bone.

In the infant hearing is the last sense to awaken. W. Preyer made observations on his own child. For the first three days of the infant's life he could get no sure reaction to sound, but on the fourth day he was convinced that his child was not deaf. In the second week there was no doubt that the infant was soothed by the sound of his voice.[1] Loud noises do not seem to frighten the infant for the first two or three days after birth. The reason for this deafness is probably due to the fact that the mucous membrane of the tympanic cavity contains embryonic tissue. This embryonic tissue forms a pad or cushion which quite fills the tympanic cavity. The remaining space is filled with amniotic fluid and macerated epithelium. As the embryonic tissue in the mucous membrane and the fluid in the tympanic cavity are absorbed, hearing takes place.

The **tensor tympani muscle** changes the tension of the drum membrane and the chain of ossicles, serving to accommodate, so that sound-waves of small intensity may be heard, and probably helping to dampen sound-waves of great intensity, thus acting as a protecting as well as accommodative device. The **stapedius muscle** raises the anterior end of the foot-plate out of the vestibular window when the muscle contracts, and is probably accommodative in its action also. The stapedius muscle is antagonistic to the tensor tympani muscle.

It is known that the **semicircular canals** and the **vestibule** act as organs of equilibration, and yet, when the vestibular apparatus is completely destroyed, which condition is found in some deaf-mutes, the eyes, the muscles, and joints seem to be sufficient to maintain equilibrium, with the advantage that rotary movements do not cause vertigo or nystagmus.

[1] W. Preyer, "Die Seele des Kindes," 1905.

The arrangement of the **cochlea** is ideal for compactness; its thick bony capsule protects its delicate nerve-endings and, furthermore, these nerve-endings are suspended in fluid within a cavity, all tending to avoid irritation of any sort but sound irritation. If the organ of Corti were surrounded by air it would constantly be irritated, possibly by heat, cold, humidity, dust, and chemical vapors. If the cochlea were filled with connective tissue, could sound-waves be perceived? Such conditions have been found in deaf-mutes. Again, in this field of speculation, do sound-waves travel by way of the drum membrane, ossicles, or vestibule to the sensory epithelium in the cochlear duct (Helmholtz), or do sound-waves go directly to the sensory epithelium by bone conduction? (Zimmermann.)

The **drum membrane** is largely protective, probably as well as accommodative, through the tympanic muscles. The drum membrane prevents the entrance of water, bacteria, and insects into the tympanic cavity and, probably more important, the drum membrane prevents the varying atmospheric air from drying its delicate mucous membrane. Only the warmed, moistened, and cleansed air from the respiratory tract can normally enter the tympanic cavity by way of the Eustachian tube. Pathologic conditions, such as thickenings, calcifications, atrophies, healed perforations, and even adhesions are not necessarily indicative of diminished hearing power, so far as we are able to test by whispered and conversational voice and by the tuning-forks.

The **auricle** is a rudimentary organ in man and the least it does is to protect the side of the head from a fall or blow. In many animals the auricles serve to protect the organ of hearing from loud sounds and may be directed toward the source of the sound, but this act may be a reflex action after the attention is called to a moving object by the sense of smell or sight. The horse pricks up its ears at the sight of food and the ears lie back when in anger. It might as well be said that the auricle is an appendage for expression. In man the movement of the auricle is a rare and useless accomplishment. Individuals with large auricles hear no better than those with small auricles. It is said that the hearing is normal in individuals who have lost their auricles. No convincing proof has yet been presented which would show that the auricle is of any importance whatever.

Physiologists, as a rule, omit the study of the physiology of the organ of hearing, because experiments on this organ are most difficult. It is not possible to observe the separate complex parts in action and record their movements. It is easy to fill in the space allotted to physiology with physics and anatomy and a few theories. Most aurists are not physicists or physiologists and thus the physiology of the organ of hearing has been slighted. New facts are, however, rapidly accumulating and the functions of the hearing apparatus will probably be solved through the study of pathology and comparative anatomy.

The following is abstracted from the writings of Alfred Denker:[1] "Sound-waves can be carried from a sounding body to the end apparatus of the eighth nerve by way of the air or when the sounding body is brought in contact with the body through bone-conduction.

"**Conduction of Sound-waves.**—There are two ways to consider in which sound-waves are conducted through the air: First, the sound-waves are transferred to the drum membrane and from here, either through the ossicular chain or through the air in the tympanic cavity, to the labyrinth and the endings of the eighth nerve; second, the sound-waves go from the air to the head bones and from these are conducted either directly to the contents of the labyrinth or from the head bones through interposition of the ossicular chain to the internal ear.

"Johannes Müller has proved experimentally that vibrations traveling from the air to a stretched membrane, and from here to a freely movable solid part, and from this transferred to fluid, are communicated to the fluid much stronger than when the vibrations go from a stretched membrane to air and from air to fluid; in other words, the same air-waves act much more intensely transmitted by way of the ossicular chain to the vestibular window than they are by way of the drum membrane through the air of the tympanic cavity to the cochlea window.

"Bezold considers that the function of the ossicular chain is to admit the lower part of the tone scale from the air. Any interruption of the free movement of this chain of ossicles causes lowering in the hearing distance for whispered speech. Helmholtz, in his work on *The Mechanics of the Ossicles and the Membrana Tympani*, has clearly shown that the ossicular chain is a powerful lever apparatus which conducts great movements of little force and converts them into slight movements of great force.

"Zimmermann believes that sound-waves can travel directly from the air to the labyrinth without the coöperation of the ossicular chain, part through the cochlea window and part through the promontory. He believes that in the conduction of sound-waves we do not have to deal with molar movement, but with molecular movements.

"As to the conduction of sound-waves to the labyrinth, Bonning has published interesting investigations from observations in comparative anatomy. He found that the temporal bone of the whale was not in

[1] Alfred Denker, "Die Otosklerosis."

close bony union with the bones of the skull, but was joined by connective tissue. He believes a direct conduction from the head bones to the labyrinth is excluded, and his opinion is that sound-waves can only be conducted through coöperation of the ossicular chain.

"Against the theory that the ossicular chain has not a sound-conducting function, but only a labyrinth pressure-regulating function, is the fact that when the labyrinth is intact there is complete deafness when there is complete fixation of the stapes in the vestibular window and closure of the cochlea window. What further supports the acceptance that the membrana tympani and the ossicular chain have a sound-conducting function is the fact that in the animal series the development of the internal ear and the tympanic cavity apparatus accompany each other.

"Bezold reported the results of hearing tests of 4 cases where the labyrinth was lacking on one side and normal on the other. In these patients there was created a natural hearing tube through the empty tympanic and labyrinth cavities in connection with the external auditory canal, which went deep into the skull, nearly reaching the healthy labyrinth. If, now, the acceptation that sound-waves can be transmitted through the bones directly to the labyrinth is correct, then the sound-waves must be carried from the walls of the hollow labyrinth and be perceived by the labyrinth on the sound side. The tests showed that the whole lower half of the tone scale up to the third octave was not heard even when the tuning-fork was violently struck and placed in the ear where the labyrinth was lacking. We know that it is impossible to occlude the perception of higher tones even when the sound ear is tightly closed so that the higher tones could not be considered. This positive observation is against the acceptance of direct bone conduction of sound-waves and we know that without the ossicular chain the hearing of the lower tones of tuning-forks up to the third octave by air is, on the whole, impossible.

"The manner by which sound-waves are communicated to the labyrinth from direct contact with the bone to a solid swinging body has not yet been solved.

"**The Function of the Intrinsic Muscles of the Ear.**—Helmholtz showed that a contraction of the tensor tympanic muscle caused an inward movement of the umbo and at the same time an inward movement of the lenticular process of the long arm of the incus, so that the foot-plate of the stapes was pressed into the vestibule.

"Tension of the tendon of the stapedius muscle causes a slight inward movement of the foot-plate on the posterior lower periphery of the vestibular window, at the same time the anterior pole and its upper periphery, on account of its broad annular ligament, is drawn out laterally. This causes a lessening of the labyrinthine pressure.

" If there is diminution of the air-pressure in the tympanic cavity, such as occurs in catarrh of the Eustachian tube, the tensor tympani predominates and the foot-plate of the stapes is pushed inward. Again, if the membrana tympani is destroyed, with both malleus and incus, then the stapedius muscle draws the foot-plate outward. Both muscles, considered by their action on the foot-plate, are antagonistic. If both muscles act at the same time, the contraction of the tensor tympani with its strong inward movement and the contraction of the stapedius muscle with its outward movement, the stapedius muscle must exert a stronger tension on the annular ligament. The tensor tympani muscle has the function of stiffening the ossicles of the sound-conducting apparatus. Both muscles are to be considered as accommodative muscles, for they are capable of the same common function, in so adjusting the membrana tympani and foot-plate through different degrees of tension that perception is favored for respective sound-waves.

" Ostmann proved on the hearing organ of dogs that in the act of listening. a contraction of the stapedius muscle took place. Persons who have fixation of the sound-conducting apparatus with lessened capability of action of the tensor tympani and stapedius muscles frequently complain that when in the company of several people speaking at once they have great difficulty in clearly understanding and in isolating a single voice. Probably both muscles take part in this accommodation.

"The Organ of Corti.—The end-organ of the eighth nerve, or organ of Corti, is suspended freely in fluid. Helmholtz knew that easily swinging bodies meeting sound-waves from sound-producing bodies were made to swing. This sympathetic swinging is called resonance. Helmholtz considered the organ of Corti to be a resonance apparatus. He still further found it was necessary to have a great series of resonators of different tones and, therefore, of different sizes, like the cords of a piano; lastly, the internal ear must be capable of resolving the tone. At first it was thought that the pillars of Corti acted as resonators, but Helmholtz found that birds and crocodiles had no pillars of Corti. Since these creatures hear, he concluded that the pillars of Corti did not act as resonators. Then Hensen discovered the cords of the basilar membrane on which the pillars were supported. Near the base of the cochlea these cords are about $\frac{1}{20}$ mm. long and they gradually increase till at the apex, where they are about $\frac{1}{2}$ mm. long. The number of the cords is from 15,000 to 25,000 and must be capable of resolving

from 15 to 20,000 vibrations. Helmholtz believed that the basil
cords were the resonating part of the organ of Corti. Helmholtz
theory of sound perception is as follows: Sound is resolved into i
different tones, which shake the basilar cords by their selective resonanc
and through the swinging of the cords the corresponding hearing cel
are affected. The stimulus is then carried to the brain through t
cochlear nerve to the cortex of the brain, where the original sound
perceived as a whole through associative tract activity."

CHAPTER III[1]

BACTERIOLOGY OF THE EAR

INVESTIGATION of purulent discharges from the middle ear began simultaneously with modern bacteriology. Most cultures were made from one to thirty days following perforation of the drum membrane. In this interval of time the middle-ear secretions could not only be infected by micro-organisms from the external auditory canal, but also secondary infection could take place by way of the Eustachian tube. Some of the early investigators examined the pus directly after incising the drum, others after spontaneous rupture of the drum membrane. The results of these investigations showed that the diplococcus pneumoniæ of Fränkel was most common; next and most frequent the streptococcus pyogenes, and lastly, the staphylococcus (albus, citreus, aureus). Later investigators tried to disinfect the external auditory canal and the drum membrane The external auditory canal was then aseptically sealed for twenty-four hours and if found sterile the drum was incised and the discharge examined. The difficulties in technic are many and it is because of these difficulties that investigators vary so greatly in their results. Taking cultures at the time of operation on acute cases of mastoiditis was first applied by Leutert. The technic at post-mortem examinations is not so difficult.

Whether the healthy tympanic cavity normally contains bacteria or is absolutely devoid of germs is a question. Citelli, Cohn, Zaufal, Hasslauer, Ernst, and others maintain that the normal tympanic cavity contains pathogenic bacteria and that these pathogenic bacteria are in a quiescent stage or few in number, and become active only when the conditions for their development are favorable. Just as pathogenic bacteria are present in the normal throat, for example, Klebs-Löffler bacillus of diphtheria is present in most throats, yet the individual does not necessarily have diphtheria, so the middle-ear cavity, which is a prolongation of the respiratory tract, may contain tubercle bacilli and yet the patient may not have tuberculosis of the ear.

On the other hand, Lannois, S. Weiss, Preysing, Stöpple, and others assert that the normal tympanic cavity does not contain pathogenic

[1] In this chapter opinions from the work of Dr. Hasslauer of Nürnberg are freely quoted.

bacteria. Lannois and S. Weiss made experiments on animals, while Preysing made his observations at autopsy on the human body.

If the middle ear contains bacteria, then the factors which would lower the vitality of the organism, allowing the bacteria to multiply, would be of more etiologic importance than the bacteria; whereas, if the statement of Lannois and Preysing be accepted, the bacteria are of great importance etiologically. In either case bacteria are important and are present in every inflammation, whether catarrhal or suppurative.

How may bacteria get into the tympanic cavity?

(a) By way of the external auditory canal in rupture of the drum membrane through direct or indirect traumatism. Karl Stöpple showed that the bacteria in the external auditory canal were mostly saprophytic and not the same composition as found in middle-ear inflammation. Probably infection cannot take place through an intact drum membrane. Secondary infection may take place after the drum membrane is incised. Sometimes a permanent opening remains in the drum membrane after the middle-ear inflammation has subsided. Here a new infection may take place, especially if water is introduced—in washing the ears, by use of the syringe, or in sea bathing.

(b) Bacteria may enter by the Eustachian tube, either by continuity or they may be forced into the tympanic cavity by sudden interruption of the air current when blowing the nose; by the act of swallowing when using the nasal douche; by sniffing fluids into the nose from the palm of the hand; sometimes in sneezing, in vomiting, or in paroxysms of coughing. Often by the Valsalva (or auto-inflation), sometimes by the Politzer air-douche, and rarely by the use of the catheter. The presence of postnasal discharge, of acute and chronic diseases of the nasopharynx, of hypertrophied adenoid tissue or tonsils which interfere with the function of the Eustachian tube, paralysis of the nerves supplying the muscles of the tube, and sudden loss of fatty tissue, as in typhoid fever— all these factors favor infection of the tympanic cavity. The infection of the middle ear is made more difficult by the length and narrowness of the Eustachian tube and by the downward movement of its ciliated epithelium; also by the presence of an intact epithelium in the middle ear.

(c) Bacteria may enter the tympanic cavity by way of the lymph and blood-vessels, as Barnick has demonstrated in miliary tuberculosis.

(d) Bacteria may enter by way of the external auditory canal in fracture of the skull, the bacteria entering the mastoid cells and the infection thus spreading to all parts of the middle ear.

(e) Bacteria may enter from the cranial cavity by way of the labyrinth, facial canal, or petrosquamous fissure.

The external auditory canal contains the bacteria commonly found in the skin (staphylococcus albus) and the bacteria which are blown or washed in from without. The staphylococcus is the most common and is usually the cause of otitis externa circumscripta. Smegma bacilli and other acid-resisting bacilli non-pathogenic in character may be mistaken for tubercle bacilli. Individuals with lowered vitality, as in rickets, anemia, or diabetes, are more liable to infection of the external auditory canal.

Aural discharges generally contain two or three varieties of pathogenic bacteria and occasionally saprophytic bacteria. Occasionally the pneumobacillus of Friedländer is found. Etienne found it 5 times in 238 bacteriologic examinations. A still rarer bacterium is the bacillus pyocyaneus. Kanthack found it once in pure culture. Kössel found the bacillus pyocyaneus in the middle ears of 3 children whose drum membranes were intact, once in pure culture, twice together with diplococci. Gerber found the bacillus pyocyaneus one day after incision of the drum membrane. J. Orne Green found the bacillus pyocyaneus immediately after incision in 3 cases. Most of the cases reported show a mixed infection and investigators disagree as to whether the bacillus pyocyaneus can cause middle-ear suppuration. Kössel believes it is pathogenic for infants, but not for adults. Kanthack believes it acts pathogenically only in combination with other pathogenic bacteria. Pes and Gradenigo assert that it can produce a general as well as a local infection of the organism. A further proof of the pathogenic nature of bacillus pyocyaneus is brought forth by Leutert, who collected 4 cases of perichondritis of the auricle where the growth showed a pure culture of the bacillus pyocyaneus. Further, Ruprecht and Helmann found the bacillus pyocyaneus in pure culture as the cause of a case of otitis externa crouposa. Preysing asserts that there is no proof that the bacillus pyocyaneus can cause otitis media in infants.

Professor Körner observed 5 cases complicated with the bacillus pyocyaneus in the course of fifteen years. In all these 5 cases the pyocyaneus had discolored the discharge the usual green color before the onset of perichondritis. This constant association of green pus with perichondritis suggested that the latter was caused by the bacillus pyocyaneus, and in a case Körner observed, this etiologic connection was confirmed.

Otitis media, in consequence of acute infectious diseases, such as scarlet fever, measles; diphtheria, influenza, etc., is designated as secondary middle-ear inflammation.

Scarlet Fever.—Marie Raskin made the first bacteriologic investigations of the so-called scarlet fever otitis; then followed Wolf, Blaxall, Pearce, Zaufal, Councilman, Thomas, and others. Marie Raskin and Leutert speak of the streptococcus as the cause of scarlet fever otitis. The otitis does not come on late in the disease, as in many cases of secondary otitis, but in the beginning of scarlet fever favored by the intense throat inflammation. The otitis of scarlet fever is, therefore, considered as a specific disease process. The streptococcus of scarlet fever soon loses its virulence and may be replaced eventually by other bacteria. Lewy describes a destructive early form of scarlet fever otitis. Acute middle-ear suppuration occurred seven days before the outbreak of the exanthem and was followed rapidly by mastoiditis with necrosis; the dura mater was exposed in the middle and posterior cranial fossæ. Necrosis of the posterior wall of the external auditory canal was present and caries of the ossicles and formation of a fistula leading into the tympano-antral semicircular canal had taken place. In a second case the middle-ear inflammation appeared in the second week of the disease, with caries of the incus and necrosis of the mastoid process. In the beginning of the disease, even on the second or third day, micro-organisms are found in the blood, either free or enclosed in the leukocytes or in the stroma of the mucous membrane, and occasionally in the lymph-cells of the connective tissue. These micro-organisms and their toxins cause suppuration and rapid destruction of the soft tissues and bone. Körner believes that the otitis should be interpreted as a symptom of the general infection and divides scarlet fever otitis into two forms: the early destructive form and the much milder late form, the latter appearing in the first stages of desquamation.

Scarlet Fever with Diphtheria.—In scarlet fever with diphtheria the bacillus of diphtheria does not appear till the ear affection has existed several days. Forbes believes it must be a secondary invasion of the bacillus of diphtheria after a true scarlet fever otitis. The secondary infection is brought about by way of the Eustachian tube. Forbes did not find an accompanying throat diphtheria in any case, but recognized the diphtheria bacillus in the discharge 32 times out of 40 cases of post scarlet fever otitis.

Measles.—The most common bacteriologic finding in measles has also been the streptococcus. Comparatively little investigation has been made of the bacteria found in the otitis accompanying measles. Otitis of measles does not appear to be caused by a specific infection as in scarlet fever, but as a local sign of the primary disease. The general disease brings about such changes of the mucous membrane of the middle ear that the pathogenic germs in the middle ear obtain a favorable field in which to develop their activity. In 100 cases of measles Nadoleczny found the middle ear affected in 59.5 per cent. Most of the cases developed within the second week of the disease. In measles a specific bacterial excitant is even less established than in scarlet fever.

Diphtheria.—Otitis media caused by Klebs-Löffler bacillus may be divided into three classes:

1. Primary diphtheritic inflammation of the middle ear, which is very rare.

2. A few cases in which the bacillus of diphtheria has made its way from the throat to the middle ear.

3. The most common form is the secondary middle-ear infection which accompanies the disease. To prove the presence of this third form Lommel found on the examination of 24 children dying of diphtheria only one normal ear, all the others showed simple middle-ear inflammation with serous or purulent exudate. Thus Lommel came to the conclusion that the otitis media belongs to the picture of a diphtheritic disease of the organ of respiration. Lewin also states that acute otitis media often accompanies genuine throat diphtheria. The aural process is not a specific one, but a local manifestation of the disease as a whole. The otitis media is not commonly caused by direct transmission. Nearly all observers have found Klebs-Löffler bacillus either in pure culture or with other pathogenic bacteria. Podak-Gerber reported a case of rhinitis fibrinosa with true bacillus of diphtheria and streptococci which developed an acute middle-ear suppuration. The culture of the aural secretion showed the pseudodiphtheria bacillus, numerous streptococci, and staphylococci aureus. From this they drew the conclusion that pseudodiphtheria bacilli were virulent true diphtheria bacilli. Pseudodiphtheria bacilli are related morphologically and in culture to the true bacillus of diphtheria; only they are absolutely apathogenic. Schilling found on incising an acute middle ear a thick white adherent membrane which acted bacteriologically as the pseudodiphtheria bacillus; it was not pathogenic for guinea-pigs, stained by Gram's method, and showed Neisser's granule stain. In the beginning of the disease the pseudobacillus was predominant, but later it was killed out by diplococci. It was, therefore, a mixed infection with two kinds of bacteria. A fibrinous exudate in the middle ear should not be diagnosed without careful bacteriologic examinations.

Influenza.—There are two groups of influenza otitis, classified according to their etiology: First, a specific, or early form, caused by the influenza bacillus, which is found in the secretions of the middle ear gaining entrance by the blood-vessels. This form usually begins on the first or second day of the disease. Second, the later variety, a secondary infection from the throat, in which are found the bacteria usually present in acute secondary middle-ear inflammation, such as diplococci, staphylococci, and streptococci. These bacteria have also been found in the early form, but they have been overgrown and completely supplanted by the influenza bacillus. The course of influenza otitis varies more or less according to the number and virulence of the bacilli and is only slightly different from genuine otitis. A special peculiarity is the intensity of the pain, which may outlast incision of the drum membrane or spontaneous rupture. Some epidemics are characterized by a hemorrhagic form of otitis media.

Typhoid Fever.—Two to four per cent. of all cases in typhoid fever have ear complications, usually in the fourth to the fifth week; or, according to Bezold, from the twenty-fifth to the thirtieth day. The typhoid bacillus is not carried by the blood; clinically the middle-ear inflammation is not typical. The mastoid process is often involved. Streptococci, staphylococci, and diplococci are found in the aural discharge in typhoid cases. Preysing found the typhoid bacillus in a case with double acute purulent otitis media in which the drum was not perforated. In another case he found the staphylococcus albus and the bacterium coli.

Cerebrospinal Meningitis.—The disease of the middle ear is generally secondary to the disease of the brain. The meningococcus intracellularis (Weichselbaum-Jager) progresses from the brain membranes to the inner ear along the auditory nerve or frequently through the aqueductus cochleæ.

Gonococcus.—The gonococcus is rarely found in the middle ear. The writer found Neisser's gonococcus in the discharge from an acute suppurative otitis in an infant who had gonorrheal ophthalmia. The right ear only was affected.

Otitis Media.—The following bacteria have been found in primary otitis media:

Streptococcus pyogenes, diplococcus lanceolatus (Fränkel-Weichselbaum), staphylococcus pyogenes aureus and albus, pneumobacillus (Friedländer), bacillus pyocyaneus, bacterium coli commune, influenza bacillus, typhoid bacillus, streptococcus erysipelatis, bacterium lactis aërogenes, Neisser's gonococcus, bacillus mucosus ozænæ, tubercle bacillus, Klebs-Löffler diphtheria bacillus, pest bacillus, meningococcus intracellularis (Weichselbaum-Jager), pseudodiphtheria bacillus, and bacillus mucosus capsulatus.

Ferreri mentions a specific form of middle-ear suppuration in cases of rhinitis atrophica with ozena which ran a long course and did not yield to treatment. Cultures in 2 cases of purulent otitis media with ozena showed the bacillus mucosus once together with staphylococcus albus.

Otitis of Infants.—Preysing found the following results at autopsy in 154 ear cases having purulent, mucous, or serous contents in the middle ears:

Pneumococcus (pure).....................................96 ears.
Pneumococcus with putrefactive bacilli.....................13 "
Pneumococcus and staphylococcus......................... 3 '
Streptococcus (pure)....................................... 1
Staphylococcus pyogenes aureus........................... 3 '
Staphylococcus and putrefactive bacilli..................... 2 '
Putrefactive (pure) .... 3 :
Sterile... 33 ``

                                                        ———
                                                        154 '

Subtracting these 33 sterile cases, Preysing found that of the 121 remaining infected ears, 112 contained pneumococcus, or about 92½ per cent. of all bacteriologic findings. Preysing says that this fact gives us the right to call the otitis media of children a pneumococcic infective disease.

Complications of Middle-ear Inflammation.—In the complications of middle-ear inflammation, such as mastoiditis, meningitis, sinus thrombosis, epidural abscess, peri-auricular abscess, extradural abscess, and brain abscess, the same bacteriologic findings are present, found in the middle ear. In two-thirds of all complications the streptococcus is the cause and in one-third the staphylococcus is the cause. This is the inverse relation found in the middle ear. Streptococci seem to melt the bone away and is the most common cause of sinus thrombosis. Gruening found pure cultures of streptococci in blood-cultures taken from 6 consecutive cases of thrombosis of the lateral sinus.

" The formation of sinus thrombosis was observed by Stenger, who carried on inoculation experiments on dogs. He injected streptococci of high virulency into the sigmoid sinus by four different methods. A tampon covered with the culture was laid on the sinus wall or carried along the sinus. Again, he injected the streptococcus into the sinus with a syringe and then he scratched the sinus wall and laid the infected tampon on the scratched vessel. Sinus thrombosis was formed only in the last method. Here an extensive sinus thrombosis with purulent destruction of the thrombosis took place. The dog died of general sepsis. According to the histologic investigation of Köster and Talker there was a gradual disease of the wall of the vein in the form of a

lymphangitis. The blood in the vein coagulated through a differentiation of the tissue fluids and was then infected by bacteria; therefore the
infection by bacteria was secondary."[1]

According to Leutert, epidural abscesses are generally caused by
diplococci. In brain abscess streptococcus, staphylococcus, and diplococcus have been found. In old abscesses of the brain the pus may be
sterile. In many cases reported sterile, anaërobic bacteria were not
looked for. J. Orne Green found in 184 cases of mastoid disease
staphylococcus in pure culture 49 times, the streptococcus 31 times,
and the pneumococcus 23 times. Green came to the conclusion that
the variety of micro-organism had nothing to do with the prognosis of
the case. Leutert found in 63 acute ears with empyema of the mastoid
streptococci in pure culture 38 times, pneumococcus in pure culture
11 times, staphylococcus in pure culture 5 times, tubercle bacillus
in pure culture twice, and the remainder, mixed infections, 7 times.

Staphylococcus is probably the most frequent cause of secondary
infections and therefore is responsible for the chronicity of aural suppurations. In chronic otitis media the pneumococcus is rarely found,
whereas the staphylococcus is always found. According to Coussieu,
middle-ear inflammation with several bacterial excitants tend to become
chronic, whereas the presence of a single variety of bacteria causes
suppuration of short duration or may cause no suppuration at all.
Acute otitis has in the beginning only one bacterial excitant. Staphylococci may be found in pure culture, but they are not so frequently the
sole excitors as diplococci and streptococci.

Streptococcus is most virulent, but soonest loses its virulency; the
diplococcus, according to Zaufal, may keep up its virulency to the
fifty-eighth day and, rarely, till the one hundred and eighty-first day.

Gradenigo found that diplococci in aural pus may take the chain
formation and, as such, represent a weakened form of Fränkel's diplococcus. These diplostreptococci possess all the peculiarities of the
diplococcus lanceolatus capsulatus in an attenuated condition and
form chains on agar. The capsule is lost. They belong to the diplococci and not to the streptococci. These diplococci have been found
by Marie Raskin, Moos, Hasslauer, and others. Probably these bacteria
have been classed as streptococci by many observers, which may account
for the diversity of results.

The pneumococcus differs from the streptococcus in three ways:

(1) The acute process runs a quicker course in the middle ear in
pneumococcus infection.

[1] Stenger, "Transactions of the German Otological Society in Berlin, 1904," p. 109.

(2) The pneumococcus has a greater inclination to extend its field of infection than streptococcus. (Epidural abscesses are more frequent.)

(3) Pneumococcus infection often remains latent a long time in the middle ear after its acute course, before it starts up an acute process in the mastoid.

Netter classified middle-ear inflammations clinically according to the bacteria and the nature of the discharge, but it is known that the intensity of an inflammation depends not only on the kind and virulence of the micro-organism, but also on the resistance of the tissues of the individual. The same micro-organism which causes a catarrhal inflammation may generate a suppurative inflammation depending on the virulence of the germ, its numbers, and the method of spreading; for example, its method of spreading in the middle ear depends on the resistant powers of the organism and the anatomic character of the tissues. It is established that certain bacteria, after remaining some time in the nasopharynx, become attenuated; and the same process takes place in the middle ear.

CONCLUSIONS

A pneumococcic suppuration is in general more favorable in its course than a streptococcic suppuration. A monobacterial infection is more favorable than a polybacterial infection. Although a pneumococcic infection seems to get well sooner, it may be latent and the inflammation may start up again in the mastoid process or meninges after apparent healing has taken place.

The same bacteria are found in empyema of the mastoid that are found in acute middle-ear inflammation.

Careful technic is essential to success. A smear should always be taken, because some of the bacteria may not grow on the culture-media. A culture should be grown and an inoculation should be made in all cases of suspected diphtheria or tuberculosis.

Blood-cultures are important in cases of suspected sinus thrombosis. Sinus thrombosis most frequently accompanies streptococcic infection. An otitis caused by a single bacterium is generally followed by no suppuration or a suppuration lasting but a short time. If one finds in the beginning of a middle-ear suppuration several infective bacterial excitors, pathogenic alone or pathogenic mixed with saprophytes, then the otitis inclines to chronicity.

Bacteria play an important rôle, but do not help always in making a prognosis or in warning us of brain complications. We should be careful not to introduce new and perhaps more virulent bacteria, and for this reason the most careful asepsis should be carried out. Strong antiseptic solutions should not be used, but such sterile solutions which cause the least irritation—*e. g.*, normal salt solution. Only sterilized sticks of absorbent cotton introduced into the auditory canal with forceps or cotton wound on cotton sticks and held in the flame should be used in cleansing the auditory canal.[1]

These conclusions are interesting from a scientific point of view; practically, the bacteriology of the ear is one of the least important aids in diagnosis of aural diseases and their complications.

[1] B. Gomperz, "Zur Sterilisierung der Tupfer Pinsel und Einlagen für Ohr und Nase." Zeit. f. Ohrenheilkunde, LI., Band, Ersten Heft.

CHAPTER IV

THE CAUSATION OF EAR DISEASES

It is not the intention to discuss here the causes of aural ailments except in that broad and general way which is necessary to give an intelligent understanding of the subject as a whole; because in dealing with each separate disease in the subsequent chapters of the work the question of causation will again be dealt with more specifically.

When collectively considered in respect to their etiology it may be said that aural affections arise from injurious agents acting from without through the external auditory meatus; from the nasopharynx through the Eustachian tube, and finally, from systemic diseases which, during their progress, and acting, no doubt, through the medium of the blood and lymph, involve some portion of the hearing apparatus.

As to the relative frequency with which each of the above influences brings about the aural affection, the causes that act through the nasopharynx by way of the Eustachian tube stand first, those acting through the external auditory meatus second, and those produced secondarily by general ailments of the system last.

Chief among the agents that cause aural disease by entering the auditory meatus may be mentioned:

Loud Noises.—The explosion of a gun or a blast of any kind when occurring near the ear may, by the sudden impact of air against the tympanic membrane, be sufficient to injure and sometimes to rupture this structure. It is believed that an explosion of moderate intensity will never cause a rupture unless there has been a previous weakening of the tympanic membrane due to a former disease of this structure which resulted in an atrophy of the part. Middle-ear injuries resulting to men who are constantly engaged in work like blasting are frequently complicated by labyrinthine deafness. The ear is injured in a somewhat similar manner to that which results from explosions by the rarefaction and condensation of the air which takes place in the auditory canal of those who work in caissons or of those who ascend to great heights in balloons. Under such atmospheric conditions the condensation and rarefaction of the air takes place less suddenly than during an explosion, and there is consequently not sufficient violence to the drum membrane to produce a rupture; but the disturbance to the circulation of the middle ear which takes place under these circumstances is productive of serous transudations, or even hemorrhage into the tympanic cavity, which may sooner or later result in either tympanic or labyrinthine deafness.

Cold and Heat.—The entrance of cold water into the meatus may cause an inflammation of the drum-head or even a suppurative inflammation of the middle ear. This is particularly true if the water enters the canal with force, as from a wave striking the ear while surf-bathing or from an individual striking the water with the side of the head in high diving. Prolonged exposure of the ear to a cold, damp wind may produce the same result. Molten metal and boiling water or steam, when entering the ear accidentally, set up a most violent inflammation, and the deep necrosis which follows may prove not only destructive to function but also to life.

Foreign bodies, if large or rough or if hurled into the ear with force, produce not only contusion and laceration of the auditory canal, but may also cause rupture of the tympanic membrane with subsequent destruction of the conducting portion of the middle ear. Awkward and unskilful efforts on the part of the physician to remove smaller and therefore harmless foreign bodies from the auditory meatus may result in serious, though entirely unwarranted, injury to the hearing apparatus.

Injuries from falls or blows are among the causes of middle-ear or labyrinthine affections. The attachment of the posterosuperior integumentary lining of the auditory meatus to the adjacent portion of the drum membrane is such that a rupture of the latter structure may occur as the result of suddenly and vigorously pulling the auricle upward and backward, as is sometimes practised as a method of punishment. A box on the ear, causing condensation of the air in the auditory canal, may rupture the membrana tympani. Falls upon the head may fracture the ossicles and rupture the membrane (see Figs. 133, 134), either with or without a fracture of the base of the skull (see Fig. 305).

General Diseases as Causative Agents.—Among the chronic diseases that cause aural affections secondarily, those of a strumous, tubercular, or luetic nature stand first. Aural discharges of tubercular origin are probably more frequent than has heretofore been realized, although a bacteriologic examination of the pus in most cases of suppurative otitis media fails to show the presence of the tubercle bacillus. In children especially the tubercular aural affection is seen in connection with enlarged and sometimes suppurating cervical glands, in which instances mastoiditis, with extensive necrosis of the mastoid, is not infrequent. Syphilis may produce an acute tubal or tubotympanic catarrh during the inflammatory manifestations that take place in the nose and throat in the secondary stage. This tubal affection may become chronic if the luetic disease progresses to the tertiary stage, when it may then affect not only the middle ear but also the labyrinth, in which case the final outcome will most probably be a greatly impaired hearing or even total deafness in one or both ears. Effusion of serum or even blood sometimes takes place into the labyrinth during the course of syphilis, and in addition to the sudden and profound deafness thus produced severe tinnitus aurium or vertigo and vomiting may occur. These aggravated results of syphilis may be accompanied by active general manifestations of the disease upon the skin and mucous membranes or, the patient having long since thought himself cured, the physician may only be able to connect the remote cause and the effect upon the ear by means of the discovery of old cicatrices in the throat, by a perforated palate or nasal septum, or perhaps by the presence of scars upon the cornea. Several acute diseases are frequently accompanied or followed by an aural affection, which seems to be the result of a toxic disturbance to the nerve or circulatory supply of the labyrinth. Among this class of general diseases, typhoid and typhus fevers and mumps are especially notable.

The exanthemata are by far the most frequent of all the general diseases in the production of the pathogenic bacteria which are essential to the development of the suppurative aural affections. The harmful action upon the hearing organ that results from these general diseases may take place through the circulatory disturbances that occur in the middle ear and labyrinth during the progress of the general affection; chiefly through the accompanying inflammation of the upper respiratory tract and particularly of the nasopharynx This inflammation often rapidly extends to the middle ear, and when infection of the latter takes place is thus primarily responsible for the many violent and destructive processes that occur in this and the adjoining cavities. The author, therefore, believes that these general diseases, when considered in their causative relation to the diseases of the ear, can be more properly considered under the following division:

Causes that Act through the Nasopharynx and Eustachian Tube.—The marked influence which congestion, inflammation, or obstructive growths in the nose and nasopharynx has upon the production of diseases in the middle ear and mastoid is recognized by all observers. Congestion or inflammation in the tympanic cavity may occur through extension of these disturbances from the throat to the ear by continuity of structure, or because a disturbed circulation in the throat may, through vascular communication, produce stagnation, exudation, and subsequent infection of the cavities of the middle ear. Growths either in the nose or nasopharynx may sometimes act mechanically to obstruct the passage of air into the tympanum; their pressure upon adjacent structures also retards the venous circulation from both nasopharynx and middle ear, causing passive congestion and exudation into the tympanum; finally, the obstruction they offer to the free drainage of the tympanum and its environs favors the growth of numerous bacteria which are ever ready to migrate from the throat to the ear, where their presence upon an already weakened membrane may be sufficient to set up the most violent and destructive inflammatory processes.

In the above ways, therefore, the presence of nasopharyngeal adenoids becomes a constant menace to the integrity of the organ of hearing. The deep fissures that penetrate or separate the lobes of these growths are constantly bathed with a thick secretion which is difficult to dislodge, and which furnishes the pabulum for the growth of pathogenic bacteria. When nasal or nasopharyngeal tumors are large enough to block the postnasal spaces and thus prevent the passage of air through the nostrils every act of swallowing rarefies the air within the nasopharyngeal space and likewise that within the middle ear, the defective ventilation resulting in impairment of hearing, tinnitus aurium, middle-ear exudation, perforation, and, finally, aural discharge with all the subsequent possibilities of mastoid and intracranial complication.

The question as to whether or not the presence of disease germs in the middle ear will cause inflammation in the absence of any pre-existing congestion or inflammation of that cavity seems not to be definitely settled. It is stated by some that in the event of pathogenic germs finding their way into the healthy tympanic cavity, they ultimately perish without having caused any local disturbance. However this may be, all observers are agreed upon the fact that in the presence of a congestion or inflammation within the tympanum, with perhaps resulting exudate, the addition of certain bacteria are the prime factors in the subsequent suppuration and destruction of tissue. If we add to the list of the causative relations already attributed to adenoids and other growths in the production of aural disease the additional ones that the patient usually sleeps badly, is often poorly oxygenated, and frequently suffers from stomach and intestinal derangements, it may be better understood how much more easily the preceding causes may become effective.

Acting in a systemic manner certain drugs produce disturbances of

audition, and if their use be continued for a great length of time permanent effects on the function may result. A list of the more active medicines of this class includes alcoholics, salicylates, opium, and especially
quinin, which latter, when given in large doses, as is the custom in
malarial districts, produces marked and permanent effects on the
hearing power.

In addition to the above division of causes, certain others, which
do not come under any one of the classes, are nevertheless sometimes
present. Among these are age, predisposition, and environment.
Each period of life seems to bear some relation to the frequency with
which certain aural ailments are met. Thus in childhood the catarrhal
and suppurative diseases are commonest. This fact is accounted for
largely because the exanthematous diseases are most common in early
life, because of the greater frequency of adenoids at this age, and because
of the anatomic differences in the structure of the nasopharynx and
Eustachian tube. Adhesive and dry forms of middle-ear inflammation
which are often accompanied by labyrinthine complications are most
often seen in adults and those advanced in years. In old age the walls
of the external auditory meatus and also of the mucous membrane of
the Eustachian tube sometimes become flaccid, collapse, and occlude
the respective channels to the extent of seriously interfering with their
proper functions.

Predisposition or heredity has an undoubted influence in the production of some cases of adhesive aural catarrh, and families are not infrequent in whom several members are similarly affected, the disease
beginning at about the same age in each and continuing to old age.
A peculiarity of heredity as a causative factor in diseases of the ear
is noted in the fact that the children of parents afflicted by this type of
aural disease may escape with good hearing, whereas the succeeding
generation is likely to develop the ailment in the original form and at
the corresponding age at which the grandparents became affected.

Mode of life and social position are factors in the causation of many
forms of ear disease. Children who are badly nourished and who
are poorly clothed and filthily housed suffer most frequently from
skin affections of the auricle and external auditory meatus; and a life
spent under these latter conditions also predisposes to suppurative
disease at all periods.

CHAPTER V

DISEASES OF THE EXTERNAL EAR

DISEASES of the auricle may be congenital or acquired. Among the congenital affections the most important are the various defects or abnormalities of the several portions of the auricle—entire absence of the auricle, excessive size of one or both pinnæ, irregular shape of outline together with thinning of the cartilage which comprises the auricle, and more or less obliteration of the folds which constitute the helix and antihelix. The conditions known as polyotia and microtia are also congenital. Chief among the acquired affections are the various skin eruptions and tumors which occur upon the outer ear, and also the deformities of the auricle which are the result of injuries to this portion of the hearing organ.

Since the auricle in man plays but a small part in the production of hearing, its diseases and deformities do not, as a rule, produce any degree of deafness except, when through lack of development, there is a coexisting absence or incompleteness of the conducting or perceptive portions of the ear, or unless the swelling, growth, or deformity of the pinna is of such nature as to block the auditory meatus and prevent the entrance of the sound-waves. The treatment of this class of diseases is, therefore, necessary only on account of the unsightly appearance produced by the auricular deformity or disease, or for the purpose of relieving pain and itching or possibly to arrest the progress of some malignant growth and not for the improvement of impaired function.

MALFORMATION OF THE AURICLE

Undeveloped Helix.—The helix is sometimes ill developed and does not turn forward and downward into its normal scroll. In many such instances the whole pinna is abnormally large, while the cartilaginous framework is unusually thin; the whole, especially if pointed at the upper extremity so as to form the so-called satyr ear, much resembling that of an animal (Fig. 58). On the contrary, the helix may be thick and the upper portion of the auricle may be turned downward and forward to an unusual extent; the helix may even be adherent to the anterior surface of the pinna. When these conditions are found the ear

84

is usually small and the cartilage abnormally thick, the whole condition comprising that known as "lop ears" (Fig. 59).

Absence of Lobule.—The lobule may be absent (see Fig. 62) or may be greatly hypertrophied. The latter condition is most common among the negro races, in some of whom the lobe is enormous in size. This portion of the auricle is sometimes enlongated in those women, chiefly of foreign birth, who wear large and heavy earrings. Occasionally the earring cuts its way through the lobe or it may be suddenly pulled through it, and in either case a divided lobule is the result.

Cartilaginous projections from the tragus or near it are sometimes congenitally present (Fig. 60). These are commonly about ¼ inch wide at the base and from ¾ to 1 inch in length, gradually tapering from the base to a blunt point in an upward, forward, or downward direction.

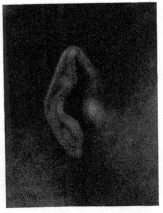

FIG. 58.—DEFORMED AND POINTED HELIX OF AN INSANE INDIVIDUAL. Satyr ear.

Treatment.—The large, thin, ill-shaped "animal ear" usually occurs in individuals who care little concerning the deformity, and

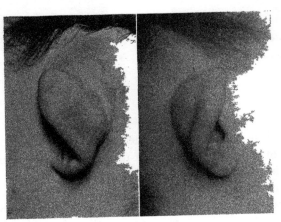

FIG. 59.—LOP EARS, RIGHT AND LEFT, OF SAME PERSON.

since no pain or other inconvenience accompanies the deformity the surgeon is not often consulted concerning it.

In the case of lop ears a correction is more often sought, and may be secured by a plastic operation in which a section of the skin covering the posterior surface of the auricle and including the underlying cartilage is included. The technic of the operation consists in the usual aseptic preparation of the field of operation, hands, and instruments, and the administration of an anesthetic. An incision is made on the posterior surface of the pinna, beginning near the furrow marking the superior attachment of the auricle to the head, and continuing downward parallel to the border of the ear, and at a distance from the border which varies according to the amount of " lopping " which is to be corrected. The length of this incision is governed entirely by the extent of the anterior folding of the cartilage. Likewise the width of the elliptic piece of skin and cartilage which is to be removed is governed

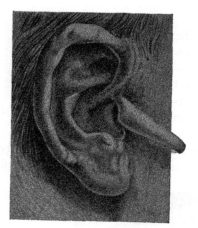

Fig. 60.—Cartilaginous Projection from the Tragus.

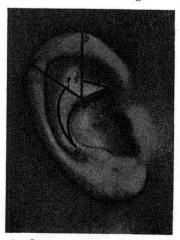

Fig. 61.—Lines of Incision for Reducing Abnormally Large Auricle.

Lines *a, b, c* indicate incisions for reducing the vertical diameter; lines *d, e* and *f, g* the incisions necessary to narrow the transverse diameter.

by the extent of the deformity to be overcome. When the elliptic piece of cartilage is dissected from the skin which covers the corresponding portion of the anterior surface of the ear care must be exercised not to injure it in any manner, since if this part of the auricular integument be injured more or less visible scar will result. Three or more interrupted catgut sutures, which should be passed through the cartilage, are subsequently employed for bringing the edges of the wound together, after which collodion is applied to the line of union, a pad of gauze is placed behind the ear, and a roller bandage is applied to hold the auricle in a fixed position until healing occurs. If judgment has been used as to the size of the piece of skin and cartilage which has been removed, and if skill and cleanliness were employed in the execution of the same, a very gratifying result may be obtained by the above method.

Cartilaginous spurs (Fig. 60) which spring from the vicinity of the tragus may be easily removed by forming an outer skin flap, which is dissected down to the base of the growth, which latter is at this point excised, and lastly by stitching the flap over the stump, using fine cat-gut sutures. Practically no scar is left when the spur is carefully removed by this method. A greatly enlarged lobule could be easily removed by plastic methods, but the surgeon is seldom requested to perform this operation.

In case the auricle is larger than its fellow and protrudes from the side of the head in an unsightly manner, both the redundant size and abnormal position may be satisfactorily corrected by a plastic operation. To successfully reduce both the vertical and horizontal diameters of the ear, triangular pieces including the entire thickness of the ear are removed (Fig. 61), after which remaining parts of the auricle are accurately adjusted and held in place by interrupted sutures. The completed dressing is made after the manner designated in the operation for lop ears. When this operation is performed on an individual in whom the opposite ear is normal both in size and position, a satisfactory outcome, in so far as the esthetic effect is concerned, will depend very much on the accuracy in judgment which is exercised by the surgeon as to the size of the wedge-shaped pieces which are removed; for if these be too large it is obvious that the resulting auricle will be too small, whereas if the wedges are not large enough, the operation will not completely correct the deformity. An error in either direction will result in disappointment.

Microtia and Entire Absence of the Auricle.—Microtia, as its name indicates, is a congenital defect of the auricle in which the ear is without definite form, often amounting to nothing more than a tab of skin at or in the vicinity of the site of the normal ear (Fig. 62). Sometimes this fold of skin contains cartilage, and the whole may be compressed and adherent to the side of the head, the same covering the site of the external auditory meatus. This class of auricular malformation is usually associated with a lack of development of other portions of the auditory apparatus. Thus, in a case of microtia, the external auditory canal may be entirely wanting or a depression only may mark its normal situation. In patients who are old enough to give reliable information as a result of tuning-fork tests it is frequently ascertained that bone conduction is deficient or absent, which fact would indicate a lack or even a complete failure of development of the internal ear. This defect may include one or both ears. It is often associated with defective mental development and with malformation of the face and mouth.

Treatment.—Correction of this class of malformation is usually impossible. The position and shape of the skin-tabs representing the auricle are often such that the individual's appearance is improved by their complete removal, in which case the attempt may be made to substitute an artificial pinna.

Various operative measures have been suggested for improving the hearing in this class of cases, but none have ever succeeded in doing so with any considerable degree of satisfaction. In case the patient is old enough to give reliable information concerning the functional examination, and it is positively ascertained that the impaired hearing

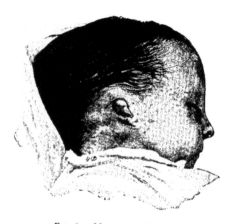

Fig. 62.—Microtia. (Dench.)

is due to a defect in the conducting portion of the ear, operative measures should always be advised in the hope that it is possible to restore the auditory meatus and thus admit sound-waves to the perceptive portion of the ear. The first step of this operation is performed by removing all tabs of skin, then making a crucial incision over the presumed site of the external auditory meatus, and, finally, lifting each of the four flaps from the bone by means of a periosteal elevator (see Fig. 161). The exposed skull surface should always be of sufficient extent to enable the operator to see clearly any landmark upon the temporal bone that may be present, and to discover any opening which may lead into the cavium tympani. If no such opening is present the operation should be abandoned for the reason that in operating without any such guide injury may be done to the brain, lateral sinus, or facial nerve. Should, however, a fistulous tract be found leading to the middle ear, the same should be enlarged by means of small gouges, which are used in the manner advocated in doing the radical mastoid operation (see p. 385). When the operation is undertaken the same anatomic knowledge should be available, and the same care and skill should be exercised as when performing the radical mastoid operation. After the intervening osseous tissues have been removed, and the newly constructed auditory meatus has been honed perfectly smooth by means of the curet or dental burr, the triangular skin flaps are tucked into the newly formed meatus and are held snugly against the osseous walls by means of a light gauze packing until adhesion takes place. Much of the raw surface is in this way lined with skin, from which the epithelium will soon grow and cover the remaining denuded areas.

Supernumerary Auricles. Polyotia.—Instances of the presence of more than one ear on each side of the head have been recorded (Fig. 63). Wilde saw a case having four auricles, two in the natural position, while the additional two were located on the neck. In this case it was stated that there were also two petrous portions for each temporal bone. The supernumerary auricle may be unilateral or bilateral; it may be more or less perfectly formed or may be nothing more than a tab of skin, as in the case reported by Birkett, in which a young girl had a large growth resembling a lobule which sprang from the middle of the neck over the sternomastoid muscle. The mass

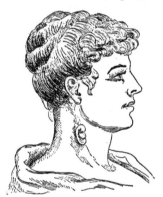

FIG. 63.—POLYOTIA.

contained fibrocartilage. Multiple auricles are always found over the lines of the branchial clefts and, according to Paget, may be considered as cutaneous growths, which though abnormal are homologous with the natural auricles.

Treatment.—The supernumerary auricles may be removed surgically. A flap of skin sufficiently large to cover the base of the auricle after the excision is performed is first dissected from the appendage, and this flap is then stitched into place by the requisite number of fine catgut sutures. If the auricle which is located in the normal situation is malformed, attempts may be made to correct the malformation by the plastic method already described. If the external auditory meatus is closed and the functional examination proves that the perceptive apparatus is not involved, the same operation which was advised under microtia for the establishment of a tympanic communication may be undertaken (see p. 88).

Congenital Fistulæ.—These are usually found just in front of the tragus or upon the face immediately in front of the attachment of the helix. The orifice leading into the fistulous tract is often so insignificant as to admit only the smallest probe and the depth of the fistula is usually not greater than 5 or 6 mm. The channel represents the position of the second branchial cleft and is not in any way connected with the middle ear. Its presence may be entirely overlooked except upon the most careful inspection, for the mouth is often hidden by a fold in the adjacent skin. Such fistulæ give rise to no inconvenience whatever unless, as sometimes happens, there is an accumulation of cystic material or unless some foreign body has entered the channel. In either case an inflammatory swelling may result. No treatment is usually necessary. Should a cyst formation take place the fistula should be laid open and its path be cureted or cauterized, after which the parts are held in contact by a compress, when complete obliteration of the cleft promptly occurs.

CHAPTER VI

DISEASES OF THE AURICULAR PERICHONDRIUM

PERICHONDRITIS

INFLAMMATION of the perichondrium may result from an injury to the auricle, may be due to the outward extension of an infection of the auditory canal, or may develop without any known cause. Numerous cases have been reported in which a perichondritis has occurred subsequently to the radical mastoid operation, during the performance of which the cartilage is necessarily wounded in the formation of the skin flaps.

Symptoms.—Following a blow upon the ear or a furunculosis of the external auditory meatus, a gradual tumefaction takes place upon the anterior surface of the auricle. At first the surface is red, the local temperature is elevated, and sooner or later the characteristic folds of the convex surface of the ear are obliterated. Since this disease involves only the perichondrium, the lobule is not included in the swelling. The swelling is due to the effusion of a serous exudate beneath the perichondrium, which dissects the latter from the cartilage and creates a cavity of varying size which is completely filled with serum or blood. This exudate may later become infected and purulent, in which event it will finally rupture through the skin, leaving a discharging fistula which may persist indefinitely. The affection resembles othematoma, but may be diagnosed from the latter by its slower formation and greater transparency. In perichondritis and tumefaction due to an exudate, if a diagnostic electric lamp be placed behind the ear in a perfectly dark room the tumor will be thoroughly transilluminated; whereas, in othematoma, in which the swelling is caused by a collection of blood beneath the perichondrium, the transillumination will show a dark area over the anterior site of the tumor.

Treatment.—Since unsightly deformity will most probably result in any case which is left to nature, prompt measures should be instituted at the earliest possible moment after the reception of an injury to the auricle which is likely to result in the affection in question. If the patient is plethoric a saline purge should be administered, the artificial leech should be applied posterior to the auricle (see p. 126), and an ice-bag should be subsequently kept in contact with the affected part for twenty-four or thirty-six hours. Since the inflamed and swollen auricle is exquisitely tender, the presence of the ice-bag will not be tolerated by the patient unless the ear be properly padded by placing a suitable roll of cotton behind the auricle. The ice-bag itself should be of a size much greater than is necessary to cover the auricle and should be only partially filled with finely crushed ice. By the exercise of all these precautions but little weight will necessarily rest upon the affected part, and therefore no considerable pain results from the treatment itself.

Should these early measures fail to prevent the effusion, surgical means should be employed before the exudate has spread and has caused extensive separation of the perichondrium from the cartilage, an event which may result in death of the latter, and consequently greater is the liability to deformity of the auricle. At an early date and before the effusion has become purulent the fluid may be removed by aspiration. It usually returns immediately, however, and some means of causing the adhesion of the separated cartilage and its perichondrium, and therefore of obliteration of the cavity, should be employed immediately after the cavity has been thus evacuated. For this purpose a stiff wire spring may be used. The auricle is padded by one or two layers of absorbent cotton on each side, and over this the expanded ends of the spring are placed and allowed to remain from twenty-four to thirty-six hours. Care should, of course, be exercised not to cause sufficient pressure to retard the circulation in the part and thus invite sloughing of the affected area.

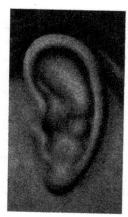

FIG. 64.—DEFORMITY OF THE AURICLE RESULTING FROM TRAUMA.

In most cases it is better to incise the tumefaction freely and by this means most thoroughly evacuate the exudate. When incised early a small iodoform wick should be inserted into the cavity to serve as a drain, an abundance of loose gauze is placed upon each side of the auricle, and a roller bandage is then applied over all with moderate pressure. When the exudate is purulent the interior of the cavity should be cureted with a sharp spoon in order to clear away all granulations and necrotic débris; the space is then loosely filled with iodoform gauze and the dressing is completed as above directed.

Some deformity of the ear (Fig. 64) may be expected in cases that have come late to operation, but if in the beginning of treatment the swelling is freely incised and is aseptically cared for afterward, the normal outline of the auricle should usually be restored.

OTHEMATOMA

Othematoma, or hematoma of the auricle, occurs as the result of an effusion of blood between the perichondrium and the cartilage. The cause of such a hemorrhage may be either traumatic or spontaneous, about three-fourths of all cases resulting from some injury to the auricle, whereas about one-fourth occur without any assignable reason. The affection is more frequently found upon the left than upon the right side, no doubt principally for the reason that the injury which causes it is often the result of a blow from the fist or open hand of an opponent in fighting or boxing, and since such blows are given by the right hand of the antagonist, the left ear must inevitably suffer most.

Excepting professional boxers, othematoma is probably more often seen in the insane than in any other class. Occurring in those with mental defect the hemorrhage is perhaps as frequently of spontaneous origin as it is due to injury, and this frequency of spontaneous hemorrhage has been explained on the ground that it is due to tissue changes in the auricle, which are somewhat common among the insane. An ingenious theory for both the tissue changes in the auricle of the mentally degenerate and of the consequent hemorrhage beneath the perichondrium has been based upon the physiologic discovery of Brown-Séquard, to the effect that a hemorrhage occurs in the auricle of animals after the restiform body has been severed.

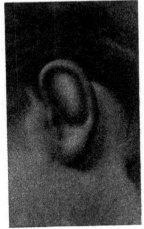

FIG. 65.—CASE OF OTHEMATOMA. TRAUMATIC. (Hematoma auris.)

Symptoms.—Whether the result of an injury or of spontaneous effusion, the hematoma auris suddenly appears upon the anterior surface of the auricle as an irregular, doughy, red, or bluish-red swelling, which obliterates the underlying folds of skin and cartilage (Fig. 65). Othematomata due to injury are usually larger than those which result from spontaneous causes. The latter variety may be multiple. Either kind may spring from the concha or near it, and when so located the hearing is impaired because of the obstruction thus offered to the passage of the sound-waves. When located elsewhere upon the auricle the hearing is in nowise affected by the swelling. The sudden onset of the hemorrhage causes considerable tension upon the adjacent tissues and hence much pain is experienced, especially in traumatic cases, in which latter a feeling of intense local heat may be present and add greatly to the suffering of the individual.

Diagnosis.—Othematoma is liable to be mistaken for only angioma of the auricle, new growths, or perichondritis. Angiomata and other tumors of the auricle are slow of growth and are often many months in attaining any considerable size, whereas the othematoma appears suddenly. Perichondritis, while of more rapid formation than new growths of the auricle, is nevertheless much less sudden in making its appearance than is the case when an effusion of blood is responsible for the auricular swelling. The tumor following perichondritis is uniformly illuminated by transmitted light, whereas transillumination of the othematoma shows a dark spot over the area of the blood-clot.

Treatment.—Small othematoma when of spontaneous origin may for a time be left to nature's process of removal by absorption, since local applications, the employment of compress bandages, and massage all have a tendency to cause a renewal of the hemorrhage and hence to increase the size of the tumor. In case the swelling does not disappear after two or three weeks, and especially if it should become larger, the same surgical measures should be employed that are advised below for the large blood-tumor of traumatic origin.

The treatment of the recent, large, and painful othematomata should for a few days be expectant. The auricle may be coated with a 15 per cent. ointment of ichthyol, soft pads of absorbent cotton may be placed on either side, and an ice-bag be applied over all, as has already been directed in case of traumatic aural inflammation. Should, however, the pain and swelling show no tendency to subside as the result of this treatment after its continuance for a period of two or three days, the best results will be obtained from a free incision of the swelling and the complete removal of the clot. In case the difficulty is of long standing and infection of the clot has taken place, the cavity must be thoroughly cureted after the pus is evacuated, in order to clear out all granulations and necrotic tissue that has formed. When the injury which causes the hemorrhage of the ear has been of a severe nature the cartilaginous framework of the auricle is sometimes fractured or perhaps comminuted, in which case necrosis of the fragments of the cartilage may occur. In this event any necrotic portions of the cartilage should be removed, along with the general riddance of all other questionable structures both in and about the seat of the abscess. When the wound has been cleansed from all disease, a loose packing of iodoform gauze is inserted and the roller

dage is lastly employed with the intention of securing moderate
ssure upon both sides of the auricle. In those instances in which
as been found necessary to remove more or less of the auricular
tilage during the operation, a through-and-through drainage is often
re efficient than that just described, and this can be secured by
tly packing the wound with sterile gauze after a plan that will allow
h end of the strip to project from each side of the opening—one upon
postauricular surface and the other upon the anterior.

CHAPTER VII

TUMORS OF THE AURICLE

NEW formations of the auricle are either of a benign or malignant character. Of the former, those most often seen on the external ear are sebaceous cysts, fibroma, papilloma, and angioma. Sarcoma and epithelioma constitute the chief varieties of malignant growths in this locality.

BENIGN TUMORS OF THE AURICLE

Sebaceous Cysts.—This variety of tumor occurs most frequently on the lobule or posterior to or below the lobule (Fig. 66). It is a variety of retention cyst, and is the result of an inflammatory occlusion of the mouth of one of the sebaceous glands and the consequent accumulation of the normal sebaceous secretion. The size of the resulting enlargement depends upon the amount of sebaceous material the adjacent structure is capable of retaining before a rupture through the skin takes place and the fluid is discharged. Thus, if the sebaceous contents accumulate slowly and the skin and areolar tissue of the lobule are gradually put upon the stretch, a tumor of considerable dimension may finally be produced. Should a rupture occur, an intermittent discharge of thick creamy or cheesy material takes place, the rupture closes temporarily, the cavity refills and again breaks through, the cycle being indefinitely repeated.

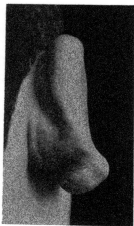

FIG. 66.—CYST OF LOBULE OF AURICLE.
Case of Dr. Wales, Mass. Charitable Eye and Ear Infirmary.

A sebaceous cyst is slightly movable under the skin, feels elastic to the touch, and is not painful when moderately compressed. The tumor gives rise to no pain or disturbance of any kind unless it ruptures and discharges. The unsightly appearance of deformity or, perhaps, the fear of malignancy are reasons which usually cause the individual to seek the advice of the surgeon.

Treatment.—Removal of the tumor by surgical methods constitutes

96

the only effective means of treatment. This may be accomplished under local anesthesia, Schleich's plan being preferable, although freezing the growth by means of the ether spray or kelin may also be employed for this purpose.

Following the established rules of asepsis in the preparation of the affected part for the operation, an incision is made through the skin down to the cyst wall, after which a dull dissector is used and the cyst is hulled out, if possible, without rupture of the sac or the evacuation of its contents Should the cyst have ruptured previously to the operation or should it be accidentally broken into during the attempt at its removal, the sac should be completely dissected out subsequently to the discharge of its contents. When successful in removing the cyst unbroken or, if ruptured, if successful in dissecting the sac out in its entirety, nothing further remains to complete the operation except the insertion of a necessary number of sutures to accurately approximate the cut edges of the wound. If the operator is uncertain as to whether or not he has completely removed all the cystic walls, the interior of the cavity should be cureted in every direction by a sharp instrument, after which carbolic acid and iodin solution is mopped over the interior and the wound subsequently closed by sutures except at its lower angle. An exterior pad of loose gauze and a roller bandage completes the dressing. Refilling of the cyst does not occur unless the sac or some portion of it has not been removed. No deformity results from the operation.

Fibroma.—This class of auricular tumor may occur on any portion of the ear, but the most usual site is the lobule. Race seems to be an important factor in the causation of fibroma, since it is seen with greatest frequency among negroes. The size of the fibroma may vary from that so small as to be scarcely distinguishable to a growth the size of a hen's egg. It is usually smooth, hard, and regular in outline, but may occasionally be nodular and even pedunculated, the latter variety sometimes being long enough to reach the patient's shoulder. The irritation to which the lobule is subjected from wearing heavy earrings, especially when these are made from base metals, constitutes the immediate cause of the growth in many cases.

The *prognosis* is good, the tumor often persisting indefinitely without degeneration and change to a malignant nature. After the most complete removal the tumor may return a second, third, or even a fourth time, and in such instances may ultimately become malignant.

Treatment.—Operative measures constitute the sole treatment. When the growth is small and consequently produces no unsightly deformity, the rule should be to allow it to remain unmolested. Should the fibroma be growing rapidly or should deformity result, its complete removal should be advised.   The technic of the removal when located on the lobule consists in making a V-shaped incision over the site of the tumor, the apex of the V pointing toward the concha, the angle and length of the two extremities of the V depending, of course, upon the size of the growth.   After the extirpation of the neoplasm the flaps should be approximated and held in place by fine catgut sutures.   When fitting the flaps preparatory to introducing the sutures a comparison of the size and shape of the affected lobule should be made with that of its fellow of the opposite side, and any redundancy of tissue in the flaps should be trimmed off to an extent that will insure a lobule which is as nearly as possible symmetric with the opposite ear.

Papilloma.—Benign epithelial excrescences may spring from the auricle either in the form of common warts, in which case the growth seldom exceeds the size of a split pea, or they may be of a conic, horn-like shape, of considerable size, and of a dense and horny structure. Horny growths of the auricle have been reported by Pomeroy [1] and Buck.[2] In all 4 cases reported by these two authors the horny growth sprang from the upper and posterior rim of the helix, varied in length from $\frac{1}{2}$ to $\frac{3}{4}$ inch, and one was about $\frac{3}{4}$ inch in diameter at its base of attachment to the helix.   The apex of the excrescences were dense and hard, whereas the bases were of a somewhat softer structure; and, in Dr. Pomeroy's case, this portion of the growth resembled cartilage.

The *treatment* consists in excision, and recovery without a return of the growth occurred in the reported cases.   Common warts should be excised from their bases by means of curved scissors, after which the raw surfaces are immediately cauterized with nitric acid.

Angiomata.—Angiomata are of two kinds—simple and cavernous. The former discolors the skin over the site of its location, but does not project from the surface of the auricle in the form of a tumor, whereas the latter protrudes from the ear in the form of a greater or less nodular mass (Fig. 67).   Angiomata are congenital or acquired.   When present at birth the auricular neoplasm may be accompanied by similar angiomata on the face, jaw, or other parts of the body.   The cause of the acquired variety is sometimes unknown, but is most usually attributed to an injury of the part.   Dr. J. M. Warren reported the case of a large angioma of the lobule which occurred twenty years subsequent to a frost-bite of the same portion of the auricle.

The color of the growth is reddish or bluish.   It is usually soft and

---

[1] *Diseases of the Ear*, p. 52.
[2] *Trans. Am. Otol. Society*, 1871.

yielding to the touch and can frequently be emptied and temporarily reduced in size by firm pressure made upon it. The affection is or is not painful, depending largely upon the rapidity of its development; for in the rapidly growing tumor the tissues are rather suddenly put upon the stretch, thus causing a varying degree of suffering, whereas if of slower growth there is less tension of the structures involved and conse-quently less pain. In cases of cavernous angioma the patient usually complains of an annoying pulsation in the affected auricle.

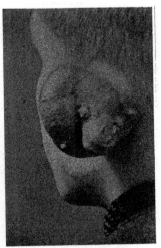

FIG. 67.—ANGIOMA OF THE AURICLE. (Hugh E. Jones.)

Treatment.—When of moderate size, removal of the angioma by means of electrolysis is convenient, bloodless, prac-tically painless, and usually successful. The platinum needle is attached to the negative pole of the battery, is passed entirely through the base of the tumor, and from 3 to 5 milliampères of current are turned on. When the parts overlying the needle are whitened, the needle is with-drawn and reinserted at a distance of about 2 mm. and parallel to the first insertion. This procedure is repeated until the whole tumor is uniformily whitened, when, if thought necessary, the needle may be passed repeatedly through the angioma at right angles to the previous insertions.

The mass of tissue thus destroyed will slough out in a few days and the wound will heal by granulation. Another and a very successful method is to perforate the tumor in all directions with a red-hot needle. The larger angiomata may be destroyed by the method first introduced by Esmarch, which is performed as follows: Small-sized threads of silk are soaked in a solution of the tincture of the chlorid of iron, after which they are threaded into a properly curved needle and passed en-tirely through the base of the tumor, each being cut off so as to project slightly from each side of the growth. The threads should be passed through the base of the angioma about 2 mm. apart, and are left in posi-tion until coagulation and sloughing has taken place. Two rows of threads, introduced at right angles to each other, may be necessary to its destruction in case the growth is large. A light sterile dressing is applied over the ear and allowed to remain until separation of the slough has occurred.

Treatment by the injection of coagulating fluids into this class of growth, with a view to its destruction, cannot be recommended, for the reason that some of the injected material may directly enter the blood-current and produce a dangerous embolus.

MALIGNANT TUMORS OF THE AURICLE

Malignant growths of the auricle are among the rarest of the neo-plasms found in this location. Affections of this nature may attack any portion of the auricle, may extend from the auricle into the auditory meatus, to the face or mastoid region; or, on the other hand, they may begin upon the face or in the auditory canal and later spread to the pinna. Of the two malignant diseases most commonly seen on the auricle—sarcoma - and epithelioma—the latter stands first in point of frequency.

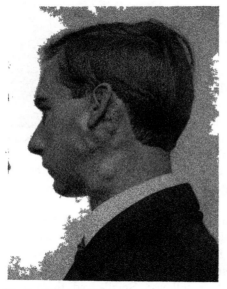

Fig. 68.—Sarcoma Affecting the External Auditory Meatus and Neighboring Soft Structures.

Sarcomata.—Malignant tumors of the sarcomatous variety rarely occur on the external ear. Most usually when found in the latter situation they are the result of an extension of the disease from structures adjoining the auricle (Fig. 68). The growth may be slow or rapid; depending largely upon whether or not it is of the small, round-cell variety or is of the spindle-cell or giant-cell type. When of round-cell structure the disease is rapid and death has been known to occur as early as seven months from the date of the onset. On the other hand, the spindle-celled sarcomata and the fibrosarcomata may be present on the auricle, as elsewhere, for years without giving rise to the symptoms of disintegration and subsequent death of the individual.

The *diagnosis* is of great importance, for the reason that when the nature of the growth is determined at an early date the institution of proper measures for treatment may not only prevent serious deformity of the ear but also the otherwise untimely death of the patient. The diagnosis is usually impossible in the very earliest stages, at which time nothing more than the fact that a tumor is present can be ascertained., At this time the integumentary covering of the growth is normal in color, there is little or no pain on pressure, and the patient is only aware of the presence of the tumor by having accidentally felt it or because of the slight deformity to which it gives rise. While sarcoma may occur at any age, it is more frequently seen in the young, during that time of life when constructive tissue metamorphosis is most active (Fig. 68). Sarcoma is unlike carcinoma in the particular that sarcoma does not usually involve the neighboring lymphatic glands, as is the case in carcinoma. Round-cell sarcomata grow rapidly and there soon appears over the integumentary covering a reddened or inflamed area which quickly disintegrates and leaves a raw, granulating, highly vascular, and sometimes fleshy-looking surface that discharges a fetid, watery, or sanious fluid. The ulceration extends both centrally and peripherally, and in the worst cases involves not only the auricle but also the external auditory meatus, the parotid gland, and the osseous structures of the temporal bone. The facial nerve is sometimes included in the ulcerative process, and as a result of its destruction facial paralysis ensues. When a sarcoma first begins actively to disintegrate and to exhibit an angry inflammatory redness over its integumentary surface, it may be mistaken for a simple inflammatory swelling. The brief duration of a swelling of the latter character and its accompanying systemic disturbances if taken into account would serve to distinguish the onset of an abscess from a beginning sarcoma. The clinical evidence obtainable by a microscopic examination of a section of the growth should, when possible, he added to that obtained from the history of the case and the physical inspection of the diseased area.

Treatment.—Any tumor of the auricle or of its immediate environs which has remained quiescent for a considerable time, but which has begun to grow rapidly, should be suspected of malignancy and should therefore be excised at once. Caustics, either of a chemical or potential nature, have no place in the treatment of such tumors. If the excision is thoroughly performed before superficial ulceration takes place and before the deeper tissues of the ear and neck are involved, the resulting scar will be less and the likelihood of a return of the growth will be greatly reduced. In case there is already a widespread ulceration and the adjoining structures, including portions of the temporal bone, are involved, operative measures are often inadvisable, and if undertaken result in the incomplete removal of the disease, which, therefore, promptly returns should the patient survive long enough. Especially is an operation for removal not to be undertaken in cases where the parotid gland is greatly infiltrated, the external auditory meatus blocked by ulcerative products, and the facial nerve destroyed, as evidenced by the presence of complete facial paralysis of the affected side. When the disease affects only the auricle, external meatus, and adjacent bone, the growth may be excised and the portions of bone which are involved may be removed by following the steps—perhaps in a modified way—which are necessary to the performance of the radical mastoid operation (see Chap. XXX.). Temporary relief may be secured in cases of this latter kind when not too far advanced, but ultimate recurrence of the growth and a fatal termination should be expected in the vast majority.

Epithelioma.—Epithelioma sometimes has its beginning in the auditory canal, but more often it originates on the auricle or in the adjoining

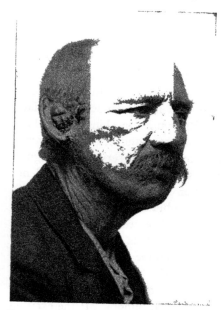

FIG. 69.—EPITHELIOMA INVOLVING THE AURICLE, MIDDLE EAR, AND LABYRINTH.
The facial nerve has been destroyed and facial paralysis is present. See also Fig. 70.

tissues, and later spreads to the meatus (Fig. 69). Its pathologic histology differs in no respect from that found in the same kind of growth when located elsewhere, but the symptoms attendant upon its development in the ear are influenced greatly by the local surroundings. In an auditory meatus that has long been the seat of an irritation from eczema, the presence of pus, or other similar affections, there may develop an abrasion accompanied by severe pain. This abrasion finally assumes the type of an angry-looking ulcer; gradually the pain takes on a more intense character and ultimately it becomes severe enough to interfere with rest at night (see Fig. 70). A scanty, foul-smelling discharge occurs, septic absorption from the abraded surface takes place, and the glands nearest the pinna are first infiltrated, and then finally the whole chain of cervical lymphatics may become involved. Necrotic sloughs take place in the auditory canal, the normal structures of which may thus be completely destroyed; ultimately the disease spreads both deeply and widely until death occurs from hemorrhage or exhaustion.

Epithelioma may be mistaken for either sarcoma or tuberculosis of the skin. Epithelioma occurs in those past middle life, whereas both lupus and sarcoma are diseases which most usually appear in the young. The ulcer which occurs in lupus is less painful than that of epithelioma, and in lupus there may be more than one ulcer present, whereas in epithelioma the ulcer is single. The ulcer of an epithelioma feels hard, its edges are indurated, everted, and whitish; the base is rough and glazed, the secretion is comparatively scanty and often foul smelling. The edges of a lupus ulcer are soft, not everted, the floor is smooth and granulating, and the exudate is abundant and free from odor. A microscopic section of lupoid structures will show the presence of the tubercle bacillus; of epithelioma, the epithelial structure and

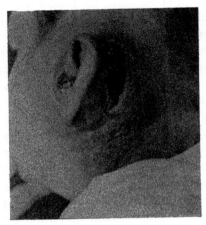

FIG. 70.—CARCINOMA OF THE MIDDLE EAR AND MASTOID.
Advanced inoperable case.

nests; of sarcoma, an embryonic structure of one of three types will be found, namely, small round cells, spindle cells, or giant cells.

Treatment.—When seen sufficiently early excision of the growth may be practised, either removing it by operating within the auditory canal or by detaching the auricle and cutting away all suspicious looking structures, including diseased portions of the temporal bone. If located upon the auricle or superficially in the auditory meatus the x-ray should be tried. When the disease has become widely ulcerated (Fig. 70) and the lymphatic glands of the neck are already infected by secondary deposits the case is hopeless, and anodynes administered internally and soothing applications applied externally constitute the chief indications for treatment.

CHAPTER VIII

CUTANEOUS AFFECTIONS OF THE EXTERNAL EAR

ECZEMA

ECZEMA of the auricle, of the external meatus, or of the skin adjoining the auricular attachment is frequently seen in aural practise. Because of its frequency, the very great suffering caused by the pruritis which accompanies the disease, and of the tendency of the acute forms to become chronic, this affection is considered of sufficient importance to entitle it to a separate chapter.

The Acute Form.—An acute eczema usually begins at some point on the auricle, just within the auditory canal or over an area behind the ear, usually that in or adjoining the furrow which marks its attachment; or the whole auricle, the external meatus, and the adjoining integument may be simultaneously involved.

Causation.—The disease may be primary as the result of some local irritation or it may be secondary to constitutional dyscrasia, in which latter instance the aural manifestation is likely to be only a part of a more general eczematous eruption. The affection sometimes arises without any assignable cause whatever, although a previous local irritation or some constitutional disturbance is usually evident. Among the local exciting agents productive of the disease may be mentioned excessive heat or cold, as exposure to the hot sun, to a low temperature in winter, or to the application to the ear of heat or cold in the form of an ice-bag or hot-water bottle for the relief of pain during acute aural inflammation. The application of certain remedies to the ear has also been followed by acute eczema. Among these may be mentioned chloroform liniments and mercurial or iodoform powders or ointments. An irritating aural discharge, if not promptly neutralized by frequent cleansing of the auditory meatus, is one of the most common local causes of eczema.

The hooks of spectacles, when allowed to hug the ear too closely, will in time set up an eczema in a susceptible individual.

The constitutional ailments that are most productive of eczema are the lithemic and rheumatic diatheses, struma, and rachitis. When due to the first-named cause the individual is usually plethoric, overfed,

104

of constipated habit, and leads a sedentary life; whereas the strumous and rachitic classes who are so affected are usually badly nourished, poorly housed, and are often compelled to perform labor in excess of their strength.

Symptoms.—A tingling, burning feeling is first felt over the affected area, and this rapidly develops into a pruritis of such intensity that the patient constantly desires to scratch and rub the seat of inflammation. In the worst forms the itching is so violent that the patient is thereby quite distracted, and in the effort to secure relief will scratch and rub the affected area so vigorously that the tissues are wounded by the fingernails to the extent that blood or serum oozes from every part of the inflamed skin. At first an erythematous redness only is seen, but soon the color is deepened and considerable swelling takes place. This is quickly followed by the eruption of numerous small vesicles which are naturally short lived, but which are commonly broken almost immediately by the vigorous scratching of the patient in his frantic efforts to secure relief. The serous contents of the vesicles, together with the subsequent serous exudate from the denuded corium, constitutes a variety of the disease commonly known as " weeping eczema." Later this exudate dries into yellowish crusts, which may be of sufficient extent and thickness to obscure the folds of the pinna or to block the external auditory meatus. When not removed these crusts confine the subsequent exudate, which latter, becoming infected, accumulates under the crusts as a reservoir of pus, and in the effort to liberate itself causes still further erosion of the underlying tissues. During its confinement under the crusts some absorption of the pus may take place, which fact furnishes an explanation for the slight rise of temperature that sometimes accompanies this stage of the eczema. No disturbance to the hearing results from the eczema unless the dried secretion and desquamated epithelium, together with the accompanying swelling of the auditory meatus, is sufficient to occlude the auditory canal, or unless the inflammatory process has involved the dermoid layer of the tympanic membrane. In either case a varying though usually moderate degree of deafness may be present.

Prognosis.—The mildest forms of acute eczema will run the entire course of hyperemia, vesiculation, and desquamation, and the recovery be complete within a few days. In this type of case the vesicles do not rupture, exudation does not take place upon the skin, and the epidermis is subsequently shed in the form of fine branny scales. The deeper skin structures not having been involved, subsequent thickening of this structure does not occur. Most cases are, however, not so fortunate.

The vesicles go on to rupture or, as most usually happens, are scratched open, the deeper structures are at the same time lacerated, and the disease runs its whole course of crust formation and pustulation; deeper desquamation then follows, requiring several days or even weeks in the worst cases for the completion of the process and a return to the normal. When some constitutional disease has been the chief causative agent in the production of the acute eczema a continuance of the disease into the chronic form is often observed. Frequent relapses may be expected in any case, and an individual who has once suffered from an eczema is thereby predisposed to future attacks.

Treatment.—The successful management of this disease must be upon a plan that will correct the continued action of the causative systemic or local irritant upon the affected parts. This should include that plan of medication which is the most soothing to the actively inflammatory state of the skin and to its highly excitable and oversensitive nerve-endings. The use of pure water for any purpose upon an acute eczematous area usually acts as an additional irritant and should, where possible, be withheld. If an aural discharge is present it is better, therefore, to mop the entire auditory canal with cylinders of cotton after the manner already given (see p. 340) rather than to cleanse the canal by syringing. Dry cleansing should be done often enough to prevent the accumulation of acrid secretions upon any part of the auditory canal. If it becomes necessary to syringe an eczematous ear for the purpose of removing dried crusts from the meatus or irritating discharges from the middle ear, the fluid best suited for this purpose is one to which 5 gr. of sodium bicarbonate to 1 ounce of water has been added, and if severe itching is present, the addition of 1 or 2 per cent. carbolic acid is indicated. Demulcent solutions, like oatmeal or slippery elm water, are also grateful to the acutely inflamed skin, and may be substituted for the alkaline solution if that should prove irritating. Each time after thus thoroughly removing all pus from the channel, a small quantity of calomel or bismuth subnitrate may be blown into the auditory canal or may be dusted over any moist surface upon the concha or pinna Powders thus employed should be known to be pure and free from lumps. Other impalpable non-irritating powders of greatest value as protective agents are starch, rice flour, talcum, oxid of zinc, and lycopodium. Under no circumstances is it wise in case of eczema of the meatus to introduce large quantities of any kind of powder, for the reason that so soon as it is saturated by the pus or eczematous exudate it forms into hard crusts, which will block the channel and retain the secretions unless the obstruction be quickly removed; and it should be remembered that the removal of such masses is often accomplished with some difficulty. When the itching is intense and the parts feel hot to the patient, especially when the whole auricle appears greatly swollen and the exudate is very profuse, the application of a wash of subacetate of lead and opium proves efficacious in many instances:

R. Tinct. opii, ℥ss;
Liquor plumbi subacetate, dilute, q. s. ad. ℥viij.—M.

A valuable astringent and sedative lotion may also be obtained by combining lime-water and carbolic acid in proper proportions to meet the requirements of the individual case. Thus the following combination may be modified and made suitable to the individual by either increasing or decreasing the amount of phenol, which, as a rule, should not exceed 1 dr. to 1 pint:

R. Carbolic acid, gr. xl;
Zinc oxid, ℨj;
Glycerin, ℨiv;
Aquæ calcis, q. s. ad. ℥viij.—M.

It is highly essential to successful treatment that some means be devised to prevent the patient from constantly lacerating his ear with his fingernails in an effort to allay the itching. Success in this direction, especially in children, is most certainly attained by first applying the local medication that is chosen, then covering the ear with a thick pad of sterile gauze, and finally finishing the dressing by the application of a roller bandage about the head, exactly as is done in the completion of a mastoid dressing (see p. 396, Fig. 255). Owing to the untiring efforts which the patient will sometimes make in rubbing the itching part through this dressing, the same will be quickly dislodged unless extra care is bestowed upon its application. The use of long strips of adhesive plaster to fasten the separate turns of the bandage as they are applied to the head is a method to be recommended in this particular dressing.

Ointments or oils frequently act better than powders or lotions, especially when the acute is passing to the subacute stage. In general, it may be said that when the parts are intensely inflamed, burning and itching, in the very beginning, and therefore before the onset of the desquamative stage, that the lotions here given may be used with good results. When the amount of the exudate is considerable but not profuse, the drying powders prove most beneficial. When there is infiltration of the skin, when crusts have formed, and underlying these the skin is denuded, zinc oxid or other non-irritating ointment has proven highly satisfactory. Carron oil, when prepared from equal parts of fresh lime-water and pure olive oil, constitutes a preparation that is non-irritating and hence quite grateful and efficacious in cases where protection of the acutely inflamed part is chiefly indicated; 1 per cent. of phenol may be advantageously added to this preparation if severe pruritis is present. The solution may be applied to the auditory canal and auricle by means of a cotton-tipped applicator, after which liberal pads of gauze are placed over the ear and a roller bandage applied, as above directed. In subacute cases, after the crusts that have been formed by the drying of the exudate have been removed or after they have ceased to form, solutions of silver nitrate are without question often of service in reducing the thickness of the infiltrated walls of the auditory meatus, and thus in restoring the lumen of the auditory canal to its normal dimensions. Silver occasionally aggravates the trouble if used in too concentrated solution at first. Hence in the beginning not more than 10 or 15 gr. to 1 ounce should be tried, but a greater concentration may be employed later if the remedy is well tolerated. The best effects are usually observed when gr. xl to gr. lxxx—$\mathrecal{z}$j are used.

Any plan of treatment which does not include careful attention to the general system of the patient will fail in a large number of cases. In eczematous children it is frequently found that the diet is faulty; that sweets, nuts, and pastry have too largely replaced the substantial foods, and that stomach and intestinal derangements are present to an extent of being largely causative of the aural or general eczema. Sedentary adults who eat too liberally of nitrogenous foods and partake too much of beer or wine are subjects of a considerable number of ailments—of which eczema is one—that are commonly covered by the terms lithemia or gout. Correction of these errors when found will usually go far toward a cure of the skin trouble at the time, and also toward its prevention and subsequent recurrence. An occasional dose of the mild chlorid of mercury at night, followed by a brisk saline cathartic on the following morning, is of value. Where lithemia is clearly present, the continuous administration of citrate of lithia for several weeks, in large draughts of pure water, is beneficial in ridding the system of the uric-acid irritant. Salicylate of methyl in combination with colchicin will give excellent results in cases of rheumatic habit or where there is a tendency for the eczema to become chronic. Arsenic should never be administered in acute eczema. The tubercular and rachitic cases must receive, in addition to the local medication, the general treatment appropriate for each of these diseases.

Chronic Eczema.—The chronic form results invariably from the acute variety, and may persist for months or throughout the individual's life. When once the chronic stage has been reached the affected area remains dry, except during acute exacerbations. The inflammatory process, which persists for a long time in the cutis and sometimes in the underlying connective tissue, results finally in an infiltration and ultimate hyperplasia of all the structures involved. Hence the lumen of the auditory meatus becomes narrowed and the auricle, if this be implicated, assumes a thickened, shiny appearance, and has a leathery feel. The epithelial covering of the affected parts is constantly shed before the cells mature, and their accumulation in the form of dry branny scales sometimes blocks the meatus completely; or if pus or other secretion is present, a foul-smelling epithelial plug is found filling the auditory canal.

While itching is seldom so violent as in the acute variety, it is nevertheless commonly present, and during the acute exacerbations of the chronic form may be very severe. The pruritus leads the patient to pick at his ears with a match, toothpick, or any convenient object that is small enough to enter the canal, with the unfortunate result of occasionally producing an acute circumscribed or even a diffuse external otitis, a full description of which is given elsewhere in this section (see Chapter IX.).

As a consequence of the long-continued inflammation of the integument of the auditory canal the ceruminous glands may be atrophied or destroyed to an extent that the ear-wax is only scantily or not at all secreted; and without this natural emollient dressing the canal finally becomes dry and presents a horny aspect, with sometimes a fissure which extends entirely through the integumentary thickness.

Treatment.—This form of aural disease is usually quite difficult to treat in an entirely satisfactory manner. The long list of remedies that are recommended by various authorities if given here would only confuse the student and would more than likely lead to an unfortunate choice in any given case. Hence it is thought best to present only a few that have proven in the author's experience more satisfactory than the rest, and to outline the circumstances under which the same should be applied.

In chronic, dry, and scaly skin affections arsenic has long been used, has proved of value, and is a proper remedy for internal administration. A convenient preparation for this purpose is Fowler's solution, which may be given to the amount of 10 or 15 drops daily, but this should be immediately withheld should an acute exacerbation of the eczema appear. The value of arsenic administered internally is probably best exemplified in cases in which the eczema is to some extent, at least, dependent upon a neurotic or trophic derangement. The remedy should never be given indiscriminately, that is, simply because a given patient is suffering from a chronic eczema. The individual case should always be studied in every particular, and arsenic be given only in those in whom it is positively determined the remedy is not contra-indicated. Sole dependence in the treatment of eczema should never be placed on arsenic, for in the most favorable cases it can only be regarded as one, and often the least important, of the means of cure. In this as in the acute form, scrofula, lithemia, rickets, anemia, etc., may be entirely responsible for the continuance of the local disease, and each case must, therefore, be studied with a view to learning the causative element and of rectifying the same according to the rules laid down in treatises devoted to the practise of modern medicine.

The local treatment should be directed toward securing comfort to the patient, toward arresting the progress of the disease if possible, and toward removing the infiltrated and thickened condition of the affected parts. For the relief of the itching of the auditory meatus the author has used no remedy that has proved so efficient and lasting in its affects as the combination of carbolic acid and iodin dissolved in rectified spirits:

R. Iodin (crystals),   gr. x ;
  Carbolic acid,   gr. x.
  Rectified spirits,   ℥j.—M.

The auditory meatus should first be cleansed by removing all loose epithelial masses, after which the walls of the canal are painted with the above preparation by means of a cotton-tipped applicator. In order that only a small quantity of the solution shall be carried to the affected parts, the amount of cotton used for covering the tip of the applicator should be small, and after it is dipped into the liquid any excess must be removed by lightly rolling the end of the instrument which carries the medicament on a piece of blotting-paper. Until the degree of tolerance the patient may have for this remedy is established, it is wise to apply the iodin-carbolic mixture rather sparingly. A single application frequently controls the itching for several days or even weeks, during which period other measures of a general or local therapeutic value may be carried out.

Bellamy uses to good advantage on other parts of the body a somewhat similar iodized fluid for the relief of papular patches of chronic eczema of an obstinate nature.

Contrary to the rule that has been given for the treatment of acute eczema, in the management of the chronic, infiltrated varieties, the best results are obtained from stimulating applications. Hence, where the skin is greatly thickened, fissured, or even widely ulcerated, these pathologic states often subside under the daily application of green soap, followed by vigorous rubbing with a coarse cloth, or even by scrubbing the same with a brush. When used in the external auditory meatus the soap is inserted with the finger and afterward vigorously rubbed into the skin with a cotton-tipped applicator. The rubbing should be continued for several minutes, following which the excess of soap is syringed away and a zinc oxid dressing immediately applied. This process may be repeated daily or even twice daily with the most satisfactory results, and is omitted only when the abraded surfaces are all healed and the thickness of the affected skin has been sufficiently reduced.

Another stimulating treatment that has proved valuable is the application of the oil of rusci, properly combined in the form of an ointment:

> R. Ol. rusci,   ℨi–ij;
>   Potass. subcarb.,   ℈j;
>   Unguent. aquæ rosæ,   ℥j.—M.

This is rubbed into the chronically inflamed and thickened parts three times a week, after first having cleared the meatus of all epithelial débris. In beginning the application of the tar preparations, like that of the oil of rusci given above, it is not wise to use the full strength, for the reason that it may prove too stimulating, and an acute exacerbation of the eczema will result. Until tolerance is established it is better, therefore, to dilute the preparation one-half or more, using zinc oxid ointment for that purpose. Dench highly praises the vinegar of cantharides, the local use of which in these cases he states will very rapidly deplete the parts and effect a disappearance of the excessive deposit of inflammatory tissue.

Whatever method of treatment is chosen, much time will be required in accomplishing all that may be desired. Should acute symptoms develop at any time, all stimulating treatment must be withdrawn, and the soothing applications which have been recommended as proper for the acute forms of eczema should be temporarily substituted. One remedy may act satisfactorily for a time in a given case, but afterward may become inert or even harmful, and hence in the course of the treatment it is often found necessary to change from one to another plan, or even to let the patient rest from all treatment for a few days or weeks.

NOMA

Noma of the fibrocartilaginous canal, the auricle, and the surrounding region is a form of gangrene of the ear similar to gangrene of the face and genitals, and occurs, as a rule, in poorly nourished children during infancy and early childhood. The disease is rare and begins in or around the ear. The ulceration rapidly spreads, attacking the parotid and mastoid regions, often with destruction of the auricle (Fig. 71).

The following report of a case of noma by Verhoeff (*Journal of the Boston Society of Medical Science*, vol. v., May, 1901) is interest-

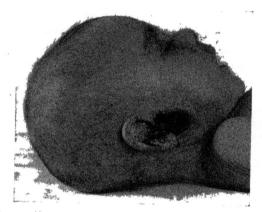

FIG. 71.—NOMA OF THE RIGHT AURICLE IN A CHILD OF FIVE MONTHS.
The gangrenous ulceration involves the tragus and lobule of the ear, a portion of the cheek, and extends into the external auditory meatus. A similar but less extensive process is present on the other side. Photograph taken six hours after death. (Verhoeff.)

ing and, together with his comments, gives a good exposé of the existing knowledge concerning this disease:

Infant, aged five months, admitted January 16, 1901. Family history unimportant. Previous history, always well and strong until present illness. For five weeks previous to admission there was a discharge from each ear. One week previous to admission the parents noticed that on the right side the discharge was irritating the skin of the external auditory canal and lobule of the ear. On admission there was a purulent discharge from both ears, the tympanic membranes were partially destroyed, and just in front of and below the lobule of the right ear there was a deep round ulcer, 7 mm. in diameter, with irregular base and slightly overhanging edges. The base of the ulcer was covered with pus. The surrounding parts were red and thickened. The left ear showed no ulceration, but on the helix there were two or three reddened spots. Despite treatment by the actual cautery and local applications of antiseptics, the ulcerative process on the right side gradually spread, involving the cheek; and on the fifth day after admission there was also a definite ulcer just below the left auricle. On the seventh day there was noted on the right side near the ulcer a reddened area about 1.4 cm. in diameter, but the ulcer seemed to spread by direct extension into sound tissue. On the seventh day it was also noticed that the left great toe, and to a less extent the little finger of the right hand, were red and swollen. On succeeding days other joints of the fingers and toes became affected in the same way. The appearance of some of the joints would vary greatly even during the course of one day, now appearing more and now less inflamed. The same thing was observed in the case of the reddened area near the ulcer of the right ear, which for two days became almost invisible, and then again reappeared as a much larger area with an ill-defined border. There was diarrhea and the child took its nourishment poorly. Both the local and general condition of the patient steadily became worse, and the child finally passed into a semicomatose condition and died on the seventeenth day after admission.

Autopsy by Dr. Verhoeff, twelve hours after death:

Diagnosis.—Streptococcus otitis media and mastoiditis, streptococcus gangrenous ulceration of the auricles and cheeks, streptococcus synovitis, streptococcus bronchopneumonia, streptococcus septicemia, croupous colitis.

Verhoeff believed there was little question that the gangrenous ulceration of the auricles and cheeks was the result of infection by the purulent discharge from the middle ear. When it is considered that the streptococcus is commonly found in otitis media, it seems remarkable that such an infection does not occur more often. In noma of the mouth there is usually a history of some previous disease, often one of the exanthemata, but in this case no such history could be obtained, thus rendering the infection less easy to explain on the grounds of lowered resistance. It is possible that the virulence of the organism is a more important factor than the lack of resistance of the patient. The streptococcus septicemia, synovitis, and pneumonia, while not, of course, alone sufficient to prove the nature of the infection in the local ulcers, nevertheless are highly confirmatory in this regard, and, in addition, indicate either that the patient possessed very little resistance toward the streptococcus or that the latter was extremely virulent.

Verhoeff was able to find 13 cases of noma auris in the literature;

8

most of them very incompletely reported. The ages varied from three weeks to four years; 8 cases were associated with otitis media, while in the remaining cases no mention was made of this disease, although in some of them it was no doubt present. In 3 cases the affection was bilateral. Death resulted in all but 1 case, that of Hutchinson, who cauterized the ulcer with acid nitrate of mercury. None of the cases were investigated histologically, and but 1 of them bacteriologically. The latter was reported by G. M. Smith, who obtained from the ulcer of the auricle and from the longitudinal sinus cultures of a short non-motile bacillus with rounded ends, often arranged in pairs or chains.

LUPUS OF THE EAR

Tubercular infection of the skin of the external ear may be classed among the rarer affections of this appendage. The disease may involve both auricles, but usually only one. Lupus is a disease occurring most frequently in early life, at a time when the developmental changes of the skin are most active, and, therefore, no doubt on this account it is more susceptible to attack by the tubercle bacillus. The cutaneous infection may be the result of the direct contact of the tubercular bacilli, or it may be secondary to a general infection in which the lungs, bones, or glandular system have been previously involved. Two varieties of lupus—namely, lupus erythematosus and lupus vulgaris—are those most frequently found upon the external ear.

Lupus Erythematosus.—This variety is much the milder of the two affections, and is perhaps most usually found associated with, rather than an integral part of, the tubercular affection which constitutes the entire essential pathology of lupus vulgaris. Lupus erythematosus occurs most frequently upon the lobule of the ear, from which point it may spread in every direction and ultimately involve the whole auricle, and possibly the adjacent skin of the face and neck. On the other hand, the lupus may begin on the face or neck and subsequently extend to the auricle.

Symptoms.—Lupus erythematosus begins as a small reddish macule upon the surface of the skin, which is slightly elevated over the affected area. This macule, in due course of time, enlarges, and after a period of many months or even years may involve more or less of the entire auricle and corresponding side of the face. These patches of lupus are of bright red, pinkish, or purplish color, and are of a somewhat circular or ovoid shape. After a long persistence of the discs the center, or point of origin of the lupus, becomes slightly depressed and faded, and in the very old cases the activity of the lupoid process ceases at the center, leaving characteristic white scars surrounded by a slightly elevated rim of advancing disease.   From the beginning the macules are covered with white or yellowish-white scales which are slightly adherent, their under surfaces sometimes having root-like projections which extend into the mouths of the underlying sebaceous glands.

The disease is most frequent between the twentieth and fortieth year.   When unchecked by treatment it often continues through the balance of the individual's life.   Although characterized by this remarkable persistency, lupus erythematosus is a disease which usually does not produce serious pain, itching, or other bodily discomfort, and may not at any time during its long course interfere with the general health of the patient.   The mental anguish due to disfigurement of the face and ear constitute, therefore, the most serious aspect of the affection.

Diagnosis.—The history of the onset and long continuance of the disease furnish strong data for a positive diagnosis.   The character of the scales which cover the discs, the elevated, circular, advancing margin of the affection, and the coexisting depressed, pale, or scar-like center of the same, taken as a whole, constitute a condition found in no other disease.

Treatment.—The fact that scores of remedies or combinations of remedies have been recommended for the cure of this disease clearly indicates its incurability or, at least, the difficulty of cure by local medicinal means.   The very acute forms of lupus erythematosus should be treated by the most soothing local applications, such as have already been recommended for the first stages of acute eczema (see p. 106). Chronic and indolent forms of this variety of lupus are more satisfactorily managed by stronger applications, the following being one of the best:

> R. Ichthyol,   ℥ss ;
>   Collodii,   ℥v.—M.

This combination should be painted over the affected area and reapplied as often as it loosens and peels from the skin.   If found too irritating, the quantity of ichthyol may be lessened, whereas in the very indolent cases advantage will be gained by increasing the proportion of ichthyol. Destructive agents are sometimes necessary and have been frequently used in the past.   Of these lactic acid, trichloracetic acid, and pyrogallic acid are preferable.   Agents of this class have recently been superseded by the methods of phototherapy and radiotherapy, and since the results of treatment by these means are more favorable than those from the use of chemical agents, the former should be recommended in any case.

As has already been stated, most cases of lupus erythematosus occur in persons who are otherwise in good health. In these general medication is not called for. When associated with tuberculosis, scrofula, or other cachectic affection, internal remedies which are proper for the associated general disease should, of course, be included in any plan of treatment. Personal hygiene and physical exercise in the open air are quite as essential to success as any form of medication.

Lupus Vulgaris.—This affection is a true tuberculosis of the skin. Like the preceding disease it may begin on the auricle—usually on the lobule—and later cover the whole external ear and auditory canal, or it may spread to the ear from the neighboring skin of the face.

Causation.—The predisposing causes of lupus vulgaris are the several cachexias which affect the poorly fed as a result principally of being badly housed and improperly clothed during the period of childhood and early adolescence. The immediate cause is due to an infection of the skin, either as the result of direct contact of the skin with tubercular matter or by the systemic infection of the integument through the blood- or lymph-channels.

Symptoms.—The appearance of small, flattened, slightly elevated macules upon an integumentary surface that had previously been in a healthy state marks the beginning of lupus vulgaris. Later these macules become nodular or papular and are elevated above the surface of the skin from which they spring. The nodules may be clearly made out by palpation of the affected area. They finally, together with the areas about their bases, become confluent, the whole forming a " patch" or " plaque." The color of such a patch is dull red or purplish and the margins have clear-cut lines of separation from the healthy integument. Sometimes the affected area is more or less marked by a covering of scales, which vary in appearance from a whitish to a yellowish brown.

Lupus vulgaris usually develops slowly and persists indefinitely. It may make little apparent progress for a long period of years, during all of which time little or no suffering or other inconvenience is experienced by the patient. On the other hand, the affected tissues may break down at any time, ulceration results, and dried crusts of pus and epithelial débris will occupy the site of the former eruption. An ulcer thus formed sometimes heals in one part while it extends in another, and hence it is not uncommon to see a case in which irregular whitish cicatricial scar tissue has already formed in the wake of an advancing ulceration. The nature and extent of the ulcer has given rise to different names descriptive of the ulcerative stage of lupus vulgaris. Thus, when it advances in a tortuous course, it is called lupus serpiginosus;

when it extends deeply, lupus profundus; when it spreads superficially, lupus superficialis, etc.

Lupus vulgaris involving the auricle most often begins on the lobule, which later becomes swollen, pendulous, and of a dark red or purplish color. When ulceration is established the lobule may become adherent to the face or neck, the entire auricle may be destroyed, and the external auditory meatus may be closed by either fungoid granulations or a cicatrix.

Diagnosis.—The earlier stages of lupus vulgaris may be mistaken for lupus erythematosus. In the latter disease the process is superficial and there are no nodules, ulcers, or thick crusts present. In lupus vulgaris, as has just been pointed out, nodules are present on the skin from the first, and ulceration and crust formation form an important part of the later behavior of the disease.

After ulceration has been established lupus vulgaris may be mistaken for either epithelioma or syphilis. Epithelioma begins at a later period of life than lupus, its course is more rapid, more painful, and more exhaustive. The ulceration of lupus may be multiple, whereas that of carcinoma is single. The ulcer of lupus may heal in one place while it progresses in another, whereas in epithelioma the progress of the ulcerative process is more rapid and without any tendency to heal. The edges of the ulcers of lupus are soft, while those of carcinoma are hard and elevated. In syphilis the history of the ulcer shows it to be of shorter duration than lupus, and if the eyes, nose, and throat be carefully examined other evidences of previous ulceration or inflammation in these localities will almost certainly be discovered. An inspection of the general integumentary surfaces of the body may also furnish other evidence in case the infection was of a specific nature.

Prognosis.—The disease may persist on the auricle for a long time without further harm than the production of an unsightly cutaneous disorder; or it may completely destroy the auricle or so completely change its normal structures as to produce a hideous deformity of the appendage. When the external auditory meatus is involved, atresia of the canal may result, in which case permanent loss of hearing on the affected side will ensue. In the deeply ulcerated varieties of lupus, systemic infection and death is the usual termination.

Treatment.—Since lupus vulgaris is frequently associated with tuberculosis, or is at least most frequently found in individuals in whom there is a predisposition to this disease, all those remedies, including personal hygiene, food, exercise, and open air, are indicated which are known to be most effective in combating general tuberculosis.

The local treatment consists in the destruction or removal of the integumentary infection. Destruction by means of such caustics as

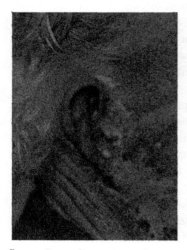

nitric acid, lactic acid, or trichloracetic acid, or by means of caustic alkalies, is now obsolete, since the resulting scar is unduly disfiguring, and since these measures are by no means certain to secure satisfactory results. If the disease has progressed to the point which makes the total loss of the auricle inevitable, the whole should be excised together with the adjacent structures which are most involved. While the dermal curet is a popular instrument for the removal of lupoid areas from other parts of the body, it is not suitable for their removal when the ear is involved.

FIG. 72.—PARTIAL DESTRUCTION OF AURICLE BY LUPUS OF LONG DURATION.
Whitish scar tissue is seen extending downward over the face, result of healing from use of x-rays.

The best results in the treatment of lupus vulgaris are to-day obtained from the use of the Finsen light, phototherapy, and the x-rays (Fig. 72). A complete description of the methods of employing electrotherapy in the cure of this disease is found in modern works on this subject, and to these the reader is referred.

HERPES ZOSTER

But few cases of herpes zoster auris have been reported. Green and Vail have each studied and reported cases (Fig. 73). Gruber found 5 cases among a total of 20,000, representing all kinds of aural affection. The author saw in 1890 a case in a man aged forty, who was the victim of a severe malarial attack.

Causation.—Most writers believe that a neurotic disturbance is the primary cause, and Head and Campbell found in 21 post-mortem examinations that inflammatory and degenerative changes existed in the ganglia of the posterior nerve-roots, in the roots themselves, and also in the peripheral nerve-fibers of these roots. Reflex irritation, as from the ingestion of certain foods, has been assigned as a cause in a few cases. Vail states that the affection is most likely an acute infectious disease, and this view is supported by the clinical fact that herpes zoster seldom occurs in the same individual a second time. Exposure to a severe cold, damp wind is an active predisposing cause.

Symptoms.—Pain of a neuralgic character and sometimes very severe precedes the herpetic eruption one or more days. This pain may be either on the anterior or posterior portion of the auricle or upon the adjacent skin. In Vail's case it was severe over the mastoid process and in the depths of the external auditory meatus. Gruber has observed the herpes in the auditory canal and upon the drum membrane, and he believes that the disease may also occur in the middle ear itself. A marked degree of deafness is present in some cases. After the pain has persisted for several days perhaps, the eruption occurs. The vesicles, like the pain, occur over the course and distribution of the sensory

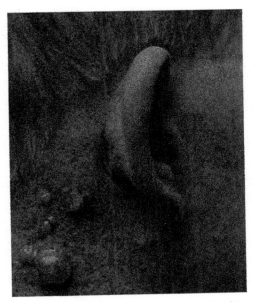

FIG. 73.—HERPES ZOSTER AURIS.   (Case of D. T. Vail.)

nerves, those most involved being the great auricular branches of the cervical plexus and the auriculotemporal branch of the fifth. Small red patches on the skin precede the appearance of the vesicles, which may be thickly set or even confluent. Since the deeper layers of epithelium are raised with the blebs, rupture does not readily take place. At first the contents of the vesicles are serous, later milky, finally purulent, and in the end dry into a scab which covers the site of a permanent scar. When the meatus and drum membrane are involved more or less deafness and tinnitis aurium are present. A high degree of fever sometimes accompanies the early period of the disease.

Treatment.—There is no known specific medication, and therefore such remedies should be administered inwardly as will best relieve pain and reduce the temperature. In the worst cases morphin codein may be given hypodermically. Phenacetin or acetanilid full doses are proper remedies to combat the high temperature.

Local applications are of little value. To protect the vesicles fr the irritating effect of the air and to avoid their accidental rupture th pads of cotton should be placed over the affected region, and th should be held in place by a roller bandage.

CHAPTER IX

ACUTE CIRCUMSCRIBED AND ACUTE DIFFUSE INFLAMMATION OF THE EXTERNAL AUDITORY MEATUS

OTITIS EXTERNA CIRCUMSCRIPTA—FURUNCLE

BOILS occur in the auditory meatus with relatively greater frequency than on most other parts of the body, somewhat, perhaps, because of the exposed situation of the canal itself, but principally, no doubt, because of the frequency with which suppurative inflammation occurs in the cavities comprising the middle ear beyond.

Causation.—Two factors may be considered chief among the causative agents productive of this disease, namely, traumatism and subsequent infection. Kirchner states that the hair-follicles of the external auditory meatus are normally inhabited by the staphylococcus pyogenes aureus and albus. The injury to the part may be so slight that the patient will have no remembrance of its occurrence, but it should be borne in mind that a trivial abrasion of the skin in the presence of the above pathogenic bacteria is ample to admit the germs, and that therefore a history of any considerable local injury preceding the onset of the circumscribed external otitis is not necessary to the establishment of the fact that a sufficient abrasion has occurred. Because of the insignificant character of the wound, evidences of the presence of the abrasion are not always visible to the examiner, even upon the most careful inspection of the parts involved.

Picking at the ear to relieve itching or to dislodge accumulated wax is probably the most frequent cause of a boil in this location. As is stated in the chapter on Impacted Cerumen, the mere presence of the hardened wax in the auditory canal for a long time will often erode the underlying parts, which are then open to the entrance of infection. A chronic aural discharge acts in a double capacity in the production of furuncle: first, the constant bathing of the canal walls with the irritating pus tends to soften and finally abrade the skin; second, the purulent material is usually laden with pathogenic material ready for absorption by any exposed surface with which it may come in contact. In addition to the causes just stated, certain constitutional disturbances, like anemia

121

and diabetes, are productive of boils in the ear, sometimes coincidently with their occurrence on other parts of the body.

Symptoms.— Usually the patient first discovers, by accidentally touching the ear, that a rather indefinite sense of soreness is present in that locality. This rapidly increases until within twenty-four or thirty-six hours it has become a pain so intense and continuous as to preclude sleep, and although apparently lessened during the day it is nevertheless constantly present and severe. Owing to the location of the boil in the outer portion of the meatus (Fig. 74), and therefore upon the

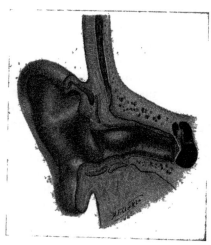

FIG. 74.—FURUNCLE.
Note its situation on the cartilaginous meatus in the outer half of the canal. Compare this location with the sagging of the inner end of the meatus due to mastoiditis (see Fig. 154).

tubular portion of cartilage which comprises the pinna, any movement of the external ear will result in very severe suffering. The whole auricle, as well as the soft structures adjoining its attachment, are swollen and edematous in the worst cases. When the furuncle is situated on the posterior wall of the meatus the amount of postauricular swelling may be sufficient to cause the auricle to stand out from its attachment to the extent of giving the whole head a lop-sided appearance (Fig. 181), much resembling that sometimes seen during an attack of acute mastoiditis.

If the situation of the boil is on the anterior wall, the tragus and the soft tissues anterior to it are usually swollen and exquisitely tender to the touch.

In the worst cases there is some rise of temperature, but rarely will it exceed 101° F. Loss of appetite, general malaise, and irritable disposition are, as would be expected, common symptoms in a disease attended by so much pain and loss of sleep.

After a period varying from two to several days from the onset, a rupture of the boil takes place and there is a slight discharge of bloody pus from the auditory meatus. Following this an immediate relief from the pain is experienced, the patient again sleeps well, the appetite returns, the temperature drops to normal, and the individual believes himself well within a few days. In many instances, however, a new infection takes place in a short time and the patient is again compelled to undergo a repetition of his former suffering. Indeed, instances are not rare in which one crop of boils follows another in the auditory meatus with such little intermission that the patient becomes quite exhausted before the disease runs its natural course or is checked by appropriate treatment.

The hearing is not seriously impaired except in cases where, because of the very considerable swelling of a single boil or of the combined tumefaction of a group of boils, the lumen of the canal is completely blocked. Occlusion of the canal to this extent may also produce tinnitus aurium and vertigo.

Diagnosis.—As a rule the diagnosis of this disease is not difficult, but cases are occasionally seen which are exceptions to the rule, and these are deemed of sufficient importance to merit special mention under the heading of differential diagnosis; first, however, the diagnosis of the simple case will be discussed.

Any case whose symptoms are such as have already been given would be suspected of having furunculosis of the external auditory meatus. Confirmation of this belief may be obtained by an examination of all parts of the auditory canal by means of the head-mirror and reflected light. Since the boil is nearly always situated in the outer two-thirds of the auditory canal it is better in all examinations where this disease is suspected not to use the speculum as a first step, for the reason that this instrument would very often conceal the area which it is most necessary to examine. The auricle is, therefore, retracted in the usual way, the canal is illuminated, and its walls are inspected first by sight alone and later by means of the cotton-tipped applicator. If a circumscribed inflammation is present it will be found necessary to handle the auricle very gently while retracting it, and to touch all suspicious areas lightly with the probe, since otherwise so much pain will be produced by these manipulations that few patients will be found who possess the fortitude to tolerate them. In its incipiency no swelling of the canal will be seen, but if the cotton-tipped probe be used and all parts of the outer two-thirds of the external meatus are carefully examined for tender areas, the location of the boil may thus be discovered in the very beginning. Later, when the swelling is approaching its height, the lumen of the canal will be more or less occluded and will appear somewhat crescentic in shape.

When it is seen by the above method of examination that the occlusion of the auditory meatus is not complete and that the tumefaction lies deeply in the canal, the aural speculum should be used during the subsequent steps. Even when moderate swelling of the canal walls is present it is often impossible to inspect the drum membrane when the usual short speculum is employed. In these cases, therefore, a longer and narrower instrument, such as is shown in Fig. 99, is most useful.

Differential Diagnosis.—Furunculosis may be mistaken for ether acute or chronic mastoiditis, for an exostosis, or for induration or abscess of the parotid gland, which latter occasionally finds an exit through the slit which exists in the cartilage of the external auditory meatus, and thence discharges through the canal itself. An exostosis is situated in the bony meatus and hence lies more deeply than is commonly true in circumscribed inflammation, which is nearly always in the cartilaginous portion. Moreover, an exostosis is painful only when the skin which covers it is ulcerated and inflamed—a circumstance which must be rare. A careful examination with the probe should leave no room for question as to the real nature of the obstruction within the canal. An inflammatory swelling of the parotid gland is usually a sequel to some general infective or other ailment, and therefore the history of the case, taken in connection with the evidence obtained by an examination of the ear and of the external swelling, should be sufficient to clear the diagnosis. It is, however, with the differentiation between a boil in the meatus and mastoiditis that the physician is most often concerned, because cases are not infrequent in which, unless one possesses considerable knowledge concerning the possible behavior of each disease, and is skilled in the examination of the deeper parts of the ear, mistakes in diagnosis with unpleasant consequences may be made. The following symptoms and conditions found in each ought to enable the examiner to distinguish the one from the other ailment:

FURUNCLE.	MASTOIDITIS.
Pain.—Always present and severe.	*Pain.*—Often present, not always severe.
Aural Discharge.—Infrequent and scanty.	*Aural Discharge.*—Present in nearly every case, often profuse.
History.—Exceptionally preceded by exanthematous disease, throat affection, or middle-ear abscess.	*History.*—Usually preceded by exanthemata, la grippe, throat affection, and nearly always by middle-ear abscess.
Postauricular Swelling.—May be present.	*Postauricular Swelling.*—May be present.
Tumefaction within Auditory Meatus.—Is present in outer two-thirds of the canal, and may occur on anterior, inferior, or posterior portion of canal wall.	*Tumefaction within Auditory Meatus.*—Is present at fundus of canal, and only in one situation, namely, the posterosuperior canal wall.
Pain on Moving the Auricle.—Very severe.	*Pain on Moving the Auricle.*—None.
Pain on Pressure over Mastoid.—Absent unless the auricle is moved or touched during the manipulation.	*Pain on Pressure over Mastoid.*—Present at tip, over site of mastoid antrum, and sometimes over whole mastoid area (see Fig. 151).

Treatment.—If the case is seen in its incipiency, efforts should at once be directed to the abortion of the inflammatory swelling. If the individual is plethoric or if the local congestion is very active, the abstraction of blood either by means of the artificial or natural leech will not only give temporary relief, but will often be the means of arresting the painful affection. The blood should be taken from a point nearest to the seat of the inflammation, and hence if the furuncle is located on the anterior wall of the meatus the depletion should be performed in front of the tragus, whereas if it is upon the posterior wall the region of the mastoid is the preferable site for the application of the leeches. Since leeching is employed in the treatment of several acute aural affections, sufficient detail concerning the principles of its use and the necessary technic in the methods of its application can be most appropriately given here.

Abstraction of blood in cases of local congestion and inflammatory states is of greatest benefit in the earliest stages of the disease; but its usefulness as an abortive or curative measure diminishes rapidly as the congestion becomes actively inflammatory, and the procedure is of no value whatever when the suppurative stage has been reached. Hence, the abstraction of blood can be recommended only in the earliest stages of an inflammatory aural affection. Natural leeches provide a well-known and efficient method of local depletion, and are preferred by many otologists to the newer methods in vogue. Some knowledge of the behavior of the natural leech is essential in order to insure its efficient service. It is perhaps overparticular concerning the kind of skin on which it is willing to operate. Hence, it is a first necessity that the area to be leeched must be thoroughly scrubbed and cleansed, for the purpose of removing the smell and taste of any poultice, liniment, or other medication that may have been previously applied. The last cleansing previous to applying the leech should be made with pure or distilled water, so that the skin may be absolutely clean and free from all features that might be objectionable to the animal.

Before attempting its application the auditory canal is filled with cotton to prevent the leech from crawling into this passage, a thing it has often been known to do when the precaution above mentioned had not been taken. When all necessary preparation has been made the leech is placed in a small glass cylinder, like a test-tube, by which means it is brought into contact with the exact spot from which the blood is to be withdrawn. If it does not readily fasten itself to the skin, the latter may be pricked with a needle to the extent of causing slight bleeding, when the leech will more energetically seize the abraded spot. In this way four or six leeches, as may be indicated by the severity of the disease, can be applied, and all should be left on until they fill themselves with blood and drop off of their own accord. ·

Because of the difficulties frequently experienced in obtaining and applying natural leeches, and the great amount of time consumed by this method, the artificial leech has come into very general use. It is more certain, more efficient, always ready, can be sterilized, and, indeed, possesses every advantage over its older rival. Preceding its application the area to which it is to be applied is rendered sterile, after which the multiple incisions are made with the spring lancet (Fig. 75) and the suction-bulb (Fig. 76) is at once applied. The small amount of

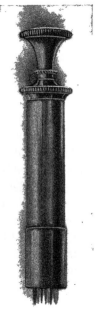

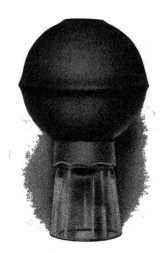

FIG. 75.—BACON'S SCARIFIER, SHOWING LANCES PROJECTING.

FIG. 76.—CUPPING GLASS FOR USE IN ABSTRACTING BLOOD AFTER SCARIFICATION BY MEANS OF THE BACON LEECH.

pain resulting from the punctures, which are made by the little lances of the instrument, can be greatly lessened by previously placing a pad of cotton saturated with 10 per cent. carbolic acid in glycerin over the part to be incised, and allowing it to remain ten minutes before the incisions are made. By the use of the artificial leech 2 or more ounces of blood, as may be indicated, can be easily and quickly withdrawn.

Should hardened ear-wax, dried pus, or other foreign material be found in the auditory canal during the formation of a boil, the same should be completely syringed away. After the canal is dried the pain can be lessened in many cases by applying a neatly shaped cone of cotton, which has been previously saturated with ichthyol ointment, directly into the auditory meatus and against the swelling. This should be heated before it is inserted and should be left in place for twenty-four hours, unless the pain is meanwhile increased. Solutions of menthol also act locally as an anesthetic and often prove more beneficial in this respect than ichthyol. Solutions of morphin, cocain, and kindred preparations have no effect on the pain when applied locally and are unworthy of trial. The continuous application of the hot-water bottle to the ear is grateful and relieves the pain in many cases. Incision of the boil constitutes the best treatment in the majority of cases, but since the procedure is exquisitely painful many patients prefer a trial of the milder measures, at least until the continued suffering convinces them of the wisdom of submitting to a more radical measure. Incision, when performed at the onset of a boil, if made deeply and extensively enough, will abort or at least cut short the subsequent course in the majority of instances, and when employed thus early takes the place of and is vastly superior in efficiency to the local abstraction of blood by leeches. Preparation for the incision is made by cleansing the canal by means of syringing if neces- sary, and then by applying a cone of cotton which has been saturated with 10 per cent. carbolic acid in glycerin directly to the meatus and against the swelling. After a few minutes it will be found that the affected area is somewhat anesthetized. The amount of pain produced in

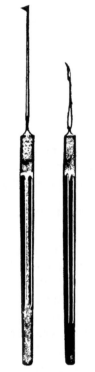

FIGS. 77, 78.—FURUNCLE KNIVES.

lancing a furuncle is dependent very greatly upon the method of making the incision. The furuncle knife (Fig. 77 or 78) should be in perfect order, the patient's head should be firmly supported between the two hands of an assistant, the auricle should be retracted, and the field of operation should be well illuminated. If the patient be a child or a nervous adult, the hands of the patient must be held by an assistant. The knife is inserted into the meatus to a point beyond the tumefaction, and is then turned so that the cutting edge is perpendicular to the latter. By firm pressure upon the handle of the knife, the point is driven as deeply as the bone or periosteum, and at this depth the blade is pulled outwardly through the whole length of the furuncle, thus draining not only the accumulation of pus, but also the congested tissues that surround the pyogenic space.

The after-treatment consists in antiseptic cleansing and the application of emollient medicaments to the inflamed area. The cotton cone, saturated with ichthyol ointment, when applied hot into the external meatus proves valuable in allaying subsequent pain, in reducing the tumefaction, and from its action as a local antiseptic.

The general health of the patient sometimes needs attention. Derangements of the digestive system are particularly active as factors in keeping the local inflammation alive. When this is the case the regulation of the diet and mode of life, in connection with the administration of salines, will be found especially helpful. Anemia, when present, is an indication for the administration of iron. The tendency toward a recurrence of the furuncle and ultimate chronicity of the disease may be caused by diabetes, and an examination of the urine is therefore imperative. Should sugar be found, diabetic diet and general treatment for that disease should be at once instituted.

DIFFUSE INFLAMMATION OF THE EXTERNAL AUDITORY MEATUS—OTITIS EXTERNA DIFFUSA

As a result of an injury to the canal or of the previous existence of some other disease in this locality, the resulting inflammation sometimes involves the whole channel instead of becoming localized, as in the preceding ailment.

No satisfactory explanation can be offered as to why the one disease is more extensive than the other, except in those cases where the initial irritation of the canal is widely distributed in one and not in the other.

Causation.—The cause of the affection can usually be traced to the entrance into the canal of irritating fluids or of foreign bodies with sharp edges which deeply lacerate the integument of the meatus, or which otherwise involve the integrity of the auditory canal to some considerable extent. The foreign body may have been smooth and may have entered the canal without any injury whatever to the parts, but the subsequent unskilful efforts to remove it have caused the injury which has resulted in the diffuse inflammation. Likewise the unskilful use of instruments in the meatus for any purpose may cause an injury which will result in the disease under consideration.

An eczema of the canal often persists a long time with no more discomfort than itching, but upon exposure to severe cold or as the result of rudely scratching the parts to relieve the itching, an otitis externa diffusa may be started. Irritating discharges from the middle ear have been known to set up the disease without any other assignable cause being present. Infection at the point of injury by the staphylococcus pyogenes aureus or albus is no doubt an essential in all instances to the establishment of the disease.

Symptoms.—The pain resulting from the swelling and tension within the canal varies from that which amounts to only an uncomfortable soreness to that which is so severe as to be almost unbearable. As is true in most affections of the ear, the suffering is worse at night. The hearing is not greatly impaired except when the inflammation is of such severity that the auditory meatus is blocked or unless the drum membrane is involved—thickened or perforated and covered with an exudate.

In addition to the hyperemia and swelling of the canal walls, ecchymoses sometimes occur, and in thirty-six or forty-eight hours a discharge which is at first serous and afterward purulent will be observed. This discharge finally dries into crusts which encase the meatal walls, and these when removed often represent partial or complete casts of the canal. Since the dermoid layer of the drum membrane is involved in the inflammatory process, and is later cast off along with the epidermal layers of the outer canal, an examination of the canal and fundus by means of reflected light shows obliteration of all landmarks of the drum membrane. After this exfoliated portion of the drum membrane is shed or has been removed the underlying structures look moist and angry, the junction of the tympanic membrane with the canal walls cannot be made out, and in severe cases the drum membrane is found to be perforated, with a discharge from the middle ear.

The discharge from the meatus is often corrosive to the parts with which it comes in contact, and hence the auricle is not infrequently eroded and swollen as a result. There may also be present an enlargement and tenderness of the lymphatic chain of glands in the neck, as a result of the absorption of septic material from the external meatus.

Differential Diagnosis.—The affection may be mistaken for a boil in the canal or for otitis media. As previously stated a boil causes swelling from one side of the canal only, and hence on examination the lumen of the meatus is crescentic during furunculosis, whereas in the disease under consideration the lumen is about equally encroached upon from all sides and, therefore, the opening of any channel yet remaining is in the center line of the meatus and continues to be more or less cir-

9

cular in outline. The history of the onset and the physical examination should serve to distinguish a suppurative otitis media from an acute diffuse external otitis.

Prognosis.—In the milder cases and those of uncomplicated traumatic origin the outcome is generally good. Cases of this character usually pass through the stages of exudation, exfoliation, and crusting, and end in complete cure in from two to four weeks. In ill-nourished or tubercular subjects the disease may persist much longer or may even become chronic. Those cases in which the inflammation of the canal is due to a previously existing eczema, or perhaps those in which both an eczema and a purulent discharge from the middle ear have been present, the prognosis is less favorable, the disease may require a much greater time for its cure, and is much more likely to become chronic. Should the active inflammation persist in the narrow or, perhaps, occluded auditory canal for any considerable time the result may be an adhesion and permanent narrowing of the lumen of the canal at some point; or interstitial infiltration and thickening of both the osseous and soft parts of the canal may take place to the extent that the external auditory meatus is ultimately occluded throughout its whole length. Stricture of the meatus from any cause may do no further harm than to seriously impair the hearing, but in case suppuration previously existed in the tympanic cavity or was brought on by the external inflammation, serious danger to the life of the individual may result from the hindrance thus offered to the drainage, and the consequent liability of extension of the suppuration to the cranial contents.

Treatment.—When the case is seen early the indications for treatment are to relieve the pain and, if possible, to abort or check the inflammatory progress. The same measures that were recommended in the incipiency of the circumscribed variety of external otitis are equally valuable in the diffuse variety. These include the administration of salines, the local abstraction of blood, the application of anodyne substances locally, and deep incision of the tumefied part (see p. 125).

When the secretion appears it should be frequently removed by syringing. When this secretion is highly irritating its reaction should be tested, and the lotion which is used for cleansing should be rendered slightly alkaline or acid, as may be necessary to neutralize the discharge. After syringing, thorough drying of the canal is essential, following which the causation, as well as the exact nature of the present wounded or inflamed canal, must be carefully considered in order to determine the most appropriate medicament to be applied. Many of the moist cases are most efficiently treated by the application to the canal of a drying powder,

> ℞. Pulv. amyli,   ℥iij;
>   Zinci oxidi,   ℥j;
>   Columnæ,   ℥ss.—M.
>   Dusting-powder.

after first syringing away the discharge and subsequently drying the inflamed area.   Solutions of nitrate of silver are highly beneficial in cases where the infiltration is great, but the secretion scanty.   Such a solution should not be stronger than gr. xx to ℥ j to begin with, but may be increased to four times this strength if well tolerated.   Should silver nitrate prove irritating or ineffectual, the cotton plug saturated with a compound mercury ointment may be inserted, and is often most beneficial:

> ℞. Hydrarg. ammon.,
>   Hydrarg. oxidi,   āā gr. ij;
>   Adipes benzoate,   ℥iij;
>   Oleum olivæ,   ℥j.—M.

Constitutional disturbances of whatever nature, especially those pertaining to the digestive tract, should be corrected.   Lithemia is particularly influential as a factor in the continuance of an inflammatory state that originates from an eczema, and hence both an antilithemic diet and antilithemic drugs are frequently indicated.

When septa or stenosis of the auditory canal results from the violence of the inflammation or as a sequel to its long continuance, the deformed canal may require mechanical or surgical treatment to restore the hearing or to prevent the retention of pus or other secretion in the cavities of the middle ear should suppuration be already present there or should it subsequently take place.   Membranous septa that are found in the canal may be cut away, and in order to prevent their re-formation the opening should be filled with a properly shaped plug of dental wax; or a sponge tent may be used for this purpose, but must be frequently replaced until healing has taken place.   This, like other scar tissue, has a tendency to re-form again, and much trouble is sometimes experienced in keeping the canal patent even after the most thorough removal of the obstruction.   If the canal is closed on one side of the head only, if the hearing is good in the opposite ear, and if there is no suppurative process going on in the middle ear of the affected side, it is best not to interfere with the obstruction in the meatus.   If, however, the hearing in the opposite ear is greatly impaired or completely lost, and the tuning-fork tests show the labyrinth of the ear on the obstructed

side to be normal, the auricle should be detached almost exact
advised in the performance of the first step of the radical ma
operation, and a groove should be chiseled from the mastoid c
sufficiently wide and deep to furnish an ample opening for a
auditory meatus after the posterior meatal integument is turned
ward into its new position.

In case a chronic suppuration exists in the middle ear of an indiv
who has complete or nearly complete cicatricial or other obstru
in the auditory canal, the radical mastoid operation is indicated
should be performed without unnecessary delay (see Chapter XX

CHAPTER X

CROUPOUS AND DIPHTHERITIC INFLAMMATION OF THE EXTERNAL AUDITORY MEATUS

CROUPOUS INFLAMMATION

THIS name has been given to that form of diffuse inflammation of the auditory meatus in which there is a deposit of a membranous exudate over more or less of the integumentary lining of the external auditory canal. This false membrane is at first pearly white and filmy in appearance, but later may become thick, opaque, and of a grayish or dirty color. It lies accurately in contact with the underlying skin, but is not firmly attached to it, and hence the examiner will be able to lift up the presenting edges with a spatula or probe, or to remove the entire cast from the meatus by means of a dressing forceps or by syringing the canal.

According to Politzer, the membrane is confined entirely to the osseous portion of the auditory canal and to the dermoid layer of the drum membrane. The membranous deposit is composed of coagulated fibrin and white blood-corpuscles, from which have also been isolated the staphylococcus pyocyaneus and the streptococcus pyogenes.

The **cause** of this affection is most probably the presence in the auditory meatus of these two varieties of pathogenic bacteria.

Pain accompanies the onset of the exudate, persists during its presence, and subsides soon after it is exfoliated. Recurrence is frequent, but under proper treatment the entire trouble promptly subsides without any impairment of hearing or other injury to the auditory apparatus.

The **treatment** of the affection is simple and consists in the removal by antiseptic syringing of all retained pus together with the membrane itself. If syringing is not effective in the removal of the membrane the small aural dressing forceps may be employed for this purpose, but the latter must, of course, be guided by the eye and a good reflected light. When the affected parts are clean and free from the membrane and have been dried by the introduction of cotton cylinders into the external auditory meatus, the dressing is completed by dusting the meatus lightly with boric acid powder.

133

DIPHTHERITIC INFLAMMATION

This is a more common and a much more serious disease than the preceding, and may be either primary or secondary to a similar diphtheritic deposit in the fauces, nasopharynx, nose, or middle ear of the same individual. It is scarcely probable that a diphtheritic membrane is ever primarily produced in the auditory meatus unless there already existed abrasions or excoriations of the skin in this locality. Hence, the disease is found primarily only as a complication of irritating aural discharges, after the skin has been denuded of its protective epithelium.

In diphtheritic inflammation of the external auditory meatus when occurring as a complication of nasopharyngeal diphtheria, the specific bacillus finds its way into the middle ear through the Eustachian tube, throughout which tract the characteristic exudate takes place. As a combined result of the pressure due to the inflammatory swelling of the tympanic mucous membrane and of the inflammatory exudate which speedily occurs, rupture of the membrana tympani takes place and an irritating discharge flows through the auditory canal, the integumentary lining of which becomes at once excoriated and infected.

At first white and thin in appearance, the membrane rapidly spreads and thickens until it may involve a part of the auricle and occlude the meatus by its own thickness and the increased swelling of the under-lying tissues. The lymphatics behind the ear become tender and swollen, and, together with the infection of the glands of the neck that has previously taken place from the faucial diphtheria, produces a tumefaction of the neck of considerable extent. Unlike the membranous exudate which takes place in the auditory canal in the croupous variety, that which occurs in diphtheria is closely adherent to the underlying skin and cannot be syringed away or removed without injury to the skin itself. Should some part of it be forcibly pulled away, the surface to which it was attached is left raw and bleeding, and another membrane is immediately formed to cover the denuded spot. In addition to this important difference in the behavior of the two classes of exudate, the fact that in the diphtheritic variety the disease is usually secondary to a throat attack should lead to an easy differential diagnosis. If, however, any doubt should exist concerning this point, a bacteriologic examination should be made to settle it.

The **treatment** should be directed to the cure of the general diphtheria, of which that involving the ear forms only a part. If antitoxin has not been administered before the process is recognized in the ear, injection of this remedy should be made at once, and repeated one or more times daily as may be indicated to limit the further spread of the membrane, to secure its exfoliation, and to prevent its recurrence.

The external meatus is treated by antiseptic syringing and by the instillation of solutions to dissolve and loosen the membrane and to soothe the inflamed canal. When the disease is primary, Gottstein advises filling the auditory canal with lime-water, which he states will favor the separation of the membrane. Efforts to remove the diphtheritic deposit by means of instruments before it is loosened by remedial or natural processes are always harmful, and result in injury to the underlying tissues; such efforts are also productive of great pain, and even if successful are not of benefit, for the reason that the membranes are re-formed at once, and usually to a greater extent than before their removal.

CHAPTER XI

PARASITIC INFLAMMATION OF THE EXTERNAL AUDITORY CANAL—FUNGOID OTITIS EXTERNA.—OTOMYCOSIS

SEVERAL varieties of vegetable parasites have been discovered in the external auditory canal, each of which has been exhaustively studied and described by a number of observers.

Causation.—While the conditions that lead to the development of this disease cannot be stated in every case of otomycosis, several factors will usually be found present in the meatus which are contributory to the origin of the growth. In the first place, the mycelium, like all other types of plant life, cannot live on an absolutely dry skin, and hence one essential for its existence in the auditory meatus is that there be present a moisture or discharge of some kind upon which the growth may subsist. A very profuse purulent discharge, however, seems to be prohibitive of the development of the fungus, owing perhaps to the fact that the spores are washed away before they can attach themselves; or that they are quickly drowned in the excess of fluid present. Bezold, Dench, and others state that the use of oils in the ear for any purpose predisposes the individual to the development of the fungus, but in view of the frequency with which patients suffering from aural diseases apply fatty mixtures to the auditory canal it would seem that fungi should be seen oftener in this situation than is the case at present if oils were a potent factor in the causation. The deeper portions of the auditory canal are most often involved. Adults are affected more frequently than children and males oftener than females. The disease is most common among those living in crowded tenements, particularly in damp places. Pain of varying degree, seldom intense, is usually present, but cases are sometimes seen in which no complaint of any kind is made by the patient.

Diagnosis.—The character of the disease may be suspected from the symptoms, but can only be definitely determined by a physical examination of the auditory canal and drum membrane, and if then in any doubt, by a microscopic examination of any suspected foreign material that may be removed from the meatus. If the parasite is of the

136

variety known as aspergillus niger, the walls and fundus of the meatus will appear blackened as though coated with a fine coal-dust, whereas if the aspergillus flaveus is present it presents, under illumination, a yellowish aspect and the canal looks somewhat as if it had been dusted with iodoform or the pollen of certain plants. Under the microscope the aspergillus niger, the fungus most frequently seen, appears as a mass consisting of numerous long transparent fibers which ultimately divide into two branches and end in a head containing the reproductive parts of the plant (Fig. 79). The fibers comprising the stems of the

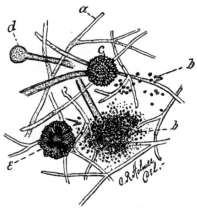

FIG. 79.—ASPERGILLUS NIGER.
a, Mycelium fiber; b, spores; c, sporangium; d, receptaculum; e, sterigmata. (Holmes.)

growth lie in close contact with the superficial epithelium of the skin, interlace each other, and embrace in their loops the intervening epithelial cells to such an extent that when the growth is pulled or washed away from its skin attachment the underlying surface is left somewhat raw and bleeding.

Eczematous or other inflammatory diseases of the canal may cause an exfoliation of the epidermal layers which can be readily mistaken for a fungoid accumulation, but the microscope, if used for the examination of the exfoliated structure, will leave no doubt concerning its nature.

Treatment.—The diagnosis having once been made with certainty, proper and efficient treatment becomes an easy matter. As a preliminary to the measures which are intended to kill the growth, as much of it as possible, together with any hardened wax or other foreign material that may be present in the canal, is first syringed away with an antiseptic fluid or is withdrawn from the canal by means of an aural forceps. Warm rectified spirits or alcohol-boric acid solution is then instilled into the canal and allowed to remain for ten minutes.[1] This is repeated one or more times daily for a few days, at the end of which time, if the fungus shows no sign of returning, the patient may be dismissed with instructions to repeat the instillations at home once or twice a week. Should either of the above solutions be painful to the ear the same may be diluted with distilled water, after which the former strength is again gradually restored as toleration is established. Sometimes the alcohol-boric acid solution fails to act satisfactorily, and then mercury bichlorid may be substituted for the boric acid and be added to the alcohol in the proportion of 1 : 800.

After the cure of the disease by the above means, recurrence is apt to take place unless any disease which may be present in the auditory meatus or middle ear is at the same time cured and the meatus restored to a normal condition. Hence, any discharge from the tympanic cavity or any inflammatory thickening of the walls of the external auditory canal should receive treatment appropriate to the existing ailment.

[1] The alcohol-boric acid solution here referred to is prepared by adding gr. xx boracic acid to ℥j commercial alcohol.

CHAPTER XII

FOREIGN BODIES IN THE EXTERNAL AUDITORY MEATUS

FOREIGN bodies in the auditory canal are, in the large majority of instances, lodged there by the individual himself. Children at play with objects of any kind seem to possess a natural desire to introduce the same, when small enough to permit it, into the mouth, nose, or ear. More rarely the lodgment of a foreign body in the ear results accidentally, as when a person picks at the canal with a toothpick, match, or other like implement for the purpose of removing hardened wax, or to scratch the meatus during the torturing itch of an eczema in this locality, and a portion of the object is broken off at a depth beyond the ability of the patient to recover. Portions and even the whole of small hairpins and parts of toothpicks and matches have in this way been lost in the canal. Various objects may enter the ear by being in some way hurled from a distance. Thus, seeds may fly into the farmer's ear during the process of threshing grain; chips of stone or scales of iron or other substance with which various artisans work may likewise accidentally enter the ear, being cast off from the chisel or other implement in use. Of a more violent and rarer origin may be mentioned gun-wads or even bullets that have been shot into and lodged in the canal, or possibly imbeded in the deeper structures of the ear beyond.

Bugs and insects are frequently met with in the auditory meatus, among which bedbugs, ticks, roaches, and the like are most often observed. In some localities, usually in warm countries, where outdoor life is almost perpetual, insects sometimes enter discharging ears and there deposit their eggs, from which larvæ are subsequently hatched in numbers sufficiently large to fill the canal. Calhoun, of Atlanta, reported the case of an ear in which he found several live maggots, which had presumably crawled into the ear of the patient from the horse stall in which he had been sleeping.

Otoliths sometimes form in the external auditory meatus. Godivin[1] reports the extraction of such a formation from the meatus of a woman aged thirty. The concretion consisted of a mixture of calcium phosphate,

[1] *Brit. Medical Journal*, March 5, 1905.

cerumen, and epithelium. The author removed an otolith from the external meatus of a negro, in 1894, which was large enough to fill the entire canal and to greatly impair the hearing on that side. It was molded exactly to the shape of the meatus and greatly resembled the petrified twig of a tree.

Symptoms.—The symptoms of a foreign body in the canal may vary from those so trivial that the individual is entirely ignorant of its presence to those in which there may be great disturbance or even total loss of function, severe pain, and marked general disturbance.

It is not an uncommon occurrence to remove some small foreign body, as a bead, pebble, or like substance from an ear at the first examination for another ailment, when the patient will deny all knowledge of its presence, it having given rise at no time to any inconvenience. If the object is large enough to fill the canal and block the passage of sound-waves, the hearing is impaired and tinnitus aurium and a feeling of fulness in the same side of the head will be complained of. Pain may or may not be present, depending much upon the size and shape of the foreign body, upon whether or not it is organic, alive, or is of inorganic structure. Its position in the canal in relation to the drum membrane is also a factor as to the presence or absence of suffering. In general, it may be stated that the presence of smooth inorganic substances like pebbles, beads, or buttons give rise to no pain unless they are so large as to make pressure on the canal walls or unless they have entered the auditory meatus far enough to lie in contact with the tympanic membrane. As is well known, this membrane is exceedingly sensitive and pressure upon it from a foreign body is quite intolerable. If the object is angular or rough and of sufficient size, the skin of the meatus is lacerated during the entrance of.the foreign body, and this, together with the inflammatory reaction that follows, is usually productive of considerable suffering.

The presence of live insects is intensely painful only when they are impacted against the drum membrane or crawl about over the same, when their small size enables them to do so. Insects with long tentacles, which spear the membrana tympani with each movement of the head in their efforts to extricate themselves from the auditory meatus, cause an agony to the patient probably equalled by few other accidents. The leguminous seeds, like peas and beans, and certain dried fruits, like currants, usually cause little disturbances at the time of their lodgment in the auditory canal, but subsequently, when moisture from the adjoining tissues is absorbed, the object swells very greatly with the result of impairment of function and the production of tinnitus and pain.

Whereas a moderate-sized smooth body may lie in an otherwise healthy auditory canal indefinitely without apparent injury, should there be present a discharging ear at the time of the lodgment of the same, the drainage may become so impaired that retention of pus in the middle ear may result and severe pain be the inevitable consequence. Such an obstruction to the drainage also favors an extension of the suppurative inflammation to the mastoid antrum and cells, where all the dangers incident to mastoiditis may subsequently develop.

Diagnosis.—There is but one safe rule to follow in making a diagnosis, and that is to actually see and feel with a probe if necessary the object which lies in the canal.

Unfortunate mistakes have been made by physicians who have ignored this one certain method of making a diagnosis.[1] In the case of children, the mother has perhaps learned from the playmates that some object has been put into the child's ear. In her excitement she may, on her journey to the nearest doctor's office, forget which ear and therefore insist that the foreign body is in the wrong ear; or possibly the object which is presumably in the canal is small and has consequently dropped out before the surgeon is reached. In either case, if the physician does not actually see the object himself, he may make the error of attempting to remove the body from the wrong ear; or, what is equally bad, he may attempt the blind extraction of an object which has already fallen from the meatus.

The surgeon's first duty is to quiet all feeling of excitement on the part of those most concerned. The child that has, perhaps, been snatched from its play and hurried to the physician's office by an unduly anxious parent, sometimes accompanied by an entire household, naturally expects severe treatment, is usually much frightened, and therefore tact on the part of the physician and an explanation of the fact to the parents that all should end well, and a quiet kindly demeanor toward the child are great aids toward securing the confidence of the patient and enabling the surgeon to make a painless examination.

If seen before rude methods of extraction have been practised by which the object has been pushed deeply inward, very commonly the reflection of light into the meatus at the same moment of the retraction of the auricle will show the foreign body lying in the outer portion of the canal. If not so superficially located the speculum is introduced

[1] An instance is recorded (*British Medical Journal*, 1877) of a physician who explored an ear for a half-hour in his efforts to dislodge a foreign body supposed to be in the auditory meatus. Pieces of bone, but no foreign objects were extracted. The child died from hemorrhage in an hour and a half as the result of the rude and unnecessary efforts of the surgeon.

in the usual way and the canal illuminated, when every portion of the deeper parts should be seen without difficulty and the nature and position of the object is discovered. When small, it will most likely lie at the bottom of the canal, near the annulus tympanicus at its lower portion; but if large it may obscure the greater portion or even all of the membrana tympani. If any doubt as to the nature of the object should arise, assistance may be obtained by using a probe or other instrument as an aid to the inspection. Should the patient be an unruly, frightened child, the insertion of any instrument either for the purpose of examination or extraction is often wisely withheld until the patient is under the influence of a general anesthetic.

Where unsuccessful efforts to extract the foreign body have been previously made, the diagnosis may be difficult or impossible, for the reasons that blood may be oozing from the canal as a result of injury from the rude manipulation, or the walls of the meatus may be so swollen as to partly or wholly occlude the lumen of the auditory canal. Under such circumstances it is more humane and expedient to make no further efforts at diagnosis except under a general anesthetic.

Prognosis.—The prognosis as to life is, with rare exceptions, good and as to function is also good in the vast majority of cases, the hearing being preserved unless the injury is severe or attempts at removal have been unduly rude. Numerous instances are recorded in which foreign bodies have remained in the ear for many years without causing any disturbance whatever. In such cases the objects were usually small, smooth, inorganic substances, such as pebbles, pieces of pencil, beads, etc.[1] Death may result from the lodgment of a bullet or other substance which fractures the skull by its entrance or which opens the jugular bulb, lateral sinus, or carotid artery, all of which vessels approach the auditory canal closely at some portion of its course (see Fig. 304, p. 550). Permanent impairment of hearing may result from the impaction of a foreign body against the drum membrane with such force as to partially or wholly destroy the structure and perhaps dislocate the ossicles. Following such an injury inflammation of the tympanic mucous membrane with suppuration quickly follows, and because of the impediment to the

[1] *The Medicinische Zeitung*, 1842, No. 32, speaks of a girl in whose ear a piece of pencil remained harmless for seven years. Haug narrates a case in which two glass beads remained harmless in the auditory meatus for twenty-eight years, while Winterbotham (*Medical Times and Gazette*, 1866) cites an instance of a cherry-stone which remained harmless in the auditory meatus for about sixty years.

Numerous deaths have been reported to follow efforts made for the extraction of foreign bodies from the auditory meatus. Poulet cites three such deaths in which meningitis followed the extraction. Clermont recites a case in which death occurred very soon after the removal of a pin from the auditory canal.

outflow of pus produced by the blocking of the foreign body, mastoid or intracranial complication sometimes quickly ensues, and death from one of these affections may ultimately result. In case the labyrinth is involved the hearing suffers greatly and total deafness in the affected side may result.

Treatment.—Briefly stated, the treatment consists in the removal of the foreign body. As previously mentioned it is entirely possible for such a body to remain in the canal indefinitely without the slightest discomfort or danger, and therefore in any case, if it is known to be of only moderate size, inorganic in structure, and smooth in contour, the case can scarcely be classed as an emergency, and hence will not require such precipitous haste in the removal of the body as to preclude the selection of a time when all necessary preparations may be made to execute the work most easily and safely.

When the object to be removed is small and perhaps lies deeply in the canal, its removal is best and most easily accomplished by syringing with warm sterile water. For this purpose a piston syringe (see Fig. 84) should be used which holds at least 2 ounces. The auricle is retracted

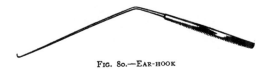

FIG. 80.—EAR-HOOK

in the usual way, but the syringing should be done with more force than is employed when the procedure is used for the removal of pus when a perforation of the membrana tympani is present. When the above simple technic is followed the foreign body will be dislodged and washed from the canal in practically all cases of this class.

If the preliminary examination has shown the substance to be a wad of paper, cotton, or other similar substance, it may be most conveniently withdrawn by any slender dressing-forceps such as are shown in Fig. 214, p. 348. A flat button or other similarly shaped article, which is so placed that the edge presents itself toward the concha, may likewise be removed with these instruments. A button having either a ring or an eye may be so situated that any conveniently shaped tenaculum or hook (Fig. 80) can be inserted into the ring and the object be thereby easily removed.

Whatever the object may be, it should be the aim of the operator not to push it farther into the meatus during any attempt at removal. Every manipulation should be made under the full illumination of the object by reflected light, and both foreign body and instrument must be seen by the operator at all times during the progress of the removal.

In the case of round, smooth bodies, like beads or beans, whose size is sufficient to entirely fill the meatus, it is particularly unfortunate to push them beyond the isthmus during awkward efforts at extraction, because while they yet lie in a position external to the narrowed portion of the canal (Fig. 81, a), they are comparatively easy to dislodge, whereas, if pushed beyond this point (Fig. 81, b), the difficulties are greatly multiplied, and sometimes detachment of the auricle may be necessary to remove them from the deep and impacted situation. Objects of this character, which are spheric or ovoid and whose surfaces are polished, cannot be grasped in the jaws of any forceps, and it is not wise to attempt the use of this instrument in their extraction because the result

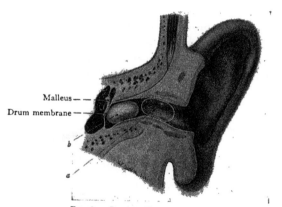

Malleus

Drum membrane

b

a

FIG. 81.—BEAN IN EXTERNAL AUDITORY MEATUS.
a Shows most usual location of large foreign body before unskilful attempts at extraction have been made; b shows body after it has been pushed beyond the isthmus of the canal.

is always the same, namely, that when the jaws are closed upon the surface the foreign body only slips out and is thereby pushed the farther inward, until finally it is unfortunately jammed through the tympanic membrane and against the inner tympanic wall. The only kinds of instruments that can be used successfully in such cases are tenacula with short, sharp hooks, which in the case of objects like beans can be imbedded directly into the substance (Fig. 82) and their removal accomplished by traction; or those with a mechanically movable distal extremity (Fig. 83), which can be passed along the canal wall to a point beyond the object, after which an elbow is constructed at the innermost end of the instrument by compressing the spring at the outer end, and then traction is efficiently made against the object, which is thus easily and safely removed.

The removal of live insects is immediately imperative because of the intense pain their presence and movement causes, and also because if the insect is large and powerful and is armed with tentacles, as is

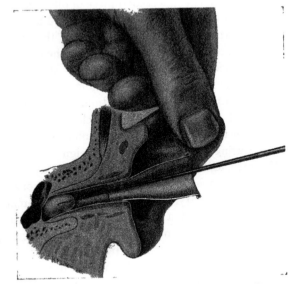

FIG. 82.—REMOVAL OF FOREIGN BODY BY MEANS OF A DELICATE TENACULUM.
The auditory meatus is straightened by upward and backward traction upon the auricle. The deep situation of the object requires the insertion of the aural speculum.

sometimes the case, much injury and subsequent inflammatory reaction may result to the drum membrane. If not impacted the insect can be successfully syringed from the canal just as in the case of any other

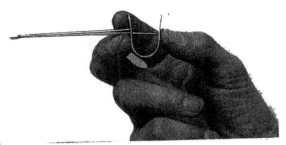

FIG. 83.—QUIRE'S FOREIGN BODY EXTRACTOR.

foreign body. If this does not succeed or if impaction has occurred, the insect should be quickly killed, or at least stupefied, so as to prevent its further painful movement. Chloroform vapors or chloroform itself is sufficient for these purposes. Some thick oil, like melted vaselin, should

10

first be poured into the ear, after which a pledget of cotton large enough to fill the meatus is saturated with chloroform and inserted into the canal against the insect.   In order to confine the chloroform so as to obtain its rapid and more certain effect, a second piece of oiled cotton is inserted air-tight on top of that containing the chloroform.   The melted vaselin is used to coat the drum membrane and walls of the meatus, and to thus prevent irritation or blistering of the parts by the chloroform which is subsequently inserted.   The insect is quieted almost at once and can then be removed by the forceps either whole or piecemeal.

The question as to the necessity for the administration of an anesthetic sometimes arises and must be settled in each case according to the probable behavior of the individual and the suffering or difficulties that are likely to arise during the removal of the foreign body.   In a patient of ordinary self control and one in whom the foreign body is not impacted in a position beyond the isthmus of the external auditory meatus, an anesthetic is never necessary.   If the patient is apprehensive and highly nervous, particularly if a child, or if previous unsuccessful attempts at extraction have been made during which the canal has been injured and is now swollen, the administration of ether or chloroform is undoubtedly indicated.   Under its influence the use of all instruments should be guided by a good illumination from a head-mirror and the manipulations should be conducted as skilfully and as gently as if the patient were wholly conscious, for only by this amount of care is it possible to avoid wounding the skin of the canal or perforating the drum membrane.

In rare instances the object is found so firmly impacted that it is impossible to remove it through the auditory meatus, in which case the auricle is detached by steps quite similar to those followed in the first stages of the radical mastoid operation (see Fig. 238 and p. 382). This operation is safe, successful, and results in practically no scar.

CHAPTER XIII

IMPACTED CERUMEN

A COLLECTION of ear-wax in the external auditory meatus is frequently observed. The cause of such an accumulation is either a retention of the normal amount of secretion or an excess of secretion. The ceruminous glands are found almost wholly in the cartilaginous portion of the canal and the wax is normally expelled by the motions of the lower jaw, the articulation of which lies immediately under the cartilaginous portion of the external auditory meatus. Since this portion of the meatus slopes downward and outward from within, the expulsion of the secretion is somewhat facilitated by gravity. When the cutaneous lining of the meatus is inflamed from any cause, it becomes roughened because of the exfoliation of its superficial epithelia, and this forms not only a barrier to the outward progress of the wax, but the epithelia are also incorporated with it, increasing its consistency and thus in a twofold way favoring its retention.

A long-continued eczema or other inflammation of the canal often results in contracting the lumen almost to the point of stricture. An exostosis or foreign body lodged in the external auditory meatus may narrow or even obliterate the passage. All these and other causes of obstruction to the canal are causative factors in the retention and subsequent impaction of cerumen.

Symptoms.—Collections of cerumen of very considerable size are often observed in the auditory canal of an individual who makes no complaint whatever of any aural disturbance. Indeed, if the organ of hearing is otherwise normal, the accumulation of wax creates little or no inconvenience, as a rule, until it completely blocks the lumen of the passage, or unless it is dislodged and carried inward against the drum membrane. Patients frequently state that a few hours previously they heard normally and thought they had no aural ailment of any kind, but that, while cleansing the ear during the morning toilet, sudden deafness and dizziness came on, and that as a result great apprehension of damage to the ear is felt. In all such instances the auditory canal had previously been almost completely filled with a ceruminous mass through which an opening persisted sufficiently large to permit the passage of sound-waves and of air for the equalization of pressure upon the outer side of

147

the drum membrane. While the patient was cleansing the ear water had entered the meatus, had caused softening and swelling of the ceru- · minous mass, after which the manipulations of the finger, hand, and towel in and about the ear had spread the wax across the opening of the canal, had thus sealed the fundus of the ear from external influences, and had in this way brought on the sudden deafness.

Another class will state that the deafness has been coming on grad- ually for months or years, but that at times the symptoms are much improved only to relapse again into a worse condition. This variation of symptoms is due to the fact that there is present a middle-ear or labyrinthine deafness, as well as an obstruction to the sound-waves by the wax plug.

Whatever may be the causation, when the canal is once tightly blocked certain similar symptoms will always develop at once. These are marked deafness, tinnitus aurium, a feeling of heaviness on the affected side of the head; and less frequently vertigo, mental depression, and vomiting. A dry, hacking cough is sometimes produced by the presence of hardened ear wax. Pain is seldom present except in cases where · the wax has become greatly hardened and has lain in the canal under a pressure sufficient to cause ulceration of the adjoining walls. Pain may also result from the dislodgment of a hardened mass, which is later driven inward and becomes impacted against the tympanic membrane.

Diagnosis.—The diagnosis is nearly always easily made by follow- ing the methods given in detail for the inspection of the external auditory meatus (see p. 169). When the auricle is retracted and the reflected light is thrown into the meatus, the mass is seen as a grayish- black or brownish object which partly or wholly obstructs the passage. Inspissated cerumen may be mistaken for a foreign body which is incrusted with wax, or for dried pus which has accumulated in the external auditory meatus in cases of chronic purulent otitis media. This latter condition occurs after the discharge has diminished to a mere trifle and is too scanty to appear at the outer meatus, where it would be observed and wiped away by the patient. Such a collection of dried pus is usually found on the superoposterior wall of the canal at its junction with the membrana tympani, in which location it some- times incrusts the adjoining wall of the meatus to a thickness which may obscure the view of the whole upper portion of the drum membrane (P. 331, Fig. 189). Sometimes it becomes necessary to supplement the inspection of the canal with the use of the probe, which instrument is always safe and valuable when carefully used under the guidance of the eye and a good reflected light.

Prognosis.—Impacted ear-wax is in no sense a dangerous condition, except in very rare cases where it complicates a middle-ear suppuration, in which instance its presence, acting as a hindrance to good drainage, might lead to such serious consequences as mastoid extension or intracranial complication.

Recurrence of the accumulation after its removal is the rule. The patient should be told that a repetition of the trouble should be expected after a period of from six weeks to a year or more, so that he may in the future be sufficiently informed to seek relief earlier than he might otherwise do.

The prognosis as to hearing is always good in those cases where the impairment occurred suddenly. In all who have grown gradually worse, or who state that they are better and worse, there is usually a labyrinthine or middle-ear complication, and hence a favorable prognosis should not be given until after a thorough physical and functional examination has been made. Should all observations of the condition of the fundus, together with the facts obtained by the tuning-forks, show that there is present a disease either of the conducting or perceiving portion of the hearing organ, an unfavorable or, at least, a very guarded prognosis should be made.

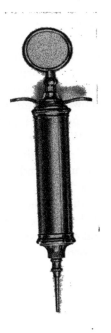

FIG. 84.—METAL SYRINGE. The sharp point is serviceable in syringing around foreign bodies and hardened wax in the auditory canal.

Treatment.—Hardened wax is, in effect, a foreign body, and therefore the treatment should consist in its removal and, where possible, in a prevention of its recurrence. When the impacted cerumen is soft and does not completely block the canal, its removal by means of syringing the canal is the simplest and safest procedure and the one to be recommended.

For the purpose of removing hardened ear-wax a large piston-syringe is preferable (Fig. 84). If the patient's ear is retracted as shown in Fig. 94 and the fluid is injected from the syringe with considerable force, the accumulation of cerumen will be quickly dislodged, and very seldom will it be necessary to have the patient return because the first attempt has proved unsuccessful.[1]

[1] Pomeroy (*Diseases of the Ear*) says, "I feel sure that the power of the syringe for removing cerumen, and a great variety of foreign bodies from the ear, is not sufficiently appreciated by the profession. As long as a considerable amount of cerumen remains in the ear to protect the membrane I have not the slightest fear of doing harm by the syringe."

The fluid used for syringing should always be sterile or antiseptic, for the reason that it can never be known beforehand whether or not the drum membrane is perforated, and should a perforatioh be present, and the operator use an indifferently prepared solution, an old quiescent tympanic inflammation may thereby be revived and suppuration follow the removal of the wax. Normal salt solution[1] or a saturated solution of boric acid is always satisfactory when properly prepared. The temperature of solutions intended for syringing the ear, especially for the removal of hardened wax, should be as high as can be comfortably borne by the back of the hand.

Neither physician nor patient should ever immerse the hand or fingers in any surgical solution for the purpose of testing the temperature. For this purpose a dairy thermometer is useful or, what is equally serviceable, is to suck up with the syringe a quantity of the solution and allow it to drop on the back of the hand. An accurate judgment as to the proper temperature will in this way soon be acquired.

When the canal is completely filled, and the surface of the cerumen has become dry, hard, and glazed, the solution cannot be thrown behind the mass, and hence syringing alone will not suffice for its effectual dislodgment. When this fact is evident, under reflected light a small spatula or hook may be inserted between some portion of the canal wall and the wax, and the latter so separated from the former as to make a passage through which the injected fluid can pass. During subsequent efforts at syringing, the nozzle of the instrument is pointed toward the crevice thus produced and the stream of water is injected somewhat forcibly through it. By this means the ceruminous plug is often quickly brought away in a mass, which retains the shape of that portion of the auditory canal in which it lay.

If not successful in the removal by the above means, other portions of the wax may be still further separated from the canal until, possibly, the whole circumference has been thus detached. Then the syringing may again be resumed or, if thought best, the outer end of the mass may be grasped in the jaws of an aural dressing-forceps and the whole be by this means withdrawn.

Cases are sometimes seen in which these methods fail or seem injudicious because the ulcerated underlying skin is too sensitive to tolerate even the most gentle manipulations. In such instances it is proper to provide the patient with an antiseptic alkaline lotion, with instructions

---

[1] Normal salt solution contains 0 65 per cent. of sodium chlorid or 49.9 gr. to ℥xvj. For practical purposes in aural treatment it may be quickly prepared by adding a level teaspoonful of common salt to 1 pint of boiled water.

to drop the same into the meatus twice a day for one or more days. At the return visit of the patient the wax will usually be found so much softened that it may be readily syringed away, as above directed.

A satisfactory lotion for softening inspissated cerumen consists of:

R. Acid. carbolic.,   gr. ij ;
   Sodium bicarb.,
   Sodium biborate,   *āā* gr. x ;
   Glycerin,   ℥ss ;
   Aquæ destil.,   ad qs. ℥ss.—M.
   Sig. Warm and drop 10 drops into the ear twice a day and allow to remain.

Following the removal of the plug, an examination of the canal walls and fundus of the ear is essential for the purpose of determining the amount of damage its presence may have done, and also to ascertain whether or not the drum membrane is perforated or otherwise diseased. Hence the parts should be thoroughly dried by the introduction into the canal of cotton cylinders (Fig. 203), and if ulcerations are anywhere detected they should be touched with silver nitrate, after which the whole canal may be lightly dusted with boric acid powder. The dressing is completed by inserting a gauze wick or a pledget of cotton into the canal, either of which may be removed after twenty-four hours. Neglect of these precautions, as to treatment after the removal of impacted cerumen, will sometimes result in an acute general or circumscribed inflammation of the canal (see Chapter IX.).

CHAPTER XIV

EXOSTOSES OF THE EXTERNAL AUDITORY MEATUS

WHILE osseous outgrowths from the walls of the bony meatus are not of common occurrence, yet every physician who frequently examines the ear must occasionally see this class of tumor.

Symptoms.—In most instances when the bony outgrowth is small, the patient will have no knowledge of its existence, and will make no complaint whatever concerning the ear in

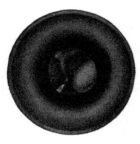

FIG. 85.—SMALL PEDUNCULATED EXOSTOSIS TWICE ENLARGED.
Viewed through speculum.

which it grows (Fig. 85). Even if it is large enough to greatly occlude the canal its presence may not have been recognized, unless some other disease attacks the middle ear or the auditory canal itself. Should suppuration occur in the middle ear, the growth when large becomes an obstruction to the free outflow of pus, pain will result from the retention of the latter, and ulceration and swelling of the delicate integument of the meatus will likely occur from the same cause.

The effect on the hearing depends entirely upon the size of the exostosis and upon whether or not it is complicated by some inflammatory disease of the canal or middle ear. When too small to occlude the lumen of the canal, and when uncomplicated by any other aural ailment, an exostosis has no effect whatever on the function. When the growths are multiple or when a single one is of great size, the auditory meatus may be so blocked that sound-waves no longer reach the membrana tympani, in which instance a high degree of deafness in the affected ear may result.

Physical Examination.—No external swelling or deformity of any kind accompanies an exostosis of the meatus. If situated at the outer end of the osseous canal a view of the tumor may sometimes be obtained by placing the patient in a strong light from a window and simply retracting the auricle. However, a satisfactory view is usually obtainable only by the use of the head-mirror, a good light, and, if the growth lies deeply, an aural speculum. Most usually osteomata appear

152

as hardened outcroppings from the walls and are covered with skin that is much thinner and paler in color than the surrounding integument. They may be somewhat pedunculated, may have a broad base, and may be single or multiple. The multiple variety will usually be seen to occupy opposing positions around the meatal walls in such a manner that the summit of each projects toward the summit of the others (Fig. 86); in the worst cases may touch each other, and, because of the pressure-contact, may become inflamed, ulcerated, and adherent to the extent of completely occluding the canal. If the exostosis is single, and moderate in size, a portion of the membrana tympani may be seen (Fig. 85), and the important information obtained as to whether or not there is suppuration going on within the middle ear. A delicate probe may be used advantageously in determining the extent of the base of the growth, and whether or not the same is sessile (Fig. 87) or pedunculated.

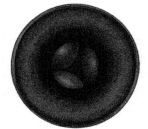

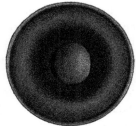

Fig. 86.—Multiple Osteomata viewed through an Aural Speculum. Twice enlarged.

Fig. 87.—Large Sessile Exostosis viewed through a Speculum. Twice enlarged.

Prognosis.—Exostoses are of themselves never dangerous to life and they impair the hearing only when large enough to completely occlude the auditory canal. It is only when suppurative processes of the middle ear are coexistent with the growth in the canal, or when suppurative diseases subsequently ensue, that the real element of danger arises from their presence, because then, on account of the obstruction they present to the free outflow of the pus, they are apt to favor a burrowing of septic material toward the cranial cavity.

Treatment.—The smaller osteomata need no treatment in so far as the growth itself is concerned, but such cases often retain the cerumen to an extent that this may require frequent removal at the hands of the physician. If the growths become an obstruction to the canal to the extent that the hearing is greatly impaired; if by their pressure upon each other they become ulcerated, painful, and adherent; and particularly if a purulent process exists in the middle ear or mastoid antrum, their total ablation is indicated and often imperatively demanded. The smaller pedunculated ones may be removed by means of a cold wire snare or, better, by the employment of a long delicate gouge. This latter is placed in proper position against the neck of the tumor at its junction with the wall of the meatus, under good illumination and the guidance of the eye of the operator, when a few gentle strokes of the mallet made by the assistant will be ample to cut through and dislodge the little mass, which can then be removed by means of a dressing-forceps. It need scarcely be stated that great precaution must be taken in the removal of these growths, by any method that may be chosen, not to drive the instrument too deeply and thereby do violence to the drum membrane. The dental drill has been used successfully to hollow out or entirely grind away exostosic masses. However, no one should undertake the operation of this instrument in the depths of the auditory canal unless his previous experience, with less harmful tools, has given him full assurance of his capability of using the burr without doing violence to adjoining healthy structures.

The question of a general anesthetic must be considered in the above operations. Local anesthesia is inefficient and ether or chloroform should be administered, if the growth is of any considerable size or if it is of the sessile variety. For the larger and multiple exostoses the removal may be much better, and certainly more safely accomplished by detaching the auricle and exposing the growths to the extent that the field of operation is always visible, under which conditions the ablation can be more efficiently and safely performed. Since the operation of displacement of the auricle is performed not only for the removal of exostosis but also, sometimes, for the extraction of impacted foreign bodies from the fundus of the canal, and for the removal of fibrous septa or adhesions, a description of the technic of its performance is here given, to which reference will subsequently be made when clearness of description may demand.

Detachment of the Auricle.—The hair is first cut short and then shaven around the auricle for a distance of 2 inches in every direction or, if great objection is offered to the loss of hair, it may be combed as much away from the pinna as possible and then covered by the application of collodium for a distance of 3 inches around the pinna. The external auditory meatus is syringed with an antiseptic fluid, and the skin over the exposed area is scrubbed and sterilized just as in the preparation for the mastoid operation (see p. 290). The patient is anesthetized by the administration of ether or chloroform. Every antiseptic precaution should be taken in the way of protecting the operative field from infection, just as would be done were a much more extensive surgical procedure contemplated, because it is highly desirable to secure a union by first intention of all the incised tissues. The initial incision is made exactly as shown in Fig. 158, p. 292, and the underlying bone is uncovered to the extent that is shown in Fig. 240, p. 383. It will be noticed that the skin, cartilage, and periosteum of the posterior, posterosuperior, and posteroinferior walls of the external meatus is detached entirely from the bone in these locations to a point in depth beyond the growth or object to be removed. The skin covering the osteoma may be adherent, in which case it will require an extra amount of care to detach it without breaking it through. As the operator approaches the depth at which the drum membrane lies a still greater caution should be exercised not to injure this structure. When the dissection of the auditory meatus is satisfactorily completed, every bleeding point must be secured and the whole wound subsequently dried by firmly packing it with gauze. The bleeding having ceased, the edges of the flaps are widely retracted (Fig. 240, p. 383), and with a small gouge and mallet the exostoses are chipped away not only down to, but somewhat beyond, their bases. It has been found that the auditory canal has some tendency to contract after these operations, and hence it is wisest to remove the bone deeply, rather than to err in the opposite direction and thus run the risk of a subsequently narrowed meatus. It is sometimes advisable, in cases of osteosclerosis of the whole bony meatus, to hollow a channel throughout the whole length of the osseous portion of the posterior canal wall, and then to line the same by first splitting the posterior meatal tissues of the soft canal, and afterward tucking the flaps thus produced backward into place, and holding them there by means of a gauze packing inserted into the auditory meatus until they adhere to their new position in the enlarged auditory canal. The cases in which extensive removal of bone is practised are much more likely to result satisfactorily than are those in which a contracted canal is left subsequently to the operation.

If detachment of the auricle is performed for the purpose of removing either a foreign body or adhesions within the canal it is necessary, after completing the dissection of the soft structures from the bone, to slit the former lengthwise to a sufficient distance to permit the extraction of the impacted object. In some cases, where the foreign body is large and therefore very firmly wedged into the fundus of the canal, it may be necessary to chisel away a portion of the posterior osseous canal wall before extraction is possible. Any necessary enlargement for this purpose adds nothing to the subsequent gravity of the case, and should be made at once when seen to be required, rather than to persist in efforts at unsuccessful extraction through the contracted channel.

After the accomplishment of the purpose for which the detachment of the auricle was performed, the postauricular structures are accurately replaced into the bony meatus, and a strip of gauze ¾ inch wide is inserted into the auditory canal with sufficient firmness to hold them in snug contact with the denuded surfaces. This dressing need not be changed for three or four days, at the end of which time the adhesion of the dissected portions of the canal walls should be complete. The postauricular incision is stitched throughout its entire extent, exactly as is described on p. 395, Fig. 253, and it will unite by first intention if the surgical technic has not been faulty. If the hearing was previously good it will remain so after this operation, unless unnecessary damage has been committed by some step of the procedure. If the hearing was previously impaired or lost, and the middle ear and labyrinth were not involved, the hearing should be greatly improved by the removal of the obstruction from the auditory canal.

CHAPTER XV

CARIES OF THE WALLS OF THE EXTERNAL OSSEOUS MEATUS WITH FISTULA LEADING INTO SOME PORTION OF THE ADJOINING TEMPORAL BONE

CARIES and fistula are sometimes seen in the auditory canal of an individual who has had a long-standing suppuration of the middle ear and subsequent involvement of the mastoid cells, which latter has resulted in the death of some portion of the bony structures that separate these cells from the posterior segment of the auditory meatus. A complete description of the condition belongs, therefore, more to the chapter on Chronic Mastoiditis than to one dealing exclusively with the diseases of the auditory meatus. Nevertheless, the importance of this condition can be profitably emphasized by a brief mention at this time.

Violently infective aural suppurations of the acute variety are sometimes productive of osseous necrosis in this location, but whether the result of acute or chronic aural suppuration, the leakage of pus through the carious wall of the antrum or mastoid cells in the direction of the meatus at once sets up an inflammation of the periosteal covering of the bone with accompanying pain and tumefaction in the auditory canal (Fig. 74). The abscess thus formed quickly ruptures into the meatus, leaving a fistula, one end of which lies deeply in the mastoid portion of the temporal bone, the other in the external auditory canal. The presence of this fistula constitutes one of the diagnostic points in chronic mastoiditis, and it may always be considered as pathognomonic of an advanced state of that disease (see p. 373).

A discharge of bloody pus from the meatus takes place at the time of the rupture of the abscess into the canal, and this, together with the relief of pain that then occurs, may lead the physician who still clings to empiricism in the practise of otology to the belief that any danger that may have been present is now passed and that recovery will quickly ensue. Every fact connected with the pathology of these cases disproves the foundation for such a belief, and whereas the patient will be temporarily improved by the rupture of the abscess and the discharge of pus into the canal, very soon polypi will spring out from the mouth of the fistula and these will in time fill the meatus and obstruct the drainage both from the fistula and the suppurating middle ear. As a consequence the retained pus becomes foul smelling and irritant, the meatal walls are excoriated, and the glands of the neck are sometimes infected and swollen. Intracranial complication is not an uncommon occurrence in these neglected cases.

The presence of a fistula in the posterior wall of the auditory meatus, which leads to sequestra or necrosis in the mastoid structures, should, therefore, be regarded as among the gravest of otologic occurrences, because it has become a common experience with operators of large opportunity for observation to find, on opening the mastoid antrum and tip of the mastoid process in such cases, that the osseous necrosis has been extensive, involving all the cellular structures of this region, and not infrequently laying bare the dura mater over the tegmen antri, tegmen tympani, or over the groove containing the lateral sinus. It is in this class of cases that brain abscess, localized or general meningitis, or sinus infection with thrombosis most frequently takes place, and no doubt can be entertained concerning the belief that through causes acting as here stated a great mortality has resulted in the past without the attendant realizing the connection that existed between the aural affection and the reported death.

Treatment.—The treatment is essentially surgical. Poultices, powders, and lotions are useless and consume time that should be employed in a more rational practise. If the case is a mild one, and particularly if the fistula and underlying necrotic area are found in any other part of the canal except that which lies in contact with the mastoid cells—namely, the posterosuperior—the ear may very properly be syringed, the granulations and polypi be snared or cureted from the canal and mouth of the fistula, and an effort be made to extract any sequestrum that may be found lying loosely in the channel, with the hope that the entire disease may in this way be reached and removed. Success, however, rarely follows these trivial measures and if the fistula enters the meatus upon its posterosuperior wall, and if it is found by probing to extend in the direction of the mastoid cells or antrum, either the radical mastoid operation or the operation described as appropriate for acute mastoiditis is, beyond question, indicated (see Chapters XXV. and XXX.).

CHAPTER XVI

OTHER CONDITIONS OF THE EXTERNAL AUDITORY MEATUS THAT ARE MORE RARELY ENCOUNTERED

HEMORRHAGIC EXTERNAL OTITIS

This affection consists in the effusion of blood under the epidermal layers of the skin of the auditory meatus, as a result of which elongated, bluish-colored blebs appear in the canal. The most usual site of the blebs is upon the inferior and posterior walls, and Politzer states that the bony portion of the meatus only is involved. The tumefactions occasioned by these hemorrhagic effusions may extend from the outer margin of the osseous meatus inward as far as the attachment of the drum membrane, and small vesicles of the same character are sometimes seen upon the membrane itself.

The **symptoms** depend upon the extent and severity of the vesiculation. If the drum membrane is involved and the blisters are large enough to fill the auditory canal, more or less deafness and tinnitus aurium will be present. A moderate deafness and some pain are complained of in the beginning, but these disappear at once when the contained fluid is evacuated either by puncture or spontaneous rupture of the vesicles.

Politzer states that the affection occurs oftenest in young persons and in those suffering from an otitis media due to influenza, but Bacon has reported cases which occurred independently of any middle-ear inflammation.

The **diagnosis** can be readily made by an examination of the deeper portion of the auditory canal, where one or more blistered surfaces will be seen as obstructive, bluish tumors. When these are touched with a probe they are found to be soft and to contain fluid of some kind. To make certain as to the nature of its contents one of the blebs may be incised and the fluid obtained for closer inspection. The disease reaches its height in three or four days and terminates in a cure spontaneously within two weeks.

Treatment.—Little treatment will be necessary further than to cleanse the meatus with antiseptics, to dry the affected areas with cotton

159

cylinders, to incise each bleb freely, to mop its contents away with gauze or cotton, and then to complete the dressing by the insufflation of a small amount of powdered boric acid. Daily cleansing and the application of boric acid powder to the canal may be subsequently required for a few days or until the parts have returned to normal.

SPONTANEOUS HEMORRHAGE FROM THE AUDITORY MEATUS

A few cases of free hemorrhage from the canal have been reported.[1] In these cases the observers could assign no cause whatever for the occurrence of the bleeding, and all state that the most careful and repeated examination of the canal failed to detect the presence of any wound or abrasion. Most instances of this kind have occurred in young girls of a nervous or hysteric habit. von Stein, however, reported a case in a boy thirteen years old. The fluid discharged from the ear is never pure blood, but is rather of a serosanguineous character and in some cases is foul smelling. More or less deafness accompanies the discharge. The flow of blood was not a vicarious hemorrhage and a hemorrhagic diathesis could not be made out. While the hemorrhage from the ears was sometimes quite free, it never became dangerous and recovery always took place. Cases of spontaneous bleeding from the auditory canal are cited rather as curiosities than otherwise and the diagnosis is the only point about which the physician need seriously concern himself. Therefore in every instance of aural hemorrhage the inspection of the meatus should be thorough, and the decision as to whether or not a diseased condition is present or whether a spontaneous hemorrhage is going on must be based upon the facts obtained by an actual observation of the parts in question. Spontaneous hemorrhage of the auditory meatus should also be distinguished from that which occurs in malingerers, in which latter the individuals themselves injure the canal, or put into the auditory meatus blood, or other fluid resembling blood, for the sole purpose of deception.

[1] Goldstein, in the American Academy of Ophthalmology and Otolaryngology, reports a case of spontaneous bilateral hemorrhage in a girl aged twenty-two. The case was under the immediate and frequent observation of the doctor for more than one year. During this time the serosanguineous fluid was seen several times to well up from the bottom of the auditory canal. No abrasion of the skin of the external auditory meatus was ever found. Goldstein believed that the hemorrhage occurred through the sebaceous follicles at the inner end of the auditory canal. Similar cases have been observed by Wheelock, Trans-Indiana State Medical Society, 1901; by S. von Stein, *Zeitschrift f. Ohrenheilkunde*, 1903; by Gradinego, *Archiv f. O.*, 1889, and several others.

SYPHILIS OF THE AUDITORY MEATUS

The occurrence of the primary, secondary, and tertiary lesions of syphilis on the auricle and within the external meatus has been recorded. The primary ulcers originate from the contact of infected towels and from the caresses or bites of syphilitic individuals. Secondary and tertiary manifestations are usually seen in connection with evidences of syphilis on some other part of the body (Fig. 88). In the auditory meatus the disease most often manifests itself in the form of condylomata, which are seen in the outer portion of the canal as grayish-red, warty, or polypoid-looking excrescences. Their presence gives rise to irritation, swelling, and fetid discharge from the canal, and when large enough to fill the lumen of the meatus, to impairment of hearing and

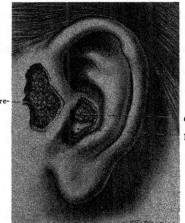

Granulating ulcer of pre-auricular region

Granulating base of ulcer

Denuded cartilage

FIG. 88.—TERTIARY SYPHILIS OF THE PREAURICULAR REGION, CONCHA AND TRAGUS.

tinnitus aurium. Pain may also be present as a result of the inflammatory swelling or from the ulceration of the canal, which is one consequence of the presence of the condylomata.

A primary ulcer of the auricle or meatus might easily be mistaken for similar lesions of an entirely different character. The diagnosis must, therefore, necessarily be made from the history of the occurrence, from the appearance of the lesions, and, in short, upon the same points from which a diagnosis of primary syphilis would be made if the genital organs instead of the ear were the seat of the ulcer. Condylomata may be mistaken for warts, granulation tissue, or polypi. Their structure is less firm than that of warts and they are more resisting to the probe than granulation tissue. Condylomata have also a paler appear-

11

ance than granulations, and their bases of attachment are commonly much nearer to the concha than in case the growths are polypi.

Treatment.—The administration of potassium iodid or mercury or of the two combined, according to the stage of the disease, is indicated in all cases when once a positive diagnosis of the specific nature of the disease is made. Increasingly large doses of these remedies should be given until the limit of tolerance is reached. Locally the parts should be kept antiseptic. Condylomata may be removed by cauterization with chromic acid or pure silver nitrate. More frequently, however, clipping them off with delicate curved scissors and afterward cauterizing the base of each will be found more expedient. After cleansing and drying the auditory meatus any moist or ulcerated surface that remains after the removal of the granulomata is often quickly healed by the application of calomel powder. Most writers, however, prefer to touch the ulcerated areas with diluted tincture of iodin, repeating this treatment frequently until all the sores are healed.

VICARIOUS HEMORRHAGE OF THE EARS

This sometimes occurs in the female at the same time as the menstrual function or it may entirely take the place of the menstruation. The diagnosis should be easy, particularly after the first attack, when it will be found to recur each month or at least with a degree of regularity that can be connected with menstruation. The treatment is gynecologic, and should be directed to the reproductive organs and the systemic condition of the individual rather than to the ear.

TRAUMATIC HEMORRHAGE FROM THE AUDITORY CANAL

As the result of either direct or indirect injury to the cutaneous lining of the external meatus, to the deeper osseous structure of the temporal bone, or to the middle ear or labyrinth, severe or even fatal hemorrhage may occur from the auditory canal. These injuries result from knife or bullet wounds, from the forcible entrance into the ear of any foreign body, and from fractures of the base of the skull which involve the petrous portion of the temporal. The entrance of corrosive chemicals, molten metals, or of live steam into the ear has been known to result in deep ulceration which lead ultimately to a fatal hemorrhage. When the fracture extends into the cranial cavity through the mastoid antrum, middle ear, or external auditory canal cerebrospinal fluid and blood may be discharged from the external auditory meatus to the amount of several ounces in the twenty-four hours. Since these injuries may involve the entire hearing organ, their full consideration is given under the heading Injuries to the Hearing Apparatus.

EAR COUGH

While ear cough can scarcely be called a disease, nevertheless it is a symptom which is so often met with while examining the external auditory meatus that its occurrence is deserving of some mention. It is not an uncommon occurrence to find an individual in whom a distressing or even violent cough is brought on every time an attempt is made to introduce the aural speculum or to probe or otherwise manipulate the instruments in the canal during an examination or treatment. This cough is dry, spasmodic, and often continues for a few seconds after withdrawing from the ear the irritant which has produced it. The presence of a foreign body, hardened ear-wax, or of inflammatory swelling of the canal may give rise to a dry hacking cough which may be mistaken as a symptom of serious pulmonary disease, and hence in any individual whose cough is of this character, and for which a definite cause is not elsewhere discovered, an examination of the auditory meatus should not be neglected.

CHAPTER XVII

THE METHODS OF THE EXAMINATION OF THE PATIENT

PREVIOUS to the establishment of accurate methods for the examination of the ear, the history of an aural disease given by the patient was regarded of such importance that upon it was based both the diagnosis and the subsequent treatment. While at present the tendency in aural practise is to base the management of any aural ailment largely upon an actual inspection and recognition of the pathologic conditions which are present, nevertheless the personal history of each case is of importance and should by no means be ignored. Such a history should include a statement of any hereditary tendencies toward deafness, tuberculosis, syphilis, or catarrhal disease, and of all the serious ailments from which the patient has at any time suffered, especially the infective diseases of childhood, meningitis, and typhoid fever. The influence of climatic changes upon the aural affection, the amount and nature of any discharge in the past or at present, the presence or absence of tinnitus aurium, and the degree of present impairment of hearing, are all subjects upon which the patient should make his own statement.

THE PHYSICAL EXAMINATION

The successful practise of modern otology must depend largely upon the acquisition of that knowledge concerning each individual case which can only be acquired by the most painstaking and thorough physical examination of the diseased ear. Neither a reliable diagnosis nor prognosis can be given nor a rational treatment instituted until it is definitely known what particular part of the ear is affected, and what the nature and extent of the given disease may be. Inference concerning the character of aural ailments should no longer receive consideration in the practise of otology, but instead definite knowledge must be ascertained by the employment of every scientific means toward the discovery of the degree and nature of the departure from the normal. The means and methods of conducting such an examination is, therefore, given here somewhat after the order pursued in actual practise.

The Light and Its Employment.—A good light is a first essential to a satisfactory aural examination, because the different parts of the ear which are to be examined must always be clearly seen and sometimes manipulated by the examiner under direct illumination.   Sunlight, the light of a candle, gas, oil, or electricity can each be successfully employed, but it is obviously best to become accustomed to one source of light, used in a given way by means of the same apparatus, in order to be the better able to judge the appearances of health or disease under a uniform illumination of the fundus of the ear.   After a trial of the other sources of light in common usage the author found that gas, used in the Argand burner with a bull's eye condenser (Fig. 92), best served his purpose, and for a number of years he has made constant use of the same for all office examinations and treatment.   During the past five years a gas mantel has been used on this lamp with the greatest satisfaction.

A most excellent examining light, and one which the author used exclusively during his early practise, may be obtained from the student's lamp.   When this lamp is used the bull's eye condenser is not wholly satisfactory, owing to the added difficulty experienced in regulating the flame.   The employment of a frosted chimney greatly protects the eyes of the examiner from the bright rays which, if not thus subdued, would interfere with that perfect vision essential to accurate inspection.

Electricity, when available, is convenient and second in choice. It has the decided advantage of not producing an uncomfortably high temperature near the patient's head.   It may be used in a condenser, in which a 32- or even a 50-candle incandescent lamp is placed.   An electric lamp consisting of only the conducting cords and bulb swung in any convenient place near the patient's head may furnish a satisfactory source of light.   However used, some provision must be made to cover the incandescent wires of the bulb, since otherwise their image will often be reflected across the field under examination in such a way as to greatly interfere with exact appearances of the parts undergoing the examination.   To obviate this occurrence the bulb should be frosted or the lens of the condenser may be of ground glass.

Sunlight or candle light are oftener used from necessity rather than from choice.   A candle gives an illumination too weak for accurate inspection and should be employed only when other sources of light are not procurable.   On the other hand, sunlight, if softened by absorption from surrounding bodies to an extent that its greatest intensity is lost, becomes an admirable medium for examining the depths of an ear.   The objection to the use of sunlight is that all conditions necessary to its use are seldom such that it can be depended upon for the purpose in question.

Since aural examinations must often be made in the home and with the patient in bed, the otologist must provide a source of light for

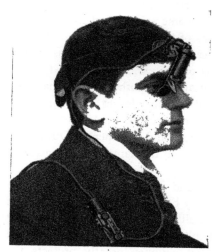

FIG. 89.—KIRSTEIN'S ELECTRIC HEAD LAMP.

illumination under such circumstances. If the residence is supplied with an electric current the head lamp shown in Fig. 89 is preferred. Such an instrument is conveniently carried in the instrument bag and during its use may be carried to any required position near the patient's head— a point of recommendation when the position of the patient must be recumbent. A pocket electric light (Fig. 90) can be used for the examination, provided it has a lens which will properly focus the rays upon the mirror which is worn upon the forehead.

An examination at the home of the patient may also be made by the use of an Argand, a student's, or other oil lamp; but when either gas or oil lamps are employed for the illumination it becomes necessary for the patient to sit erect in bed or, preferably, in a chair, since otherwise it would be difficult to reflect the rays of light to the depths of the ear.

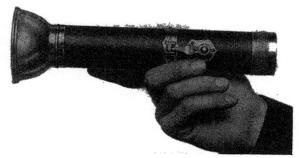

FIG. 90.—ELECTRIC LIGHT, CONVENIENT TO CARRY IN THE BAG FOR MAKING EXAMINATIONS AT THE HOME.

Whatever source of light is selected, it is necessary to employ a proper mirror to reflect it into the auditory meatus. Such a reflector was formerly held in the hand, but since this required the use of one of the operator's hands which could be more advantageously employed otherwise this method of reflection has been discarded and the reflector is now either worn upon the examiner's head or is supported from an arm at an exact focussing distance from both the light and patient. The head-mirror is given preference chiefly because any movement of the head of the patient can be immediately followed by the operator without that loss of time which would be required for readjustment if the reflector is stationary; hence when the mirror is worn on the head the field to be examined can be constantly illuminated and the examination proceeds without interruption.

Both the reflecting mirror and the head-band should be carefully selected. The size and focussing distance of the mirror are of great

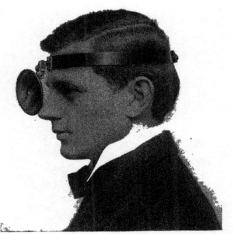

Fig. 91.—The Head Mirror with Celluloid Head-band and Proper Movable Joints of Attachment. Note that the mirror has a double ball-and-socket joint.

importance. A mirror with a diameter of 3 inches and a focussing distance of not more than 10 inches is preferable. A focussing distance greater than 10 inches renders the illumination indistinct and one less than 10 inches would necessitate such close proximity of patient and examiner as to interfere with the necessary manipulation of instruments in the ear. A head-band of celluloid fits more accurately, feels more comfortable on the head, wears longer, and is more sanitary than any other (Fig. 91). A simple ball-and-socket joint at both the attachment to band and mirror are all that can be desired. The nasal and forehead supports, which instrument-makers sometimes attach to the head-band or mirror, are a hindrance to the employment of the reflector, and are, therefore, objectionable features.

The light to be used is placed to the right of the patient, on a level with the ear to be examined and a short distance behind it. The patient is seated in a chair in front of the examiner, who is also seated. Although a good examination may be made while the patient occupies any ordinary straight-backed chair, yet certain features in the construction of the chair shown in Fig. 92, which has been made as a result of the needs of the otologist, add not only to the comfort of the patient but also to the ease with which the examination or treatment is conducted. The ideal chair has a seat which can be quickly raised or lowered according to the height of each patient. It should rest so

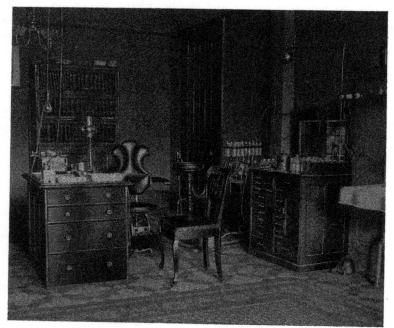

Fig. 92.—Convenient Arrangement of Furniture and Instruments for Office Examination and Treatment.

securely upon the floor that no tilting motions are possible. The back should be straight and have a head-rest which will enable the examiner to change the position of the patient's head frequently, easily, and without discomfort as the examination progresses. Should giddiness suddenly seize the patient a chair that may be quickly tilted to the horizontal is both convenient and useful. The chair represented in Fig. 92 combines a commendable number of these features.

When the patient, light, head-mirror, and examiner are ready as above described, the external auditory meatus should be examined before an aural speculum has been introduced. This precaution will prevent overlooking any abnormality or disease which may be located in that portion of the canal which is commonly covered by the speculum when the latter is in place. Boils of the auditory canal are located just within the meatus, and should one be present, it will not only be thus concealed, but the introduction of the speculum against it would give rise to very considerable pain.

To accurately reflect light from a head-mirror into a narrow cavity like the external auditory meatus requires much practise. Before the student of otology attempts the illumination of the depths of the ear he will do well, therefore, previously to practise its reflection into the cavity of an ear model (Fig. 39); or, if such a model is not accessible, a valuable experience may be obtained by reflecting the light upon a spot on the wall. Persistent practise in the management of reflected light will prove highly profitable to the student or physician because the art of its employment is not only of use in ear examinations but also in the inspection and treatment of all the accessible cavities of the body.

Aural Specula, Their Selection and Methods of Use.—The drum membrane lies at the bottom of a crooked canal and at a depth of about 1½ inches. It is only in exceptional cases, there-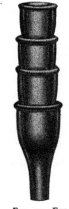fore, that the examiner is able to see this structure without the aid of an aural speculum, to separate the walls of the auditory meatus, and to assist in straightening the canal. Aural specula are constructed of silver, vulcanite, or aluminium. The two former materials are preferable, silver being given choice, first, because it can be sterilized by heat; second, from this material the speculum walls can be made very thin, thus giving the instrument the largest possible lumen, a feature of great importance in both diagnosis and treatment, since the larger the opening through the speculum the better the view of the parts to be examined (Fig. 93). Hard-rubber specula may be steril-ized by boiling, provided they are not handled with suffi-cient force, while they are yet hot, to distort their shape.

FIG. 93.—EAR
SPECULA.

Specula are constructed with either a cone or a funnel shape and the one or the other can be used equally well according to individual preference or experience of the examiner. Since the shape of the external auditory meatus is somewhat oval, some operators prefer a speculum with an ovoid instead of a circular contour. During an examination of the fundus of the ear the examiner often finds it desirable to rotate the speculum, and specula of circular construction are obviously easier of rotation.

The length of the aural speculum is of importance. When properly inserted into the external auditory meatus it should project from the concha no further than is necessary to enable the operator to grasp its outer extremity firmly and to manipulate it with that perfect ease which should characterize every step of an aural examination. If the speculum is too long, proper illumination of the deeper portions of the auditory canal and ease of instrumentation within the ear will be hindered.

Retraction of the Auricle.—Since the cartilaginous and bony meatus join each other at an angle (Fig. 81), it becomes essential to

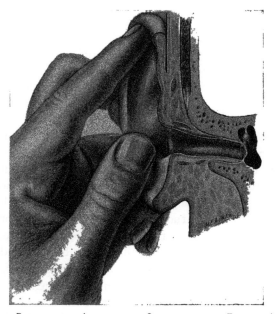

FIG. 94.—METHOD OF RETRACTING THE AURICLE AND OF STRAIGHTENING THE EXTERNAL AUDITORY MEATUS. Compare the direction of the canal shown in this illustration with that shown in Fig. 81, in which the external auditory meatus is in its position of normal repose.

straighten the meatus and thus to render the two portions of the auditory canal coincident with each other before it is possible to illuminate and inspect the fundus. From without inward the auditory canal runs first inward, upward, and backward, and then inward, downward, and forward. To efficiently straighten it, therefore, the cartilaginous or movable part must be lifted upward, backward, and outward. The left hand of the operator is sufficient to manipulate the speculum, retract the auricle, and to some extent support and secure the desired

movements of the patient's head.   Fig. 94 shows this position ready
for the illumination and inspection by the examiner, who now properly
focusses the light upon the drum membrane, which may be found
normal or abnormal.

The Membrana Tympani.—(a) The *normal drum-head* presents a
characteristic and rather pleasing appearance (Fig. 95).   Its oval
contour, irregular surface, and its color, lights, and shadows form a
picture not easily mistaken for other structures after once having been
recognized.   Certain landmarks are always clearly distinguishable
upon its surface, the most prominent of which is the short process of
the malleus (Fig. 96).   This tiny osseous promontory projects outward

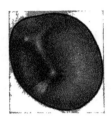

FIG. 95.—NORMAL DRUM MEM-
BRANE AS VIEWED THROUGH A SPEC-
ULUM BY REFLECTED LIGHT.[1]

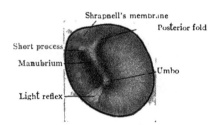

FIG. 96.—LANDMARKS OF NORMAL DRUM MEMBRANE.

from the point of juncture of the anterior and posterior folds, and is
cloaked by its covering of tympanic membrane.   Under illumination
the rays of light which are strongly reflected from its summit give an
appearance resembling a minute ripe pustule.   The long process of
the malleus extends downward and backward from the short process,

[1] One of the most difficult tasks with which the author has had to deal in the preparation of this book has been that of producing a satisfactory representation of the normal
and pathologic drum membrane, as seen by reflected light through the aural speculum.
A comparison of the illustrations of the normal drum heads that are given in the several
works on otology will show a considerable variation in appearance.   No doubt this difference arises from two reasons: First, the high-class artist, who alone is capable of repro-
ducing the appearance of the drum membrane when viewed through a speculum, is
unfortunately not able to see the structures intelligently in this way, and hence must
depend largely upon drawings made by the aurist.   Second, the picture of the whole
drum head, as shown above, is a complete one.   No aurist can see a whole drum membrane at any one instant, and hence to see the whole he must place the patient's head in
several different positions, as stated in the text, and it is the combination of these several
fragmentary images of the membrane that makes up the whole, as shown in Fig. 95.
Several normal membranes, figured in various text books, partake largely of the nature of
the *anatomic* membrane, that is to say, they look much as the membrane would if all the
soft parts were cut away and the tympanic ring, with its drum membrane attached, were
held squarely up to view.   Viewed through a speculum, however, the appearance of the
structure is greatly changed.   The diameters of all drum membranes shown in this
work are, for the purpose of greater clearness, twice enlarged.

producing the appearance of a ridge across the membrane as far as its center, at which point the process curves somewhat forward and ends at the umbo (Fig. 96). From the umbo a light reflex begins, widens as it extends downward and forward across the membrane, and at its base blends with the deepening shadow of the surrounding surface before the margin of the tympanic ring is reached. This cone of light is caused by a reflection from the tympanic membrane and its total disappearance or alteration from the normal denotes that a serious pathologic change of some kind has occurred in this structure.

The anterior and posterior folds may be seen to extend, the one forward and upward and the other backward and upward, from the short process of the malleus to the annulus tympanicus. The posterior fold is most clearly seen, and because of its situation in the plane much nearer to the eye of the observer appears to be the longer of the two. These folds separate the membrana tensa from the membrana flaccida (Fig. 96).

The color of the healthy drum membrane varies somewhat with the intensity and quality of the light used for its illumination. When illuminated by artificial gas, burned in a lamp provided with a gas mantel and condenser, the membrane has a pearl-gray appearance and a lustre entirely peculiar to itself. The membrana tympani is quite sensitive to the manipulation of instruments and the contact of fluids, and hence if it is examined immediately after syringing the auditory canal, or after prolonged retraction of the auricle and repeated insertion of the speculum, there will probably be observed a blush of redness over the greater part and a deep injection of the vessels running parallel with the manubrium.

(b) *The Diseased Tympanic Membrane.*—A description of the pathologic appearances of this structure which characterize its diseases will be given in subsequent chapters devoted to the inflammatory affections of the middle ear, and therefore mention of them will be made here only in a general way. In all examinations of the fundus of the ear the landmarks of the membrane should, if present, be made out, and any change in their position or size should be noted. Absence of these landmarks would indicate an inflammatory thickening of the drum-head which is sufficient to obliterate them. The light reflex and normal color are the first to disappear during an inflammation, and after these the umbo, manubrium, and short process usually follow in the order given. The short process may often be distinguished long after the others have been submerged by the inflammatory changes. Likewise, in destructive diseases implicating the middle ear, this process, owing to its abundant blood-supply, withstands necrosis better than the surrounding tissues, and it is therefore frequently preserved in the midst of the general destruction (Fig. 191).   Perforations may appear in any portion of the membrane and may be of any size, from that of a pinhole up to that including the entire drum-head (see Figs. 191, 194, p. 332).

It is not always an easy matter to determine the presence, size, or location of a perforation in the membrana tympani. Assistance in this respect may be obtained if during the inspection of the fundus the patient should employ the Valsalva method of inflation, which, by forcing bubbles of air and secretion through the rupture, will thus designate its size and position. Should the whole drum membrane be wanting this fact may not be easy of verification. However, if the membrane is entirely destroyed, the fundus will usually appear more distant, the tympanic mouth of the Eustachian tube can often be seen, and a probe can be passed into it; the promontory can be outlined and the niches of the oval and round windows are often visible. If still in doubt, Siegle's otoscope (Fig. 97) may be used to produce suction upon the fundus, during which the observer will note whether or not there is movement of any part of the suspected drum membrane. If absolutely no movement be observed at the site of the drum membrane it is probable that this structure is not present. Adhesions of the membrane to the promontory or other portions of the internal tympanic wall are also best detected by the use of Siegle's otoscope. This instrument should be provided with a suction-bulb instead of a mouth-piece as formerly. When it is used for examination purposes the air is partly expelled from the bulb, the speculum part is introduced, air-tight, into the external auditory meatus, and the auricle is retracted just as must be done when the examination is made with the common speculum. When the fundus is well illuminated and the observer clearly sees every part, the hand holding the air bag slowly releases the compression, when suction will at once be made upon all the deeper structures of the auditory canal. If the drum-head is normal it will be observed to move perceptibly outward. If it is bound by adhesions at any point the same will be shown by their lack of mobility during suction, while the adjacent membrane can be moved outward and inward at the pleasure of the observer. Siegle's otoscope should be used neither for purposes of examination nor treatment except under good illumination and the direction of the eye of the examiner, who should see every movement of the drum membrane which is produced by the manipulation of the instrument, and should note the exact effect produced by the suction upon the movable parts.   If this care in the use of Siegle's otoscope be not observed, atrophic areas in the drum membrane may be ruptured by the suction, following which, unless the proper precaution be taken, an infection and consequent suppuration of the middle ear may occur.

Granulations and polypi are frequently present in cases of chronic aural discharge.   Polypi may be small and occupy only the cavity of the middle ear or they may grow through the perforation into the auditory canal, which they wholly or partially fill, and in neglected cases may become large enough to protrude from the external orifice of the

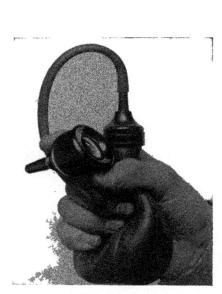

FIG. 97.—SIEGLE'S PNEUMATIC OTOSCOPE.
The illustration shows the bag partly compressed preparatory to insertion of the speculum tip, and outward suction upon the membrana tympani.

FIG. 98.—AURAL PROBE.

auditory meatus (see Fig. 201).   These growths appear red and injected when viewed through a speculum and may be mistaken for an inflamed and swollen drum membrane.   They bleed easily and the patient often gives a history of bloody discharges from the ear having taken place. Indeed, the alarm commonly produced by an aural hemorrhage is frequently the sole reason for the patient seeking immediate advice concerning the ailment.   A delicate aural probe (Fig. 98) is of much value in determining the true nature of many pathologic conditions at the fundus of the ear, concerning which impressions formed by inspection alone may have been unreliable. Polypi or other growths may be moved about by this instrument and both their character and point of attachment may thus be proved. By bending it to any required angle, the probe can be passed through perforations in the drum membrane, and necrotic areas in otherwise inaccessible parts of the drum cavity may by this means be positively determined.

In uncomplicated cases of labyrinthine deafness, of deafness due to disease of the auditory nerve, or its center in the brain, the tympanic membrane frequently appears unaltered in any way and presents all its normal characteristics.

Impediments to the Examination of the External Auditory Canal and of the Fundus of the Ear.—(*a*) In elderly persons the walls of the auditory canal are often so relaxed as to greatly narrow the lumen. Narrowing also results from both acute and chronic inflammation and from the presence of osteoma or other growths. In some individuals the channel is naturally small and the drum membrane deeply seated. Abnormality from any cause may hinder the introduction of the speculum or prevent the passage of the rays of reflected light to such an extent as to render the examination impossible or incomplete. Usually, however, it is possible by the selection of a long, narrow, and properly constructed speculum (Fig. 99) and careful retraction of the auricle to obtain a view of the deeper parts that will prove at least fairly satisfactory.

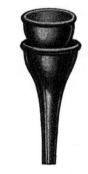

Fig. 99.—Long Narrow Specula for the Examination of the Deeper Parts of the Meatus when the Latter is Partially Obstructed by an Inflammatory Swelling or Growth.

(*b*) In some persons, usually men whose bodies are unduly covered with hair, a growth of stiff hairs is found in the outer portion of the auditory canal which is sufficient to obstruct the view of the parts beyond. A speculum can often be selected in such instances which will efficiently press the hairs from view; but if this is found impossible they should be removed by means of delicate curved scissors.

(*c*) Sometimes cases are seen in which the introduction of an aural speculum gives rise to such severe reflex cough as to render the examination difficult. A thorough inspection under such circumstances can only be made when the greatest possible care is exercised to produce as little irritation as possible from the use of the examining instruments.

Determination of the Patency of the Eustachian Tube and the Method of Inflation of the Middle Ear.—*Preliminary Exam-*

ination of the Nose and Nasopharynx.—Before the steps necessary for either an efficient examination or treatment of the Eustachian tube or middle ear can be carried out, a definite knowledge of the condition of the nose and nasopharynx should be obtained. While it is entirely

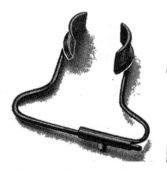

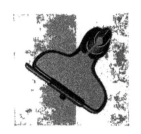

FIG. 100.—MYLES' NASAL SPECULUM.
A most convenient and efficient instrument for examining the anterior nasal fossæ. Adult size.

FIG. 101.—MYLES' NASAL SPECULUM.
Child's size.

beyond the province of this work to describe minutely the methods of conducting such an examination, nevertheless it is deemed important to emphasize the necessity for thoroughness in this respect and to briefly outline the necessary course to be pursued.

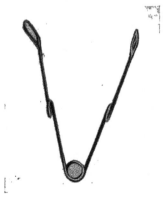

FIG. 102.—BOSWORTH'S SPECULUM.
Convenient for very small children.

Using a Myles nasal speculum (Figs. 100 and 101), first one nostril and then the other is dilated, and the lumen of each nasal meatus is carefully inspected to determine the presence of turgescences or new growths of the turbinates or of spurs or deflections of the nasal septum. This examination will be much facilitated if there is sprayed into the nostrils a 4 per cent. solution of cocain, which is followed shortly by a spray of the solution of adrenalin chlorid. Further application of a stronger solution of cocain may, if thought necessary, be made to the lower turbinate by means of a cotton-tipped applicator, which instrument should at the same time be employed for the purpose of further determining the size and nature of any hypertrophy or spur that may be present. In case of very small children or a narrow vestibule, the small size of Bosworth's speculum is most serviceable (Fig. 102).

After a few minutes the nasal tissues will have been so shrunken that the lower meatus will be opened to its fullest extent, and through it the examiner will often be able to determine much concerning the condition of both the nose and nasopharynx. In this way the experienced examiner will often be able to make out the presence of an adenoid which, on account of a sensitive throat, he is unable to see by means of the postnasal mirror. Collections of ropy mucus or dried crusts will also be seen if present, whether in the nose or in the nasopharynx.

The condition of the mouth and teeth should next receive a careful inspection. Syphilitic ulcers, either secondary or tertiary, may be found in the mouth, while the teeth by their peculiar setting and characteristic shape may indicate the inheritance of the disease (Fig. 303). The presence of healed cicatrices are most usually indicative of a previous syphilis and may account for an otherwise inexplicable aural affection. The discovery of a decayed tooth or an ulcerated gum may account for an earache that is. complained of, and therefore in any case of otalgia in which the drum membrane is found on examination to be normal, an explanation for this pain should at once be sought for in an exposed dental nerve. Ulceration of the throat, especially if implicating the tissues of the epiglottis, tonsil, or lateral pharyngeal wall, may also reflexly give rise to an otalgia. Much importance must be attached to the influence of the faucial and nasopharyngeal tonsils in the causation of aural diseases, and hence an examination of these structures should not be overlooked. This subject is considered of sufficient importance to merit a separate chapter for its consideration (see Chapter XX).

Crusts of dried secretion, such as are present in the nose and nasopharynx of those afflicted by atrophic rhinitis or ozena, must be removed before attempts are made to pass the Eustachian catheter. Likewise the thick ropy mucus which is often present as a result of acute or chronic disease must be cleared away by the postnasal syringe or atomizer (Fig. 103), since if this be allowed to remain it will block the orifices of the Eustachian tubes to such an extent as to greatly hinder or entirely prevent the passage of the air through the catheter, even when the latter has been properly placed in the mouth of the Eustachian tube. There is also a probability of blowing some of the foul nasopharyngeal secretion into the middle ear and of inciting an acute otitis media, should it not have been thoroughly removed before the Politzer or catheter inflation is performed.

It has already been shown in the chapter devoted to the physiology of the hearing apparatus that the Eustachian tube has a function most

12

essential to normal hearing. Any acute or prolonged disturbance of this function will not only impair the hearing but will also lead to pathologic changes in both the tube and tympanic cavity of an exudative, suppurative, or proliferative nature. An examination as to the condition of this tube must, therefore, be considered an important part of the aural investigation. There are three methods of determining the patency of the tube and at the same time of inflating the tympanic cavity:

(a) The *Valsalva method,* which dates back to the sixteenth century. It is performed by the individual himself, who first takes a deep inhalation, closes the mouth tightly, obstructs both nostrils completely by compressing the nasal alæ between the thumb and forefinger, and then makes forcible effort to blow the obstructed nose. The air meets with resistance at every outlet except the Eustachian tube, into which it

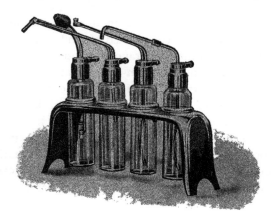

Fig. 103.—Set of De Vilbiss' Atomizers.

enters with a force determined by the resistance within the tube, and by the power with which the air-current is driven against it. Inflation through the principles involved in this method is frequently, though unintentionally, accomplished during the progress of head colds, when the nostrils are so much obstructed that great effort is required to blow and cleanse them and air is, as a consequence, forced into the middle ear. Inflation under these circumstances is thus so frequently performed during a severe rhinitis that the patient may as a result complain greatly of fulness, discomfort, or pain in the ear. Disease germs are also at times transported to the tympanum in this way, where they become the exciting cause of inflammatory or suppurative affections of this cavity. As a means of treatment the Valsalva method is not often to be recommended, since the patient is apt to employ it to an excess that is productive of middle-ear congestion or relaxation of the tympanic membrane. As an aid to diagnosis it is sometimes of use. During an examination of the drum membrane it is, as previously stated, often difficult to recognize a small perforation. If Valsalva inflation is performed by the patient while the fundus is illuminated, and there is a rupture present in the drum membrane, its situation will usually be demonstrated by the escape of air, together with any secretion that may have accumulated within the middle ear.

(b) The *Politzer method* was devised by Prof. Politzer, of Vienna, in 1863. It consists in driving the blast of air through one nostril at the moment when all the exits to the nasopharynx except the Eustachian tubes are closed. The Politzer air-bag, a short piece of connecting rubber tube, and a bluntly conic hard-rubber or metal nasal tip constitute the only outfit necessary to its performance (Fig. 104). An air-bag should be selected of such size as can be readily grasped by the operator's hand. Hence, each operator may most conveniently use a different sized bag. The caliber of both connecting tube and nasal tip should be ample to transmit the full blast of air from the bag. If the latter is to be used only for purposes of Politzer inflation, it is not necessary that it be constructed with an intake air-valve. However, it is often desirable to use the bag in connection with the Eustachian catheter inflation, and when so used an air-valve is of the greatest convenience, since it avoids the necessity of removing the nozzle from the mouth of the catheter after each compression of the bag.

Technic of Politzerization.—The patient should usually be seated. He is given a small sip of water and requested to hold it in the mouth until told to swallow. While stating this request, the operator inserts the conic tip of the Politzer air-bag into the vestibule of one nostril so that it fits tightly and blocks the opening. The wing of the opposite nostril is compressed against the adjacent nasal septum with sufficient firmness to occlude the passage. The patient is then told to swallow, coincident with the performance of which act compression of the bag is quickly made.

Inflation of the middle ear will usually result from the above procedure provided the technic has been followed and the patient has given efficient coöperation. Failure will result, first, if the Eustachian tube is greatly obstructed by mucus, swelling, or stricture; second, if the conic tip fits the nostril imperfectly, or if complete occlusion of the opposite nostril has not been effected; third, if the patient fails entirely to obey the command to swallow, or if the operator fails to recognize the fact that swallowing is taking place, and hence empties the air-bag either too soon or too late. Failure from any of the latter causes is due to the fact that the nasopharynx has not been shut off from the space below, and hence the blast from the bag enters the stomach or blows the water from the patient's mouth. A good rule is to watch the patient's "Adam's apple" at the instant the command is given the patient to swallow, and when this prominence of the larynx begins to rise, this fact is evidence that the act of swallowing is in progress, and that the proper time has arrived to perform the inflation.

In actual practise, certain modifications of the Politzer method are often found necessary. Children will seldom coöperate satisfactorily,

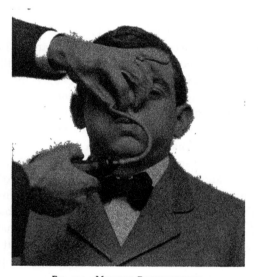

FIG. 104.—MODIFIED POLITZERIZATION.
The patient inhales deeply and then forcibly blows between the partly closed lips while the operator performs the inflation in the usual manner.

and hence his method will, in this class of patients, prove a failure. Almost every child, however, can be induced to blow out his cheeks with sufficient force to make an effective opposing current to the one driven from the air-bag, and the two, meeting in the nasopharynx, will satisfactorily open the Eustachian tube and produce the desired effect (Fig. 104). Merely puffing out the cheeks, by using the air already in the mouth, is not sufficient coöperation on the part of the patient, because the procedure furnishes no counter-current in the fauces. The child must, therefore, be shown how to perform by first filling his lungs by a deep inhalation and afterward forcibly blowing out between the partly compressed lips, just as he would do in blowing a blast from a horn.

If this plan is not comprehended by the child he may be given a mouthpiece, through which is a small opening, and told to blow vigorously through the same. When the child is observed to blow with sufficient energy, the tip of the air-bag is inserted into the nostril and the inflation can be successfully performed (Fig. 104). No difficulty should be experienced in inflating the middle ear of infants, because the act of crying shuts off the nasopharyngeal space quite as efficiently as any of the artificial methods just described. Hence, during the height of the expiratory cry the nasal tip is inserted, the opposite nostril occluded, and the inflation gently performed. Moreover, in infants and young children the Eustachian tube is proportionately shorter and wider than in the adult, and for this reason inflation is correspondingly easier.

As a therapeutic measure, Politzerization holds a middle position between the Valsalva method and inflation by means of the catheter. In children it is the only satisfactory means of restoring the normal air pressure in the tympanum, since before the age of ten it is seldom possible or desirable to use the catheter for this purpose. In cases where nasal obstruction is present or in which the mucous lining is hypersensitive, and in patients who are apprehensive concerning the use of instruments through the nose, Politzerization often becomes the method of choice.

(c) *Catheterization of the Eustachian Tube.*—In adults and in all cases where there is no nasal obstruction present which prevents its use, the Eustachian catheter should be employed in preference to either of the preceding methods, since by its employment a much greater precision in diagnosis and treatment is possible.

In cases where only one ear is diseased, it is clearly evident that none but the affected organ should be inflated, and that this desired end can only be attained by the use of the catheter. When the Eustachian catheter is employed the operator is able to accurately measure the degree of force of the air current he is using—a matter of the greatest importance when it is remembered that this force should vary according to the amount of obstruction to be overcome in the Eustachian tube and to the amount of resistance offered by the drum membrane to its replacement. When this membrane is found on examination to be atrophic or thin at any point, even a moderate force employed during the inflation might cause a rupture. On the other hand, if the membrane is thickened and bound in an abnormal position by adhesions, a pressure of 30 or 40 pounds may be used without any perceptible outer movement of the drum-head or without running the slightest risk of its rupture.   Hence, when provided with compressed air, which is governed by a pressure-regulator, the physician is enabled by the use of a catheter to employ that exact amount of force during the inflation which the preceding examination of the drum membrane may have shown to be indicated.

Eustachian catheterization is not resorted to as a means of diagnosis and treatment as often as its importance would indicate.   This is partly due to the slightly greater time required, but more largely, perhaps, because of the skill necessary to its successful and painless performance. Armed with a definite knowledge of the anatomy of the nose and nasopharynx and a proper amount of training in the steps necessary to its passage, the physician should be able to successfully introduce the catheter easily, quickly, and painlessly in any case in which the nasal

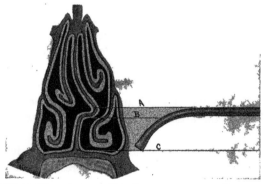

Fig. 105.—Perpendicular Section through Nose Showing one of the Difficulties in Eustachian Catheterization.
The catheter with an arc of A C could not pass through the inferior meatus the width of which is B C. In many cases like this the catheter may be easily inserted by turning the concavity of the instrument upward and causing the beak to hook under the deflection until the deformity is passed, when the guide is turned into the usual downward position.

passages are not obstructed.   Bleeding from the nose or severe pain occurring as a result of Eustachian catheterization is evidence either of the employment of unnecessary force or of faulty technic, and should be considered an inexcusable occurrence.   Catheterization must be regarded as a procedure requiring only the most gentle and painless manipulation for its performance, and it can therefore in no sense be classed as an operation.   Before attempting to introduce the catheter for the first time the nostrils should be examined by means of reflected light in order to determine whether or not they contain new growths or deformities to such an extent as to interfere with or entirely prevent the introduction of the instrument.   If, as frequently happens at this examination, the patient is unduly apprehensive concerning the procedure, it is wise to spray a

2 per cent. solution of cocain into the nostril and allow a few minutes to elapse before attempting to introduce the catheter. In case the nostrils are narrow or the turbinates are sufficiently turgescent to fill the spaces the addition of a solution of adrenalin chlorid to the cocain mixture will provide additional room in the nose, and will thus greatly facilitate the ease of the performance. Should the nasal septum be greatly deflected to one side or a spur so project across the nasal space as to obstruct the lower meatus (Fig. 105), it is often difficult or even

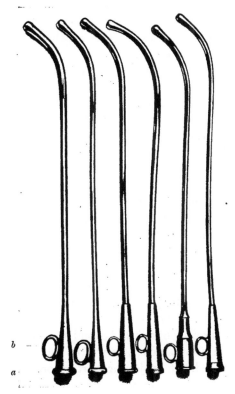

FIG. 106.—EUSTACHIAN CATHETERS.
Different-sized catheters from which a selection can be made to fit almost any case.

impossible to pass the Eustachian catheter. Hypertrophies or new growths which are large enough to partially or completely block the nasal passage may likewise render the procedure impossible. The catheter may frequently be passed through a nostril which is much occluded by a spur or hypertrophy, should the instrument be introduced in a position the reverse to that normally employed, or should the operator allow it to follow a corkscrew course through the inferior meatus.

At least three catheters of different sizes are necessary and a full assortment representing many sizes and shapes are advantageous (Fig. 106). Each should be so constructed that the largest lumen is provided that is consistent with the required strength of the instrument. The nasopharyngeal end, or beak, must have the edges of its circumference so beveled and smoothed that no injury can be inflicted on the tubal orifice or its adjacent parts. The proximal or funnel end (Fig. 106, *a*) is provided with an elliptic ring (Fig. 106, *b*), called the guide, which is attached in such manner that it always points in the same direction as the beak, a device whereby the operator may know, at any time during the insertion of the catheter, the exact angle at which the beak may be directed. This guide is of particular service, as will be presently seen, in indicating the proper position of the catheter when it has been finally turned into the tubal orifice. Eustachian catheters are usually made from pure coin or German silver or from hard rubber. Catheters constructed from pure silver are best because of the ease with which they may be bent into any desired shape. A stock instrument, constructed of inflexible material and with a standard curve at its distal or nasopharyngeal end, could not be successfully introduced in every case, for the reason that the normal width of the nasopharynx of each individual varies greatly, and therefore a different length of the arc-end of the catheter will be required to meet this variation. Hence, it often becomes necessary for the operator to change both the length of the arc and the degree of the curve before he will be able to successfully introduce the catheter.

Catheters are found in the shops varying in length from 5½ to 7½ inches. One of 6½ inches will be most satisfactory in the great majority of cases. When the instrument is properly introduced its proximal or funnel end should project but little beyond the tip of the patient's nose, for if it protrude 2 or 3 inches, as will be the case if the longest catheter has been selected, the projecting part becomes a lever of such length that even the delicate manipulations necessary to perform the inflation will produce a powerful movement of the beak within the tubal orifice, and consequent discomfort or pain to the patient.

The patient's full confidence and coöperation should always be obtained if possible, and he should be requested not to squint the eyes, make facial grimaces, nor swallow during the few seconds required for the introduction of the instrument, for as will be presently seen, under technic of catheterization, any such muscular movement at this time will not only cause the patient pain but may also defeat the purpose in view. Having obtained a knowledge of the condition within the nose, and having secured the patient's confidence by assurance that the performance is a painless one, all is ready to proceed with the introduction of the instrument.

Technic of Eustachian Catheterization.—(*a*) *First Method.*—Both patient and operator are seated facing each other. If the nasal passages have been found to be fairly normal, reflected light is not needed during any period of the catheterization. With the patient erect and his head slightly inclined forward, the fingers of the left hand of the operator rest gently against the nose and lower forehead, for the purpose of supporting the head and at the same time securing any desired change

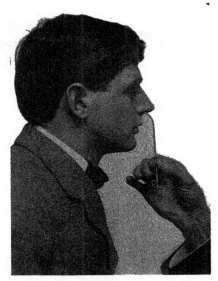

FIG. 107.—POSITION OF THE EUSTACHIAN CATHETER DURING THE FIRST STEP OF ITS INTRODUCTION. The tip of the patient's nose should be slightly elevated by the thumb of left hand of the operator during this step.

of position. The thumb of the same hand slightly elevates the nasal tip. The catheter is taken lightly between the thumb and first two fingers of the right hand and held somewhat perpendicularly, in which position it is inserted, beak downward, against the floor of the nasal vestibule (Fig. 107). The hand holding the catheter is then lifted until the instrument is horizontal and its beak rests upon the floor of the nostril, in which position it is advanced, with the most gentle effort possible, along the entire length of the floor of the inferior meatus and until the distal end is felt to move with such freedom as to indicate its entrance into the nasopharynx. It is absolutely necessary in order to insure final success that the instrument shall follow the floor of the

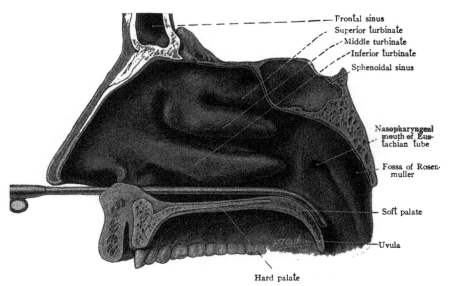

Frontal sinus
Superior turbinate
Middle turbinate
Inferior turbinate
Sphenoidal sinus

Nasopharyngeal
mouth of Eus-
tachian tube

Fossa of Rosen-
muller

Soft palate

Uvula

Hard palate

FIG. 108.—CATHETER PROPERLY INSERTED THROUGH THE INFERIOR MEATUS.
The illustration shows the position of the instrument when withdrawn until the arc of the distal end hugs the posterosuperior surface of the soft palate.   The same position of the guide is shown in Fig. 110. and of the beak in Fig. 112, A.   If the shaft of the catheter is rotated outward until the guide points toward the outer canthus of the eye of the same side, Fig. 111, the beak of the instrument will enter the pharyngeal orifice of the tube Fig. 112, C.

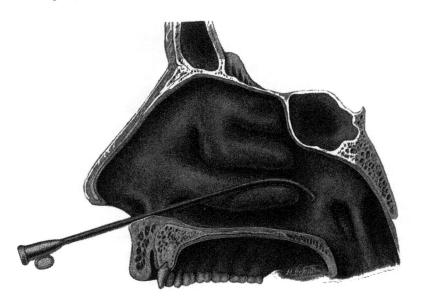

FIG. 109.—FALSE POSITION OF THE EUSTACHIAN CATHETER.
Introduction of the instrument, as here shown, is a frequent cause of failure in the beginner to properly enter the nasopharyngeal orifice of the tube.   While in the position here shown it is impossible to rotate the instrument into the mouth of the tube.

inferior meatus during this step of its passage (Fig. 108), since it must be clear that should it be directed so as to cross the inferior turbinated body as shown in Fig. 109, it could never be turned into the Eustachian meatus.

When the distal end has reached the open space of the nasopharynx, with the beak of the instrument still pointing downward and the shaft resting upon the nasal floor, the catheter should, without undergoing the slightest rotation, be gently withdrawn until the concave surface

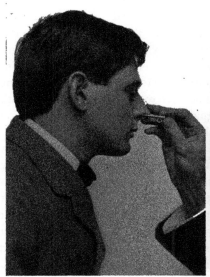
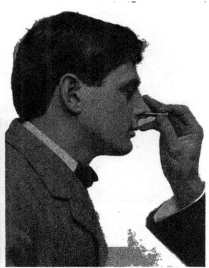

FIG. 110.—POSITION OF THE GUIDE WHEN CATHETER IS INSERTED ALONG FLOOR OF INFERIOR MEATUS, AND HAS THEN BEEN DRAWN OUTWARD UNTIL THE ARC OF THE DISTAL EXTREMITY HUGS THE SUPEROPOSTERIOR SURFACE OF THE SOFT PALATE.

This same position of the whole instrument is shown in Fig. 108, and the position of the beak is seen at point A, Fig. 112.

FIG. 111.—POSITION OF THE GUIDE WHEN THE CATHETER IS. PROPERLY INSERTED INTO THE NASO-PHARYNGEAL ORIFICE OF THE TUBE.

This position of the guide corresponds with that of the beak when rotated to point C, Fig. 112.

of the curve firmly hugs the upper posterior surface of the soft palate (Fig. 110). In this position the instrument is ready to be turned into the orifice of the Eustachian tube, the mouth of which is easily entered by the beak, provided the catheter is moved neither inward nor outward during its rotation. To provide against such movement the part of the instrument which protrudes from the nostril is grasped and held in position by the thumb and forefinger of the left hand while the remaining fingers of this hand are supported against the patient's head, in which position the catheter is rotated outward by the right hand until the guide points toward the outer canthus of the eye of the same side. Fig. 111 illustrates the position of the guide, while point C, Fig. 112 shows that of the beak at the time of the completion of the procedure.

(b) *Second Method.*—If for any reason the first method should fail, the instrument should be rotated inward until the guide projects horizontally toward the opposite side, which will bring the beak to point B, (Fig. 111). In this position it is withdrawn until the curved distal end of the catheter hooks snugly over the posterior end of the nasal septum. It is then held, as above described, by the thumb and forefinger to prevent either an outward or inward displacement, while at the same time it is rotated outward until both guide and beak occupy the position shown in Figs. 111 and 112.

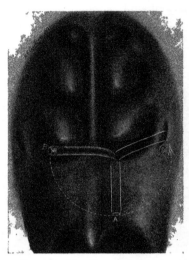

FIG. 112.—THE POSTERIOR NARES AND POSTERIOR-UPPER SURFACE OF THE SOFT PALATE AND UVULA, SHOWING THE DIFFERENT POSITIONS OF THE BEAK OF THE EUSTACHIAN CATHETER DURING THE SEVERAL STEPS OF ITS INSERTION INTO THE NASOPHARYNGEAL ORIFICE OF THE TUBE.

A, the position when first inserted; the shank of the instrument lies upon the floor of the inferior meatus, and the curve hugs the posterosuperior surface of the soft palate.

If the instrument is turned from this position toward the Eustachian orifice, C, it will usually enter this orifice when the position of the guide shown in Fig. 110 is reached. B shows the position of the beak when the catheter is drawn forward until it closely hugs the posterior end of the nasal septum (second method). If rotated in the direction of C it will usually enter the pharyngeal tubal orifice.

(c) *Third Method.*—If desired or if required by circumstances after the catheter has entered the nasopharyngeal space it may be pushed further in until the beak touches the posterior wall of the nasopharyngeal cavity. It is then slightly withdrawn and rotated until the guide points horizontally toward the side to be catheterized. In this position it is gently drawn outward along the lateral pharyngeal wall, the beak first passing the fossa of Rosenmüller, then rising over the posterior lip of the nasopharyngeal orifice of the Eustachian tube, and finally dropping into its mouth; the instrument is then rotated into the position shown in Fig. 111. This latter method, because of the irritation likely to be produced upon the nasopharyngeal structures and the consequent possibility of the patient coughing or retching, is not to be recommended except after failure of the other methods already described.

Difficulties Sometimes Encountered during Catheterization.— Undue anxiety on the part of the patient or a hypersensitive nasal or nasopharyngeal mucous membrane will sometimes incite a faucial spasm during the performance of Eustachian catheterization. If the distal end of the catheter has already entered the nasopharynx and a muscular spasm is thereby incited, the instrument is suddenly grasped by the muscular contraction with such firmness that it becomes for the time immovably fixed, and to turn it into proper position would require a force sufficient to greatly injure the surrounding soft parts and to cause the patient much needless anxiety and pain. When thus locked in the muscular grasp of the palate and pharynx non-interference is recommended until the spasm has relaxed. The instrument is, therefore, allowed to remain in the nose unmolested, while the patient should be assured that the difficulty will rapidly subside. The patient is requested to open the eyes and mouth, to inhale deeply through the nose, and to refrain from swallowing or talking. Immediate relaxation usually results when these instructions are followed by the patient and the catheter is again found free in the nostril. The uncompleted step of turning the beak into the Eustachian tube may then be accomplished or, if the patient continues to be nervous concerning the matter and the faucial muscles are still unduly excitable, the instrument should be withdrawn and no further attempt be made to insert it until a future examination.

How may the operator prove that the beak of the catheter has properly entered the mouth of the Eustachian tube? The experienced otologist recognizes the correct position of his instrument by an almost indefinable sense of touch. A more definite knowledge concerning the subject is, however, desirable on the part of the learner, and therefore the following points will prove helpful in this respect:

(a) When the catheter is in proper place the guide should, as has already been stated, point toward the external canthus of the eye of the same side of the patient's head. If the guide should point in either a higher or lower direction it is not probable that the catheterization has been successfully performed. (b) When the beak of the instrument is once in proper position in the nasopharyngeal mouth of the Eustachian tube a sense of resistance is met when the attempt is made either to advance or withdraw the instrument, the sense of lodgment of the beak within a cavity being imparted to the hand of the operator. (c) After the catheter has been successfully introduced into the tubal mouth the patient experiences no pain or discomfort should he then attempt to talk or swallow, whereas if failure to enter the mouth of the tube has resulted, any such movement of the throat will cause no inconsiderable distress. (d) By the proper interpretation of the sounds heard through the diagnostic tube by the examiner during the inflation of the middle ear.

Aural Auscultation.—Tympanic inflation, when produced by any of the foregoing methods, causes certain well-defined sounds in one or more divisions of the hearing tract, which may be perceived by the ear of the examiner, should his ear be connected by means of the auscultation tube (Fig. 113) with that of the patient.   The sounds thus produced

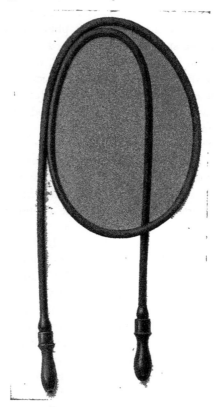

Fic. 113.—Diagnostic Tube.

are either normal or abnormal, according as the cavities through which the air passes are in a state of health or have been altered in size and shape as a result of diseased processes.   It is because of the possibility of distinguishing the abnormal from the normal sounds that aural auscultation is of importance as a diagnostic measure.

The sound perceived by the listener during the inflation of the normal ear is a compound one, and made up, first, by the rapid passage of the air through the narrow Eustachian tube; second, by its slower.

accumulation and vibration within the tympanum, and, third, by the displacement of the drum membrane outwardly. Normal auscultatory sounds, being of complex formation, are not easy of accurate description, and must be repeatedly heard by the examiner before a correct interpretation of their character is possible. Politzer compares this sound to that produced by placing the tongue against the roof of the mouth and then quickly performing expiration between the partly closed lips. Because of the small amount of secretion present in the normal tube and middle ear the auscultation sound of such an ear is always dry. The note produced is moderately low, but varies in pitch with the force used in inflation, with the lumen of the catheter employed, and with the normal differences in the size and conformation of the cavities through which the air passes. The sound which results from the inflation seems close to or even in the examiner's own ear.

The sound produced by inflation through a catheter, the beak of which has not been properly placed in the mouth of the Eustachian tube, will seem far removed from the examiner's ear and will produce no impulse upon the latter; but after having been frequently heard and compared with tubal or tubotympanic sounds, can be readily interpreted as originating from the nasopharynx. If the cleansing of the nasopharynx, which should have been done as a preparation for Eustachian catheterization, has been imperfectly accomplished the tubal orifice may contain a quantity of ropy mucus sufficient to fill it. Under such circumstances the catheter may have been properly placed, but the air would of course fail to enter the tube, and the sound produced by its passage through the tenacious secretion will be distant and discordant. Repetition of the efforts at inflation will usually displace the mucus and finally permit the air to enter the tympanum, after which the normal bruit will be heard.

Pathologic changes within the Eustachian tube or tympanum will greatly change the character of the normal inflation bruit. If the Eustachian tube is occluded by tenacious secretion, by swelling of the mucous lining, or by proliferative changes in its walls, the inflated air cannot, of course, reach the middle ear and the inflation sound will seem correspondingly distant. Should the tympanum be wholly or partially filled with polypoid or hyperplastic tissue, the normal blowing sound will be either greatly reduced or entirely absent. Accumulations of mucus, serum, or pus within the middle ear are productive during inflation of bubbling or crackling noises, due to the passage of the air through the liquid. Such sounds are, however, only possible when the exudate is sufficient in quantity to rise above the level of the tympanic

orifice of the Eustachian tube or when the patient inclines his head to
the opposite side during the inflation.

Small perforations through the membrana tympani, which are located
in any portion of the membrana vibrans, will give rise to a perforation
whistle which is usually intense enough to be heard at a distance of
several feet from the patient without the use of the auscultation tube.
Such a whistle is not produced if the perforation is blocked by polypi
or if the location of the rupture is distant from the tympanic tubal
orifice. Sometimes adhesions of the membrane to the adjacent inner
tympanic wall will shut off that portion of the middle ear which is in
communication with the Eustachian tube, and for this reason no perforation sound is heard during the inflation. Perforations in Schrapnell's membrane are, for the above reasons, not productive of this very
characteristic sound.

Fatal Results from Catheterization.—The fact that 3 deaths have
been reported as a result of Eustachian catheterization proves nothing
more than that force and awkwardness have been employed instead
of that most gentle dexterity which alone is justifiable, and which will
be entirely sufficient to insure successful catheterization in any case
where this procedure is a proper one to employ. The deaths were due
to emphysema of the tissues of the neck. The beak of the catheter
had abraded the mucous membrane and the subsequent efforts to
inflate the drum-cavity resulted in the injection of air directly into the
tissue of the neck in exactly the same manner that air is injected with
the blow-pipe when this instrument is used to facilitate tissue dissection.
Such an accident need never be feared when the catheter is used in a
skilful or even careful manner.

CHAPTER XVIII

EXAMINATION OF THE FUNCTION OF THE EAR

A GREAT majority of all the diseases of the hearing apparatus are accompanied by deafness varying in degree from an impairment so slight that it is scarcely noticeable to the individual to that in which the hearing is altogether lost.

The examiner will have ascertained, as a result of the previous physical examination, the amount and nature of the pathologic changes that have taken place in the conducting portion of the ear; but from physical appearances alone he will be unable in the vast majority of cases to state with any positive degree of accuracy the effect such changes have had upon the function of the organ. The physical examination will also fail to indicate whether the impairment is altogether one of perception or of conduction. The purpose of the functional examination is, therefore, to determine the degree of deafness, and to ascertain whether or not the disease responsible for the same is located in the conducting or in the labyrinthine portion of the ear.

The room in which a functional examination is to be made should, if possible, be well removed from street noises, since a confusion of sounds from without will greatly lessen the value of any conclusion which may be derived from an investigation conducted under such circumstances. The room should also be of sufficient length to permit the examiner to carry out some of the tests at a distance from the patient of at least 15 feet.

Since the normal ear is capable of perceiving both the quantity and quality of sound, certain sound-producing instruments in which the one or the other of these elements predominates are respectively used in the functional examination in order to determine the power the diseased organ may have for detecting the same, and by this means to form a basis for estimating the loss of function it has sustained.

The most useful quantitative tests are made by using the watch, the voice, the whisper, and Politzer's acumeter; but before describing the methods of their employment, certain precautions in their use should be mentioned.

Accurate information concerning the hearing distance of a diseased

13   193

ear can only be obtained when the patient is not permitted to see the source of the sound used in the test. This is particularly true when the voice or whisper is used in testing, because it is a well-known fact that those who are unable to hear distinctly very soon learn to read the lips of those with whom they are speaking. The patient should, therefore, be seated with the affected ear toward the examiner, which position will not only be the best for perceiving the sound, but will also guard against his obtaining information concerning it otherwise than through audition. In children all tests are often unreliable unless much tact is used in their employment. The child will often state that he hears the tick of the watch or the click of an acumeter at impossible distances; in which instance it will be found more satisfactory to use the voice test. If too young to understand and repeat some number which the examiner pronounces, the simplest words which are known to all children, as "papa," "mamma," or "brother," may be spoken by the examiner either in voice or whisper, and if the same are repeated by the child the inference concerning his hearing power for the voice or whisper may be conclusively known. It is obviously necessary to have the patient, whether child or adult, repeat the spoken or whispered words.

The Watch Test.—This ever-ready means of determining the degree of hearing is quite commonly employed, and, although it often gives rise to erroneous impressions, it is not without merit. During the examination the watch should be held at that distance from the ear at which it is known to be normally heard, and then gradually be brought nearer until the hearing distance for the ear in question is ascertained. If the watch is first held near the affected ear and is then gradually removed from it in order to learn the distance at which it may be heard, it will often be found that the hearing distance is greater for the latter than it is for the former method, for the reason that when the tick is once perceived by the patient the impression upon the impaired ear will persist, even when the watch is removed beyond the point at which it could possibly be heard.

For the purpose of recording the results of the watch test the hearing power of any individual may be described by taking the number of inches at which the watch in use is normally heard for the denominator, and the number of inches it is heard by the affected ear for the numerator. Thus, the normal hearing distance for a given watch may be 5 feet, whereas the patient hears it only 2 feet. The record for such a case should read, "Hearing power for watch equals $\frac{24}{60}$." Normal hearing in such a case would, of course, be $\frac{60}{60}$.

It should be stated that many partially deaf persons hear the watch tick comparatively well, whereas they perceive the voice comparatively poorly, and that therefore an improvement in the hearing distance for the watch, as the result of treatment, may not be a source of satisfaction to the patient, for the practical reason that it is the voice and not the watch that he most desires to hear.

The Voice Test.—A mild degree of deafness may be present and yet the patient may hear ordinary conversation with entire satisfaction. This is due to the fact that the normal perceptive power is greater than is necessary for the usual purposes of life. In cases of slight deafness the patient is annoyed by his defect only when the speaker is at a distance, as when following a lecture or sermon, or when in a company, several individuals of whom are engaged in conversation at the same time. Whatever may be the degree of impairment, it is important that the hearing distance for the conversational voice be accurately determined and recorded. The pitch of the examiner's voice should not be raised above the normal unless it is first ascertained by trial that the conversational voice cannot be heard by the patient. Many patients will hear the pure notes of the speaking voice much better than they will if the same be pitched an octave or more higher. A shrill voice is especially confusing to those suffering from certain forms of labyrinthine affection. If both ears are about equally diseased, it is easier to obtain accurate results from the voice test than in cases where only one is defective. In the latter instance it is necessary to block the auditory canal of the sound ear during the examination, which may be accomplished by the patient, who inserts his wetted forefinger tightly into the external meatus.

When the voice is heard at a distance of more than 15 feet the whisper should be employed. The patient is told to repeat what he hears. Standing at the greatest distance from the patient at which the whisper is likely to be heard, the examiner whispers at the end of expiration, using the reserve air. This method gives a more uniform whisper, according to Bezold. The examiner then whispers a word or a number of two figures. If this is not heard, the examiner gradually approaches the patient, repeating the number at each foot of the progress until the patient hears and repeats what is said. If the opposite ear is also to be examined, a different set of numbers or words should be used in the test, because when once a given word is perceived it will be heard or guessed much more readily if whispered or spoken immediately afterward. Thus the numbers 22, 46, 99, etc., may be employed in examining one ear, and 24, 57, 88, etc., for the other. It will be found that words containing a large proportion of vowels will be heard farther than those made up largely of consonants. Thus, the word

Boston, when either whispered or spoken, will be heard at a greater distance than will the word Massachusetts. This fact must, therefore, be considered in making a comparison of results obtained at the several different examinations which may be made during the course of the treatment; for unless words are used at each test which contain a somewhat similar arrangement of vowels and consonants, an erroneous conclusion as to the progress of the case will be formed.

Politzer's Acumeter.—For testing the hearing of those who are quite deaf, this instrument (Fig. 114) possesses decided advantages, but because of the intensity of the clicking sound produced by it the milder cases can be better examined by the foregoing methods. Acumeters are so constructed that they always produce approximately the same note, and herein lies their value when it is desired to compare the result of the examinations made by different observers.

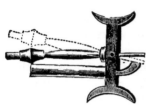

FIG. 114.—POLITZER'S ACUMETER.

A comparison of the results of the foregoing tests cannot be satisfactorily made when either the watch or voice tests have been employed, for the obvious reason that the watch used by one examiner may represent a make of instrument which ticks with an entirely different intensity from that used by another; and the voices of no two observers are likely to have an identical force or quality. The whisper test, when produced as above directed, is more nearly the same for all persons, and therefore it becomes a good test when comparisons are to be made.

Tuning-forks.—The power of the human ear for the perception of sound lies within the limits of 16 vibrations per second as a minimum, and 50,000 per second as a maximum. In the majority of individuals a rate of vibration of less than 24 or more than 16,000 per second are not perceived.[1] It is probable that those who are able to hear a rate either lower or higher than those last given, do so as a result of musical training.

The sound produced by the lower number of vibrations is designated a low note, while that which results from rapid vibrations constitutes a high note. The hearing power may be impaired for the detection of either the higher or the lower notes, and it is of great importance in diagnosis, prognosis, and treatment to be able to determine which part and to what extent the musical scale is defective in any case of deafness. For the purpose of detecting such deficiencies a series of tuning-forks whose rates of vibrating cover the normal limits of hearing

---

[1] Howell, *An American Text-book of Physiology*, 1896.

would be necessary, and Bezold has actually devised such a set of forks and whistles. These, while possibly essential to absolute accuracy, are fortunately unnecessary except in rare instances of complicated aural ailments. The Bezold set is expensive and its use requires more time than is usually justifiable.

Hartmann's set of tuning-forks (Fig. 115) consists of five instruments ranging from C = 128 to C₄ = 2048 double vibrations. This range is usually quite sufficient to obtain the information desired; and, indeed,

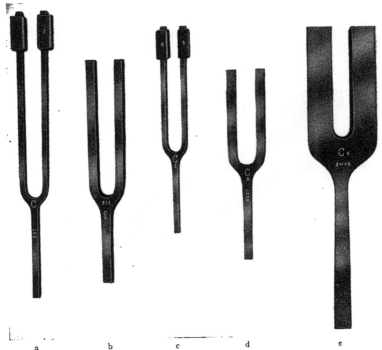

FIG. 115.—HARTMANN'S SET OF TUNING-FORKS RANGING FROM C TO C4 IN SERIES, AND FROM 128 V S TO 2048 V S.

the knowledge that may be gained from the use of the forks C, C₂, and C₄, when taken in connection with the intelligence gained through the physical examination of the ear and the history of the case, is often sufficient to justify a diagnosis as to the part of the ear affected by the disease, as well as the degree of impairment of the hearing.

For the detection of the upper tone limit the C₄ fork in the Hartmann set is not always sufficiently high. The Galton whistle is a serviceable aid in such instances. Since this instrument is constructed like an adjustable organ pipe, it is possible to obtain as low as 16 vibrations per second or as many as 50,000 per second, which latter represents the maximum normal limit. Likewise in cases where there is but slight impairment of hearing, the C fork of the Hartmann series will not be low enough to detect the defect, and in such instances the use of Dench's fork (Fig. 116), will serve a useful purpose. The three most useful tests of the tuning-fork in determining the perception of an ear for the quality of sound are:

(1) *The Schwabach Test.*—The value of this test depends upon the fact first established by Schwabach, that when there is obstruction to the passage of sound through either the external or middle ear, a vibrating tuning-fork will be heard longer when placed in contact with the cranial bones than it will through the air, if held while vibrating near

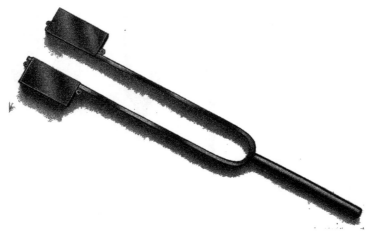

Fig. 116.—Dench Fork for Testing Low Tone Limits.
With clamps 80 V. S.; without clamps 120 V. S.

the ear. Thus, if the patient has impaired hearing and the vibrating tuning-fork is heard in both ears longer when the shank of the instrument is placed against the forehead than it is when held at a short distance from either one or the other ear, the inference should be that the disease is located in the middle ear or external auditory meatus, in which instance it is properly spoken of as an obstructive deafness or a deafness due to impairment of the conducting apparatus. Should, however, the patient who is partially deaf hear the vibrating fork longer through the air than through the bone, the fact would indicate a labyrinthine and not an obstructive aural disease.

In all the tests requiring the application of the vibrating instrument to the bone, the examiner should use a middle fork, the one most commonly selected being C_2, Fig. 115, *b*. The excursions of the slowly vibrating prongs of the lowest forks (Fig. 116) are great enough to produce a sensation upon the part against which the handle of the instrument rests, which, in view of the fact that the remaining sensibilities of those who are deaf are greatly increased, may be felt rather than heard by the patient. While the Schwabach test is entirely reliable in nearly every case, certain complicated conditions arise that sometimes render it uncertain, in which instances the results obtained by it must be compared with those of other tests, and also with the findings of the physical examination and the history of the patient, before a definite conclusion is reached.

(2) *Weber's test* depends for its value upon the physical fact that if in cases of one-sided deafness the tuning-fork is placed, while vibrating, upon the median line of the skull it will be unmistakably heard best in the deaf ear, provided the cause of the deafness is in the middle ear; whereas, if there is a purely labyrinthine affection present, the fork will be heard best in the healthy ear. Should the case be one of mixed deafness, that is, should there be disease of both the middle ear and labyrinth, the test may prove uncertain and the examiner must seek more positive information through the employment of other measures. If the implication of the labyrinth and middle ear are equal in a patient who is quite deaf in one ear the chances are that the vibrations will be best heard in the good ear; whereas, if the middle ear is the more involved the sound will be best heard in the bad ear, but for a shorter period than when uncomplicated by a labyrinthine involvement.

(3) *Rinné's Test.*—In this the experiment of comparing the length of time the vibrating fork is heard through the air when held near the ear with that for which it is heard through the bone when it is placed upon the mastoid process is performed. Normally the C_2 fork is heard twice as long by air as by bone conduction ($a c = 2 b c$). If the reverse is found to be true, this fact is indicative of middle-ear deafness. In uncomplicated labyrinthine deafness air conduction is better than bone conduction ($\frac{a c}{b c}$), the high notes are heard through the air comparatively poorly and the low notes comparatively well. When the vibrating fork is heard longest by air conduction, Rinné's test is said to be positive (Rinné+), but if heard longest when the handle is placed against the mastoid, the test is negative (Rinné−). In those in whom the hearing distance for the forced whisper is less than 6 feet, Rinné's test is not the best one to employ.

Summary of the Various Tuning-fork Tests and of the Inter-

pretation of the Results Obtained from Each, or from All Used Collectively.—(*a*) *Evidence Furnished by the Use of the Tuning-fork which is Indicative of Middle-ear Deafness.*—In any partially deaf individual the hearing for the lower tone limit by air conduction is raised; that is, if the patient does not hear C (Fig. 115, *a*) by air conduction, this fact is usually indicative of middle-ear deafness. If then Weber's test is applied, the vibrating C_2 fork being placed on the median line of the cranium, and the patient hears the vibration best in the bad ear, this fact furnishes further evidence that the disease is located in the middle ear. Should additional evidence be necessary and the Rinné experiment be performed and found negative, the diagnosis of middle-ear deafness may then be safely made.

(*b*) *Evidence Indicative of Labyrinthine Affection.*—When the examination is conducted with the series of Hartmann forks and C is heard by air conduction, but C_3 and C_4 (Fig. 115, *d* and *e*) are not so heard, or heard but poorly, labyrinthine disease should be suspected. Should C_2 (Fig. 115, *b*) be then placed upon the median line of the skull and the vibration is better heard in the better ear, the former suspicion is further confirmed; and, finally, if Rinné's test is positive (Rinné+, $\frac{a c}{b c}$), the diagnosis of labyrinthine disease should be made.

In addition to the evidence obtained by the use of the tuning-fork for the purpose of locating the disease either in the conducting or perceptive portions of the hearing apparatus, the facts obtained by the physical examination are often of great value. Thus, in cases of deafness due to disease of the conducting apparatus there may be found in the external auditory meatus obstructing growths, inspissated cerumen, or dried pus. The tympanic membrane may be found perforated, indrawn, thickened, or adherent. The Eustachian tube may be swollen and collapsed or narrow and strictured. On the other hand, when the functional examination points to the labyrinth as the sole seat of the affection, no obstruction whatever will likely be found in either the external auditory meatus or Eustachian tube, provided the internal ear disease is primary. In such instances the drum membrane may appear entirely normal in every respect. In case the internal ear disease is a complication of some middle-ear ailment, all of the above changes that were noted in the conducting apparatus may be found. Any one of the tuning-forks which is selected for use is set vibrating by holding the shank in one hand and striking one of the prongs against some object. If the latter be hard, as, for instance, the wood or marble top of a table, compound notes or overtones will be produced. These overtones may be heard by the patient, whereas, the pure tone, the ability of the patient to hear which the examiner desires to ascertain, may not be at all perceived. It is, therefore, essential that some semi-elastic substance, like the operator's knee, be struck with a moderate force, and the resulting note examined by his own ear for the purpose of detecting any overtone before the vibrating instrument is used to test the hearing of the patient. The vibrating fork, when used to test the air conduction, should be held about 2 inches from the ear of the patient and with one of the vibrating prongs directed squarely toward the meatus. If the instrument is rotated from this position a point will be reached at which the vibrations are entirely inaudible, and consequently the test might be rendered unreliable.

CHAPTER XIX

THE INFLUENCE OF NASAL AND NASOPHARYNGEAL DISEASES UPON AFFECTIONS OF THE EAR

THE anatomic and physiologic relationship of the nasal and nasopharyngeal spaces to the cavities of the middle ear is so intimate as to make it inevitable that continued disease of the former must sooner or later affect the latter.

It has already been shown that certain physiologic processes connected with normal hearing are mechanically performed. Thus the normal ventilation of the tympanic cavity takes place during the act of swallowing and is the result of a muscular traction upon the walls of the Eustachian tube which is sufficiently powerful to open this channel and to allow that free admission of air which is at all times necessary to equalize the atmospheric pressure upon the tympanic side of the drum membrane.

Any growth which is large enough to fill the nasopharynx must interfere greatly with that perfect action of the palatal muscles which is constantly taking place in the normal throat, and, therefore, with efficient ventilation of the cavity of the middle ear. Normal admission of air to the middle ear also depends at all times upon the presence in the nasopharynx of an unobstructed supply of air. Should the nose or nasopharynx be obstructed by new tissue, each act of deglutition will exhaust the air from the nasopharynx and tympanic cavity rather than replenish it.[1]

Secondary to a lowered intratympanic air pressure a distention of the vessels which supply the mucous membrane of the middle ear occurs. When continuing for any considerable length of time this vascular congestion gives rise to an exudate into the cavity of the middle ear (see p. 235), which may cause rupture of the membrana tympani, or may remain permanently and become ultimately organized into new

---

[1] This fact may be demonstrated by any one upon himself. Catch the alæ nasi between the thumb and forefinger of one hand and compress tightly. Then swallow while the passage of air through the nose is thus completely blocked. A sensation of stuffiness is immediately produced in both ears which is caused by the exhaustion of air from the middle ear and the consequent displacement of the membrana tympani inward by the unequal atmospheric pressure upon the outer surface of the drum-head.

tissue. The engorgement of these intratympanic vessels also predisposes the individual to an active inflammation of the middle ear, of either a catarrhal or suppurative variety, the inflammatory state being quickly added to that of congestion whenever a sufficient number of pathogenic bacteria find entrance to the cavity of the middle ear.

Individuals who are affected by **growths in the upper air tract** are subjects of frequent colds in the head. This is true to the extent that many children are seldom free from nasal stuffiness and discharge except during a short time each year in summer, and medicines, local applications, or hygienic management of the patient seems to have little or no effect upon this condition so long as the obstructed air tract remains.

ADENOIDS[1]

Pathogenic bacteria are now known to play an important part in the production of aural affections, and it is to some extent because adenoids and other growths of the nasopharynx form an ideal culture-field for these germs that the presence of such growths become most harmful. The mechanical irritation caused by the presence of adenoids induces an abnormal secretion of thick, ropy mucus, which, because of the obstructed condition of the nostrils, is difficult and often impossible to completely dislodge. The retention of this almost purely albuminoid secretion at a proper temperature is attractive to several varieties of bacteria which are found here in great numbers, and which are apparently ready at all times to invade the middle ear whenever certain conditions of congestion or other weakened state of the membrane occurs in that cavity. (See Chapter III.)

The author believes that nasal and nasopharyngeal obstruction due to adenoids or other growths constitute the most frequent and harmful factor in the causation of aural diseases. A very considerable percentage of all ear affections have their incipiency in childhood, and therefore at a period of life before the patient is old enough to realize the degree of his defect or to make any complaint of the impairment of his hearing. Tubotympanic congestion with resulting exudate into the middle ear is a common complication of nasopharyngeal disease. It is not often a painful affection, and parents are therefore seldom alarmed concerning its indefinite continuance; indeed, they seem to be very infrequently cognizant in any way of the existence of an affection that

[1] While the term *adenoids* is commonly used to describe hypertrophied lymphoid tissue in the vault of the pharynx, the word *adenoid* would be more correct for the reason that the several lobes of which the growth is composed are attached to but one base. When removed en masse by one sweep of the curet, as advocated in the text, the hypertrophy comes away in one piece as shown in Figs. 129 and 130.

may in the future debar the individual from active participation in social or commercial life. The listless appearance and the semi-idiotic facial expression of the child are sometimes overlooked entirely by those who are constantly with such children, and if observed are usually attributed to a habit of inattention, for which the child is unjustly faulted both at home and at school.

Earache is a frequent complaint of the child afflicted with adenoids. The most trivial exposure to cold or dampness is frequently followed by a head cold, this is often quickly succeeded by pain in the ear, and later by a serous, mucous, or purulent discharge from the external auditory meatus. The frequency of the attacks of this nature in adenoid children is sufficient to cause serious interruptions in their attendance at school; and this, together with their limited ability to hear what is said when their physical condition permits their presence in the classroom, is quite sufficient to hinder their educational progress to an extent that they are often rated as unduly stupid.

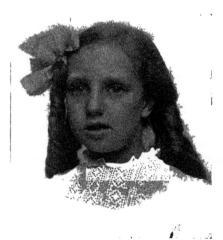

FIG. 117.—TYPICAL ADENOID FACE.
The open mouth, expressionless appearance, impairment of hearing and evil effects upon the general health have produced the condition known as aprosexia.

A dull eye, widely opened mouth, peculiar facial expression, and general appearance of impaired mentality are present in the typic adenoid case, and constitute a condition which Guye has designated aprosexia (Fig. 117). It should be remembered, however, that a large number of children suffer from adenoids who do not exhibit the above symptoms to any marked extent. Large nasopharyngeal growths of this nature are often found in children with bright faces, who possess a high degree of intelligence, and whose parents will state that they always breathe with the mouth closed. Careful investigation in such instances will show that the parents are mistaken and that mouth breathing is complete, the child keeping the lips separated so slightly as to prove deceptive to the casual observer, but nevertheless sufficiently to admit the inspired air. A painstaking physical and functional examination of this class of cases will almost invariably detect, in addition to the adenoid itself, the presence of more or less impairment of hearing. It may be stated by the parents that the hearing is perfect, and this may apparently be true in so far as the child's ability to hear common conversation is concerned, but since it is true that normal hearing is more acute than is needed for the perception of ordinary conversational tones, it is likewise true that some of the hearing power may be lost and the person or those about him be unaware of the fact, unless some unusual test is brought to bear upon the case.

In early childhood the prompt recognition and thorough removal of nasopharyngeal adenoids constitute the best known prophylactic against future deafness, as well as against future suppurative aural affections and their possible mastoid and intracranial complications. At this period of life prompt measures directed to the removal of these obstructions from the upper air tract will in a majority of instances cure the existing aural disease, and will prevent in a great measure the liability of its subsequent occurrence. Left either to nature or to medicinal treatment, the adenoid is, in the vast majority of cases, a menace to the integrity of the ear, of such harmful nature that few of those who are so fortunate as to be allowed to "outgrow" their ailment reach adolescence without serious and permanent aural impairment. In cases of deafness accompanying adenoids in childhood, the otologist is given an opportunity to do the little patient an immeasurable and permanent good, whereas the same individual, if allowed to continue untreated until adult life, will then frequently present the most hopeless condition in so far as cure or relief of the aural condition is concerned. The entire future social and commercial welfare of this heretofore neglected class of children depends largely upon the early recognition and complete removal of this comparatively trivial growth from the nasopharynx; and since the institution of compulsory inspection of the health of school children, at present attracting public interest, and already being carried out in many cities, it is probable that an earlier recognition of the causative factors in aural disease will in the future be made, and that as a consequence the percentage of deafness will, even in the next generation, be greatly reduced.

Although adenoids are most frequently observed in childhood, and the aural affections for which the growths are responsible begin in the majority of instances at this period of life, these obstructions not infrequently persist into adult life. Thus, the adenoid vegetation that blocks the respiratory tract of the child almost completely prior to the age of ten, is often believed to have disappeared entirely before the age of fifteen. The basis for this belief is the greater ease with which the individual at this latter age is able to breathe through the nose. A physical examination of the nasopharynx by means of re-flected light, the post-rhinoscopic mirror, and the palate retractor (Fig. 118) will, however, demonstrate the fact that the adenoid has not disappeared, and that the improved nasal breathing is largely due to the rapid enlargement of the nasopharyngeal space which takes place at the age of puberty.   The evil consequences of the adenoid growth, therefore, continue indefinitely to act mischievously upon the ear, although with a somewhat lessened activity.   When untreated sur-gically the adenoid slowly undergoes atrophy, and hence when the nasopharynx is examined after the age of twenty-five the remaining hypertrophy usually appears as a chronically inflamed and thickened pad of lymphoid tissue, running backward across the roof of the naso-pharynx from the vomer in front and extending downward a variable distance upon the posterior wall of the cavity.   Several deep fissures will be seen traversing the flattened mass, all of which run in an antero-posterior direction; filling these fissures, and perhaps spreading from

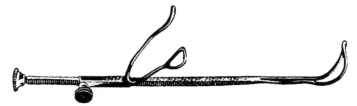

FIG. 118.—WHITE'S SELF-RETAINING PALATE RETRACTOR.

them over the entire nasopharynx and thence downward toward the pharynx, collections of thick ropy mucus will be seen.   The ex-aminer will be able to pass a properly bent probe behind the palate, and, guided by the examining mirror to explore the fissures and to note their number and depth.   The method of making the post-rhino-scopic examination is shown in Fig. 119.

After the age of thirty the adenoid will be found still more atrophied. It frequently persists, however, into old age and is the most potent predisposing factor in the causation of chronic nasopharyngitis.   It furnishes, in addition, the chief source of the thick mucous or muco-purulent secretion which drops into the throat below, and gives rise to the disagreeable desire, and even the necessity, of the patient's incessant hawking and spitting.   Hence, it may be stated as a fact that in either childhood or adult life the presence of an adenoid in the nasopharynx is a constant menace to the integrity not only of the nasopharynx but also of the middle ear as well.

The influence of the **faucial tonsils** in the causation of ear diseases is much less than that arising from the presence of adenoids in the vault of the pharynx. Enlargement of the faucial tonsils is frequently accompanied by a corresponding amount of hypertrophy in the vault, and as a matter of course when this is the case, aural complications are the rule. Even when very greatly enlarged the faucial tonsils seldom, if ever, produce direct pressure upon the mouths of the Eustachian tubes, and in their situation behind the oral cavity do not favor the

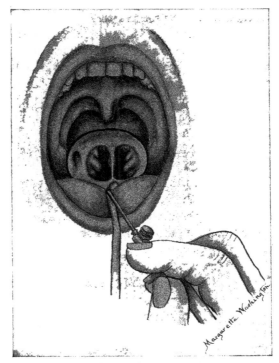

Fig. 119.—Method of Making Examination of the Posterior Nares and Nasopharynx. (D. Braden Kyle.)

The handle of the mirror should be somewhat lifted to bring the nasopharynx into view. The illustration shows the nasopharynx to be free from adenoid hypertrophy. If an adenoid were present it would obstruct the view shown in the upper part of the mirror, and the upper turbinates and posterior end of the vomer could, therefore, not be seen.

suction of the air from the middle ear during each act of deglutition, as in the case when the nasopharyngeal vault is filled with adenoid vegetations. The chief harmful influence exerted upon the ear by hypertrophy of the faucial tonsils comes, no doubt, from the fact that the greatly enlarged glands seriously interfere with the normal contraction of the faucial muscles in swallowing, and hence from the hindrance they offer to the normal method of opening the Eustachian tube and consequently to the ventilation of the middle ear. The presence of diseased tonsils also sets up a chronic pharyngitis coincident with increased and vitiated secretion of the glands of the pharynx and nasopharynx; and this, as has already been seen, is productive of middle-ear disease.

Nasal obstruction due to the presence of inflammatory or new growths may affect the auditory mechanism in much the same manner as adenoids. When the obstruction is situated in the anterior portion of the nasal chamber, a rarefaction of the air in the nasopharyngeal space follows as a result of the passive interference with the free admission of air to the cavity, whereas if the growth occurs posteriorly and extends backward into the nasopharyngeal space, it will not only cut off the free ventilation of the nasopharynx, but will in addition mechanically hinder the action of the palatal muscles, and will therefore interfere with the normal method of opening the Eustachian tube. Partial blocking of the nostrils from any cause necessitates an increased exertion on the part of the patient in cleansing the nose by blowing, and a too vigorous and frequent effort in this direction sets up a passive congestion of the Eustachian tube and middle ear. Moreover, pathogenic bacteria may also be carried from the nasopharynx to the tympanum by the powerful air blasts which the individual attempts to blow through the partly obstructed nose in his efforts to clear the stuffy nasal channels.

The dangers to which the child with adenoids is submitted are very greatly increased during an attack of scarlet fever, measles, or diphtheria. Any one of these diseases which might otherwise be quite mild and harmless to the ear in the case of a child with a normal throat, may run a violent course, and cause serious and extensive destruction of the tissues of the ear in the child whose upper respiratory tract is blocked with these growths. Undoubtedly diphtheria frequently begins in the diseased nasopharynx several hours before it makes its appearance in the fauces, where it is most commonly first detected. The author has had an opportunity to examine several cases of this disease in which there was present a well-formed diphtheritic membrane covering the adenoid tissue in the vault of the pharynx at a time when absolutely no evidence of the disease existed in any part of the oropharynx. The large extent of surface provided by the exterior of a well-formed adenoid, together with that of all the numerous and deep fissures between its various lobes, furnishes an extensive field for the deposit of such a membrane, as well as for the absorption of the pathogenic products of the disease which are produced in the crypts and upon the gland.

During the angina which accompanies scarlatina, measles, and tonsillitis the streptococcus pyogenes is very frequently and perhaps always present.[1]   The well-known fact that the occurrence of one of these diseases is a menace to the integrity of the hearing apparatus is explained on the following grounds: (a) During the inflammatory state of the tonsils and nasopharyngeal adenoids which accompanies the height of the particular disease, there is a rapid increase of the normal number of streptococci, pneumococci, or other pathogenic bacteria which inhabit these structures. (b) The mechanical stimulus produced by the presence of the pharyngeal growth, together with the inflammatory action taking place within these glandular structures, induces the secretion of a large amount of ropy mucus in the naso-pharynx, of which the patient rids himself by blowing the nose and hawking. (c) The mucous lining of the Eustachian tube, together with that of the tympanic cavity, is more or less congested and swollen in common with that of the entire upper air tract, and is therefore in a state receptive to inflammatory action so soon as the necessary bacteria are added. (d) Owing to the blocking of the nose and nasopharynx by the inflamed adenoids and tonsils, blowing the nose for the purpose of dislodging the infected, ropy mucus becomes difficult, and the powerful efforts of the patient to clear the upper air tract often drives the bacteria-laden mucus through the Eustachian tube into the middle ear, where violent infection at once ensues and suppuration and tissue destruction are the inevitable results. It must be admitted that bacteria may find their way into the middle ear by means other than that pro-vided by the patient when blowing the nose, since the inflammation accompanying these diseases in children too young to perform this act must be otherwise explained. In infancy and early childhood the Eustachian tube is shorter and wider in proportion than in adults and the bacteria, no doubt, find their way through such a channel much more readily than would be possible in the long narrow tube of the grown individual.

Children usually do not expectorate the secretions which form in the nasopharynx or pharynx until the age of puberty, and hence the large amount of mucopurulent material that forms in the upper air tract, largely as a result of the presence of the adenoid, enters the stomach, where it interferes with the digestion, and consequently with the general nutrition of the child. Partly for this reason and partly from the fact that oxygenation of the blood is imperfectly accomplished, owing to the

---

[1] Rudinger, *Journal Amer. Med. Assoc.*, Oct. 13, 1906, found the streptococcus pyogenes present in all of the 75 cases examined. In measles it was found present in 9 out of 14 cases, and it was found always to predominate in cases of tonsillitis.

difficulty with which respiration is carried on, the physical condition of these cases is usually impaired. As a result, any aural or other affection of the child yields slowly or not at all to treatment until first the diseased condition of the throat is restored to normal.

Diagnosis.—The diagnosis of adenoids may easily be made in most typic cases. The peculiar expression of the eyes, the obliterated lines about the alæ nasi, the open mouth, dead voice, noisy respiration, and history of frequent cold-taking, earache, dulness of hearing or aural discharge, form diagnostic symptoms that point unmistakably to this condition. There is, however, another very numerous class of adenoid children in which the symptoms are much less marked, although the adenoid mass, when removed, seems quite large enough to have filled the nasopharyngeal space completely. By means of a careful examination of a child of this class it will usually be possible to detect a majority of the symptoms that attend the typic case, but in a less marked degree. The child is a mouth breather, but keeps his lips so approximated that only a chink is left through which the air passes. The breathing is moderately noisy during sleep, and the child is usually so restless that the bedclothing is frequently displaced. Head colds are frequent, earaches and aural discharges are common, and a varying degree of deafness may usually be detectd when the function is carefully examined in this respect. Parents will frequently state that the child has the habit of making a low, snorting, or puffing noise through the nose. The reason for the performance of this by the patient is explained by the fact that bridles of thick ropy mucus collect upon the surface of the adenoid, stretch from it into the choanæ, and lie as a weight upon the superior surface of the soft palate. The child makes the puffing, blowing noise through the nostrils in order to displace the mucus and thus give momentary freedom of respiration as well as relief from the load of mucus which lies upon the palate. The history of the child constantly making such a noise forms one of the most reliable subjective symptoms of adenoids.

A physical examination is, however, entirely necessary to a positive diagnosis in many cases. If the child is past six years of age, if the examiner can obtain its entire confidence, and if the throat be not oversensitive to the instruments, the adenoid may be seen by postrhinoscopic examination by means of a suitable tongue depressor (Fig. 119), small postrhinoscopic mirror, and reflected light. It is also frequently possible to see an adenoid by means of an anterior rhinoscopic inspection. The nostrils of adenoid children are frequently quite wide, and, when such is the case, if a small quantity of a solution of adrenalin chlorid

(1 : 1000) be sprayed into each, and the examination be continued five minutes later, it will be found that the tissues of the lower meatus are greatly shrunken and that the adenoid mass can be seen distinctly through the widely, open nasal fossæ. In such instances it is often necessary to touch the adenoid with a probe in order to be sure that it is hypertrophied lymphoid tissue and not the posterior wall of the naso-pharynx, which is seen through the nostril. If the probe is to be used for this purpose a 4 per cent. solution of cocain should be sprayed into each nostril at the same time that the adrenalin solution is used. When the mucous membrane of the nostril is thus anesthetized and shrunken, a delicate cotton-tipped applicator can be passed through the dilated nostril, into the nasopharynx, and the adenoid mass can be lifted from side to side or moved upward by the instrument, and the

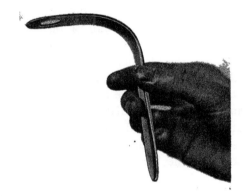

FIG. 120.—CONVENIENT, EASILY STERILIZABLE TONGUE DEPRESSOR.

diagnosis can thus be made with certainty. When the applicator is withdrawn, it will be found that if adenoids were present, the cotton on the tip of the applicator is stained with blood, even though the gen-tlest possible manipulation was made, because the epithelial covering of an adenoid is always delicate, and the ease with which it bleeds is, therefore, a good diagnostic sign of its presence.

In case the examiner is not able to see the growth by either of the above methods, the index-finger may be inserted into the nasopharyngeal space and the growth be detected by actually feeling it in this location. Before proceeding with this method the examining finger should be thoroughly scrubbed and sterilized, since otherwise the child might be infected and serious consequences result. The child is then placed horizontally across the lap of an assistant with its head toward the examiner and hanging somewhat downward. The examiner places the back of the head in the palm of his left hand, while the fingers of the same hand grasp the child's cheek and push it between the teeth in order to prevent any mishap from biting while the examination proceeds. The child's head being thus supported, the sterilized finger is quickly inserted behind the soft palate, is carried to the vault of the nasopharynx, and is swept from side to side in order to make certain the condition of this cavity. In childhood the adenoid mass feels soft to the touch, and owing to the struggles of the child at the instant and also the vigorous contraction of the soft palate around the examining finger, the contracted palate may be easily mistaken for an adenoid. If the tissue in the vault of the pharynx feels hard, and if the posterior end of the septum can be made out over its entire height, it is probable that no adenoids are present, whereas, if the whole vault seems filled with a soft, though somewhat resilient structure, the diagnosis of adenoids may be made. After its withdrawal the end of the examining finger should be inspected and also the posterior wall of the child's pharynx. If blood be found on both, and no violence was done during the insertion of the examining finger, the bleeding furnishes additional evidence of the presence of the adenoid. This method of diagnosis requires considerable experience on the part of the physician before the information gained by it can be considered reliable. Rude manipulation during such an examination is not essential and is never justifiable.

Treatment.—Medical measures by internal administration or when applied locally to the lymphatic enlargement have little or no effect on the removal or lessening in size of enlarged adenoids or tonsils, even when this mode of treatment is continued over a prolonged period.[1] Their removal should, therefore, be accomplished by surgical means, and at the earliest convenient period after their presence is discovered. When both the faucial tonsils and nasopharyngeal adenoids are simultaneously enlarged, all three of the glands may, and usually should, be removed at the same operation. The question as to whether or not a general anesthetic should be employed during an adenoid operation is one to be determined largely by whether or not the tonsils are imbedded—the "submerged" tonsil of Pynchon—and as to whether or not the child has a reasonable amount of self control. The experience and training of the operator have much to do with the question of the employment of

---

[1] The author once treated 20 cases of greatly enlarged tonsils and adenoids, each for a period of six months. Solutions of iodin and iodid of potassium in glycerin were applied to the hypertrophied tissues three times a week, and potassium iodid was administered internally three times a day. At the conclusion of the course of treatment no appreciable difference was noticeable in the condition of any case, and it became necessary to remove both adenoids and tonsils surgically.

a general anesthetic or of operating under cocain anesthesia. Undoubtedly either method may be followed with equal success by those who have been trained to do the operation thoroughly by either the one or the other plan. However, the element of danger arising from general anesthetics, when administered for this particular class of surgery,

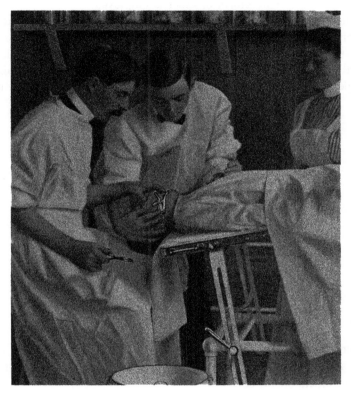

Fig. 121.—Position of Patient for the Removal of Adenoids under a General Anesthetic.
In this position the blood flows from the nostrils and thus lessens the danger of the patient inhaling it into the larynx. It is often preferable and frequently necessary to turn the patient upon one or the other side. Operations of this nature under general anesthesia are best performed by means of a curet with a bonnet (Fig. 124), or with adenoid forceps, (Fig. 123), since by either of these instruments the detached hypertrophy is immediately withdrawn, and danger from its presence in the throat is thereby avoided.

should not be forgotten, since several deaths, chiefly from chloroform, have been reported.[1] Nitrous oxid, ethyl chlorid, and somnoform have been extensively used during adenoid and tonsil operations, but their effect is of such short duration that unless the operator is very rapid,

[1] Hinkel, *Laryngoscope*, July, 1898, reported 18 deaths from chloroform anesthesia occurring during adenoid operations between the years 1892 and 1898. Hinkel states that the habitus lymphaticus, of which hypertrophied tonsils and adenoids constitute a part, renders the child particularly susceptible to death from chloroform.

has first-class assistance, and loses no time after the operation is begun, the patient is often awake before the work is satisfactorily completed, in which case a second administration of the gas is necessary. Moreover, these latter anesthetics do not thoroughly relax the palate, and hence the manipulation of instruments in the nasopharynx is more difficult than when either chloroform or ether is employed.

When a general anesthetic is necessary, ether should usually be administered because of its greater safety. It is necessary to prepare the patient by administering a cathartic on the previous day, allowing only a light diet on this day, and no food whatever on the morning of the operation, because undigested food in the stomach is sure to be

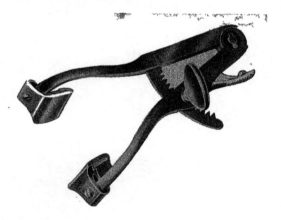

FIG. 122.—PYNCHON'S MOUTH GAG.

vomited, and this occurrence during throat operations not only introduces an unnecessary element of danger but also greatly hinders the progress of the operation.

When anesthetized the child is laid upon a narrow table with its head hanging down over the edge (Fig. 121). A mouth-gag (Fig. 122) is inserted, the mouth is thereby widely opened, and the instrument is held in place by an assistant, who also supports the patient's head in any desired position. In cases where both the faucial tonsils and adenoids are to be removed at one operation, it is easiest to remove the lower glands first, for the reason that if the adenoid is first removed the very considerable flow of blood which results will so obscure a view of the isthmus of the fauces as to make it difficult to see with accuracy the necessary steps of the subsequent tonsil ablation. The patient's throat is illuminated by the reflected light of a head-mirror (Fig. 89) worn by the operator. The tongue is depressed by an assistant, whose duty it will also be to mop blood from the throat when necessary as the work progresses.

Tonsils should always be removed deeply enough to include the bottom of all the tonsillar crypts. Therefore, if the gland is imbedded or "submerged," a satisfactory operation can only be done after it has been dissected loose to an extent that will permit the free motion of the tonsil when it is seized and traction is made upon it with a tenaculum. Several forms of tonsil knives are advocated for loosening the adhesions; the author uses the ones devised by Makuen. The dissection is made by seizing the gland in the teeth of a double tenaculum and making sufficient traction upon it to lift the gland from its bed, and thus demonstrating the points that need further loosening. The

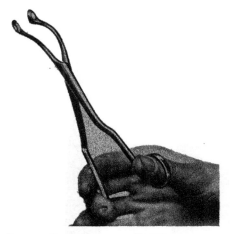

Fig. 123.—Quinlan's Adenoid Forceps.

tonsil knife is used first to sever all bands between the anterior pillar and the tonsil, then the gland is pulled forward and downward and all attachments in the supratonsillar fossæ are cut, after which traction is made outward and the knife separates the tonsil from the posterior pillar. The opposite tonsil is dealt with in an exactly similar manner.

Each gland is then quickly removed by means of the tonsillotome (see Fig. 126), the tonsil snare, or the guillotine ecraseur. If the gland contains a large amount of connective tissue, as is usually the case after repeated attacks of tonsillitis, and in adult life, the snare or ecraseur should be chosen because of their efficiency and also because less hemorrhage follows their use, whereas, if the patient is quite young and the gland is soft and protrudes without adhesions, the tonsillotome is equally safe and effective. The sharp bleeding which occurs

for a short time after the tonsil ablation often necessitates an interruption
of the operation, during which time the patient's head is lowered sufficiently to permit the blood to flow from the nose and mouth, and thus
obviate the possibility of its entering the larynx.

The removal of the adenoid is then accomplished either by the use
of the adenoid forceps (Fig. 123), the curet (Fig. 124), or by the two

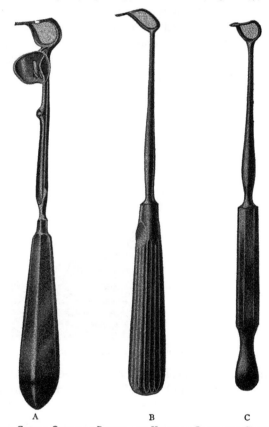

A   B   C

FIG. 124.—ADENOID CURETS, ONE WITH BASKET AND HOOKS TO CATCH THE GROWTH WHEN SEVERED,
AND THUS PREVENT THE POSSIBILITY OF ITS DROPPING INTO THE LARYNX.
The basket is especially valuable when operating under a general anesthetic.   The exact shape and dimensions
of these curets are shown in Fig. 127, b.

combined.   When forceps are employed, the operator stands at the
patient's head, his left forefinger is passed behind the soft palate as far
as the vault, and is kept in the nasopharynx and used as a guide so long
as it is thought necessary to reintroduce the adenoid forceps.   The
forceps is introduced while closed, passing along the finger as a guide,
and when the vault is reached, it is opened as widely as the cavity of
the nasopharynx will permit in order that the largest possible grasp

of the growth may be secured.   After grasping the growth firmly between the jaws of the instrument, a slight rotary motion is given the handle, and thus a large mass of the adenoid is torn and bitten away from its attachment, and withdrawn from the throat securely fixed by the blades. The forceps is quickly reintroduced and the process repeated until the examining finger no longer detects any considerable portion of the growth in any part of the nasopharynx.   The adenoid curet may then be inserted into the nasopharynx and carried forward against the upper posterior end of the vomer, after which it is caused to sweep the entire vault of the nasopharynx in such a way as to sever any remnant of the adenoid that may have escaped the forceps.

The adenoid curet (Fig. 124) is of itself entirely sufficient to completely remove the adenoid mass.   Unless, however, some means are provided by which the severed gland can be withdrawn from the throat along with the curet, there is some danger of its finding its way into the larynx and producing asphyxiation.   Therefore, when the curet alone is depended upon, an instrument should be selected which is provided with hooks and a basket (Fig. 124, A), which provides for the certain withdrawal of the severed growth.   Sharp bleeding follows the removal of an adenoid, but this persists only for one or two minutes, and it is only necessary to allow the patient's head to remain lowered until this has subsided and the patient has recovered consciousness sufficiently to expectorate the blood.   The mouth-gag should be removed just as soon as the operation is completed.

The author advocates the performance of a large majority of all tonsil and adenoid operations with the employment of only a local anesthetic.   In cases of children, where the faucial tonsils are not imbedded, both tonsils and adenoids can be completely removed in a few seconds.   The pain, although considerable, is not severe or of long duration, and the danger and nausea attendant upon general anesthesia operations are entirely eliminated.   When the operation is undertaken under a local anesthetic, a carefully planned and skillfully executed technic is necessary to a successful performance.   A 10 per cent. solution of cocain is applied by means of a cotton-tipped probe around the base of each tonsil and to the nasopharyngeal space.   This may be repeated one or more times in the succeeding five minutes.[1]   When

---

[1] The cotton applicator should not be dripping wet with the cocain solution, since the contraction of the palatal muscles around it when in the nasopharynx will squeeze the solution out, the patient will swallow it, and toxic symptoms may result.   Cocain solutions should not be sprayed into the pharynx or nasopharynx previously to operations upon the throat.   It is more satisfactory and safer to apply the drug directly to the spot to be anesthetized, and in stronger solution than could be safely used in spraying.

the parts are sufficiently anesthetized, an assistant holds the child
upright in his lap, the patient's legs are placed between the knees of the
assistant, where they are firmly held, the child's arms are placed along
its sides and across its lap, and the assistant locks the fingers of his
own hands over them. The child's head rests upon the left shoulder
of the assistant, and a second assistant grasps the head on either side
and supports it somewhat vise-like. In this position the child is held
absolutely quiet, and cannot interfere with the operator at any period

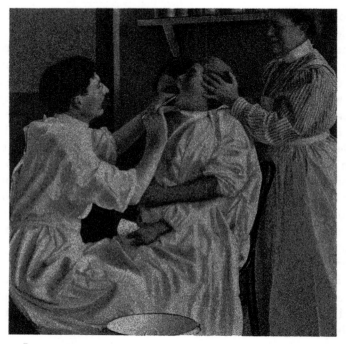

FIG. 125.—METHOD OF OPERATING FOR ADENOIDS UNDER LOCAL ANESTHESIA.
The correct size and shape of the curet to be used is shown in Fig. 127. The position of the curet in the
nasopharynx is shown in Fig. 128.

of the operation (Fig. 125). This position, which must be absolutely
maintained by the assistants, is entirely essential to rapid and certain
results, and no operator should undertake the performance of this
class of surgery unless he has at hand the assistance above described.

The faucial tonsils are first removed by means of the Mackenzie
tonsillotome (Fig. 126). The assistant who supports the child's head
allows two fingers to extend under the angle of first the right jaw and
then the left, making external pressure over the seat of the tonsil and
forcing it somewhat inward at the instant the operator is ready to

remove it.   The operator requests the child to open its mouth, then using the flat blade of the tonsillotome as a tongue depressor, slips it quickly over first the right tonsil and then the left, and removes each deeply before the child is scarcely aware of what is taking place. Without a second's delay, and therefore before the child begins to strangle from the free outpouring of blood from the excised tonsils, a curet of proper width and shape is inserted behind the palate and the adenoid is severed by a single sweep of the knife over the vault.   The child's head is then held forward, he expectorates the adenoid into a

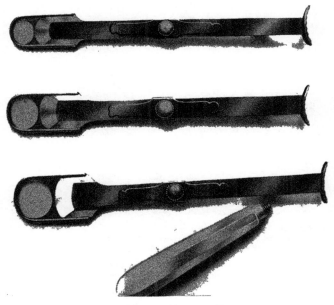

FIG. 126.—SET OF MODIFIED MACKENZIE TONSILLOTOMES.
The use of these instruments is recommended only in cases where the tonsils project well from their bases. When the glands are imbedded, even partially, they must be loosened by dissection and are then best removed by means of the cold wire snare or scissors.

basin, and blood pours from the nostrils and mouth for a minute or more.

The instruments to be used in any given case for the purpose of removing hypertrophied tonsils and adenoids must be intelligently selected at a previous examination.   The tonsillotome should be of such size that its fenestra will fit snugly over each tonsil.   The width of the adenoid curet must be governed by the width of the child's naso-pharyngeal space, and therefore this point must be noted with as much accuracy as possible, for if a curet be used which is too small it is obvious that only a portion of the adenoid can be secured at one cut, and the operation must therefore be repeated under difficulties. The fenestra should be of sufficient width in each case to require very gentle crowding of the shanks upon the lateral walls of the nasopharynx when the curet is inserted. If an instrument of proper size and shape be selected it is always possible to cut away the entire growth at one sweep of the curet (Fig. 128).

In the removal of an adenoid by this method, the child's head must be held squarely toward the operator. The operator must insert the

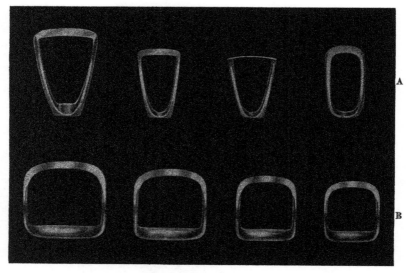

Fig. 127.—Showing the Distal Faces of Adenoid Curets. (Actual size.)

A, improper width and shape of fenestræ. With this form of curet successful removal of the adenoid, en masse, is impossible. B, curets of proper width and shape of fenestræ. Note that the narrow shanks occupy but a minimum of lateral space, and that the width of the cutting blade takes up but the smallest anteroposterior space. A profile view of the curvature of the shank is shown in Fig. 127. When selected according to the width of the patient's nasopharynx it is possible with this curet to remove the adenoid en masse at one sweep of the instrument.

instrument so that it will be kept exactly in the median line of the patient's nasopharynx. So soon as the curet is inserted behind the soft palate it must be pressed upward to the vault, and forward against the superoposterior portion of the vomer. Should the operator make a sweep of the instrument before the cutting blade is known to be in this position, only a portion of the growth will be severed. Should he begin this "sweep" at the point shown in Fig. 128, and hug the vault of the pharynx continuously throughout its course, the whole growth will most certainly be removed *en masse* (Figs. 129 and 130), provided the curet has been properly selected and is of sufficient width.

Following an operation by any method, little subsequent treatment is necessary further than to keep the patient quiet for from two days

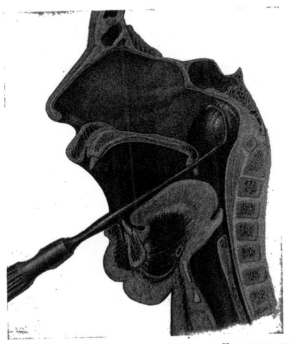

FIG. 128.—PROPER POSITION OF ADENOID CURET IN THE REMOVAL OF HYPERTROPHY BY ONE SWEEP OF INSTRUMENT.

Patient in upright position. Curet must be of dimensions ample to surround entire growth. See Fig. 127. Note that the mouth is open to its fullest extent and that the uvula and soft palate are crowded well upward.

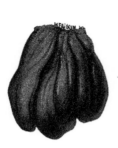

FIG. 129.—LARGE ADENOID REMOVED EN MASSE BY ONE SWEEP OF THE CURET.

Type of growth when removed by this method. Actual size; child six years old.

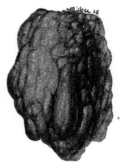

FIG. 130.—ADENOID REMOVED BY CURET FROM CASE SHOWN IN FIG. 117. Actual size.

to a week. After removal of the faucial tonsils, an astringent and antiseptic solution is prescribed:

℞. Tr. ferri chlorid,   ʒij;
    Glycerin,   ad. q.s. ℥iij.—M.

Sig. Half-teaspoonful to be swallowed every two hours first day, every four hours afterward. An appropriate prescription for children too young to gargle.

Following tonsillectomy, the character of the food must be regulated. During the first day iced milk should constitute the sole nourishment. Afterward, soups, custards, boiled rice, and the softest food in general should be directed.

ACUTE AFFECTIONS OF THE MIDDLE EAR

PRELIMINARY REMARKS

IN this division of the work are included the diseases of the membrana tympani, acute catarrhal congestion of the Eustachian tube and tympanic cavity, the acute catarrhal, and the acute suppurative inflammations of the middle ear. In all that pertains to the causation, symptoms, and pathology of these several diseases, the Eustachian tube must be considered as forming an important part of the middle ear, as, indeed, must also the mastoid antrum and the mastoid cells. Therefore in the study of the diseases incident to the conducting portion of the organ of hearing, the student should have a broader conception of the term "middle ear" than has heretofore obtained, and should always think of it as including not only the tympanic cavity but also the Eustachian tube, and, at least in a very closely associated way, the accessory cavities of the mastoid antrum and mastoid cells. With this conception of the middle ear, the rather considerable extent of mucous membrane, beginning at the nasopharyngeal orifice of the Eustachian tube and ending in the mastoid cells at the tip of the mastoid process, will be better realized and the causation, pathology, and treatment of the several affections of the labyrinth of cavities comprising the conducting portion of the hearing apparatus will undoubtedly be better understood. The environment of the middle ear, the external auditory meatus, the nose and nasopharynx should also be more carefully studied in its causative relations to the aural diseases of this portion of the ear.

CHAPTER XX

DISEASES AND INJURIES OF THE MEMBRANA TYMPANI

SINCE the membrana tympani separates the external from the middle ear, and since its inner surface or mucosa forms a portion of the tympanic cavity, while its outer surface or dermoid layer is a continuation of the skin of the external meatus, it follows that the structure may be affected by diseases involving either the middle ear or external auditory meatus. The drum membrane is, however, sometimes affected independently of any disease in the neighboring tissues, and it is evident that when this is the case the affection cannot properly be classified with the diseases of either the external or of the middle ear.

ACUTE MYRINGITIS

Acute myringitis, or inflammation of the drum-head, occurs as the result of infection or irritation of this portion of the organ of hearing. It usually results from the entrance of cold water into the ear, from the exposure of the ear to the direct action of a severe cold wind, or from the instillation of caustic or irritant fluids into the external auditory canal. Any of the causes previously enumerated as productive of an otitis externa may also give rise to a myringitis.

Symptoms.—The patient complains of an earache which may be very severe or quite mild, of tinnitus aurium, and of a full stuffy feeling in the affected side of the head. There is little complaint as to loss of hearing, since this function is seldom seriously affected. In case the patient is a child, some fever and restlessness may accompany the disease.

The appearances upon otoscopic examination are those that are characteristic of the earlier stages of inflammatory affections of the middle ear. The plexus of vessels along the handle of the malleus is first seen to be injected, and then the redness spreads over a portion or the whole of the membrane. The vascular injection together with the swelling which takes place in the structure of the drum membrane itself soon obliterates the normal landmarks. In the severest cases small dark brown spots are sometimes seen. These are caused by minute hemorrhages into the substance of the tympanic membrane. The exudation of serum or blood beneath the dermoid layer, which occasionally takes place, appears in the form of dark blue or slightly yellowish blisters upon the surface of the posterosuperior quadrant. If the observation of the membrana is made at a later period no blisters may be visible, but a slight serous or bloody discharge will be found in the auditory canal which results from the rupture of the blebs and the subsequent discharge of the exudate from the denuded areas. If examined at the end of a week from the onset, the drum membrane will probably be found dry and desquamating, and sometimes the whole or at least a considerable portion of the entire dermoid layer of the drum-head is found to have exfoliated, and to be lying, partly detached, at the fundus of the auditory canal. After the removal of this detached portion the underlying membrane may still appear uniformly red, but of a less intensity than at the height of the inflammation. Gradually the drum membrane is restored to its normal color and thickness; or more rarely the disease may become chronic. Politzer (*Diseases of the Ear*, p. 237) relates a case in which there was an abscess formation in the structures of the drum-head which finally ruptured into the middle ear and set up an acute otitis media.

Diagnosis.—The chief difficulty lies in differentiating myringitis from acute otitis media of either the catarrhal or suppurative variety. The appearance of the drum membrane during the otoscopic examination may be exactly the same in each disease. The occurrence of bullæ upon the surface is more common in myringitis than in otitis media. The pain, tinnitus, and stuffy feeling in the head are usually not so severe in myringitis as in otitis media, and the amount of deafness which results from otitis media is very much greater than that which occurs from myringitis. Indeed, it is upon this point that the diagnosis can be best made, for in any case in which there is pain in the ear, tinnitus, and fulness in the head, and in which the drum membrane shows signs of active inflammation, if the hearing is but slightly impaired the conclusion should be that only an inflammation of the drum membrane is present, whereas, if more pronounced deafness is present, the same is evidence of an involvement of the cavum tympani. Since a discharge may occur as a result of either disease, it is important to determine whether this comes from the middle ear through a perforated drum membrane, or whether it occurs from the bases of the ruptured bullæ which spring from the membrana tympani itself. This question may be settled by actually seeing the perforation during the otoscopic examination, but if uncertain concerning this point, politzerization or catheter inflation may be performed while at the same time the examiner observes the drum-head when, if the perforation exists, its location will be made evident by the escape of bubbles of air or fluids at the site of rupture. Myringitis may be mistaken for earache of a reflex or neuralgic nature unless the physical examination of the drum membrane is carefully made. In myringitis this membrane is, as already stated, highly inflamed and swollen; the landmarks are often submerged and wanting. When, however, the otalgia is due to reflex causes the drum membrane usually has an entirely normal appearance. Moreover, in non-inflammatory earache the source of the reflex pain may be discovered in a carious tooth or an ulcerated throat. An examination of the mouth and throat, including the teeth, should not be omitted in any questionable case of earache.

Treatment.—When seen at the onset, palliative measures should be at once instituted. If the pain is severe codein may be administered in $\frac{1}{4}$- or $\frac{1}{2}$-gr. doses, and repeated every two to four hours if necessary. Dry heat applied locally to the ear by means of the hot-water bottle is usually very grateful to the patient. Local depletion either by means

15

of the artificial or natural leech not only relieves the pain, but if applied early may be classed as an abortive measure. A pledget of cotton of proper size to fit the meatus snugly, if dipped in the carbolized glycerin solution (see p. 256) and applied against the drum membrane as hot as can be borne, is of undoubted assistance in relieving both the pain and the feeling of fulness in the ear.

Should one or more large blisters form in the dermoid layer of the drum membrane, the same may be incised with a delicate knife (Fig. 141). Usually, however, the blebs rupture almost immediately after they are fully formed, thus rendering their incision unnecessary. In case the knife is used to incise them, care must be taken not to penetrate the entire thickness of the membrana tympani, since this is unnecessary and a deep incision might admit some of the contents of the bulla into the drum cavity, with the result of infection and subsequent suppuration within the cavity. The serous discharge following the spontaneous rupture or the incision of these blisters is usually slight and promptly ceases. Should the areas occupied by the bases of the blebs remain raw and moist, boric acid should be insufflated into the external auditory meatus in a quantity sufficient to form a thin coating over the dermoid surface of the drum-head. In case the exudate persists and becomes purulent and foul smelling, the ear should be frequently syringed with an antiseptic solution, should afterward be thoroughly dried, and the dressing should then be completed by the insufflation of the finely powdered boric acid after the manner just stated.

CHRONIC MYRINGITIS

Chronic myringitis sometimes persists as a sequel of the acute variety. It occasionally accompanies a chronic otitis externa. Existing as an uncomplicated affection it is rare.

The **symptoms** of the disease are a moderate foul-smelling discharge from the ear and an intense itching in the depths of the auditory meatus. The impairment of the hearing is not so great as would be indicated either by the nature of the discharge or the appearance of the drum membrane. Pain, fulness in the head, and tinnitus aurium are less marked than in the acute variety. The diagnosis will be based upon the fact that the hearing is comparatively good, and that inflation of the middle ear gives rise to no perforation whistle or other evidence of ruptured drum membrane.

The appearances of the drum membrane are not diagnostic of this disease. The external surface will be dull when covered by an epidermis that is ready to exfoliate. After exfoliation the underlying membrane may look thickened, uniformly inflamed, and moist with exudate. Politzer (*Diseases of the Ear*, p. 239) describes the occasional presence on the drum membrane of small, light red papillary excrescences, singly or in groups, in which latter instance the membrane has the appearance of a purple raspberry.

The **treatment** consists in cleansing the ear of any irritating discharge by means of the syringe. Bichlorid of mercury solution (1 : 8000) is best for this purpose. The canal is then dried and a mixture of equal parts of finely powdered boric acid and oxid of zinc is insufflated by means of the powder-blower (Fig. 213). When the membrane looks raw and finely granular the alcohol and boric acid lotion may be instilled into the ear in either a pure or somewhat diluted form. This solution is prepared as follows:

R. Acid. boracis,   gr. xx ;
  Alcoholis,   ℥j.—M.

If there is much odor to the discharge, mercuric bichlorid may be added to this preparation in the proportion of 1 : 8000. Should severe pain result from the instillation of this preparation into the ear, it should

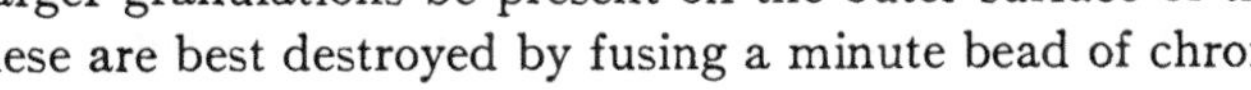

FIG. 131.—DELICATE ALUMINIUM PROBE. (Three-fourths natural size.)
Very useful as a caustic carrier in treatment of granulations and small polypi.

be diluted by the addition of distilled water, and then gradually be increased to full strength as the patient acquires a better toleration. Should larger granulations be present on the outer surface of the membrane, these are best destroyed by fusing a minute bead of chromic acid upon the end of a very small applicator (Fig. 131), and then touching each granulation separately every third day until all have disappeared.[1]

[1] In the local treatment of the exuberant granulations, which are frequently met with in the ear, especially in the chronic suppurative aural affections, the application of chromic acid, nitrate of silver, or other active caustic is often recommended. The student should, therefore, acquire the exact methods of preparing these powerful caustics so that they may be carried with ease, safety, and accuracy to the remotest portions of the drum cavity and to the most limited areas. The employment of crude instruments and bungling methods in carrying these agents to a definite spot in a situation so deeply seated may result in great harm to the ear and in intense and unnecessary suffering to the patient.

The applicator which is selected for carrying caustic agents into the middle ear should be flexible and its diameter beyond the handle should be exceedingly small (Fig. 131). If pure nitrate of silver is to be used the crystals should be melted in a small platinum or porcelain receptacle over an alcohol flame. The distal end of the cold applicator is then dipped into the melted silver, when a thin pellicle of the caustic instantly adheres. By allowing this to cool, and then again dipping it, a bead of silver of any desired size may finally be secured (Fig. 132). To prepare a chromic acid bead on the end of the

The preparation of the area in the ear which is to be touched by the caustic is no less important. Caustics have a tendency to spread rapidly in the presence of moisture and to damage the surrounding healthy parts. The ear should, therefore, be. entirely free from all secretion before the application of any caustic is undertaken.

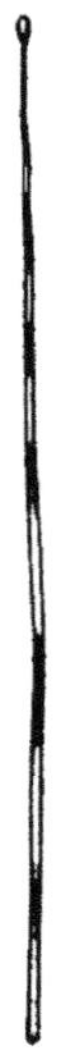

INJURIES TO THE MEMBRANA TYMPANI

The situation of the tympanic membrane at the bottom of the deep and somewhat angular auditory meatus is one that affords a maximum of protection to this delicate structure. This, together with its elasticity of structure and peculiar setting that permits of considerable inward and outward movement, accounts for the comparatively infrequent injury to this portion of the conducting apparatus.

Wounds of the drum membrane are either direct or indirect. The injury to the membrane may constitute the sole damage or the wound may be of such severity that not only is the structure of the membrana tympani completely destroyed, but also the parts beyond it—namely, the ossicles, the mucous lining of the tympanum, or even the labyrinth and adjoining osseous structures. In some of the worst injuries, that to the drum membrane itself constitutes but a small fraction of the damage done to the adjacent parts.

Fig. 132.—Very Delicate Aural Applicator with Bead of Nitrate of Silver Fused on End.

Direct injuries are the result of the impact or penetration of the membrane by some foreign body which enters the external auditory canal with sufficient force to be driven deeply into the fundus. An individual sometimes wounds his own drum membrane while picking at his ear or while scratching the canal with some pointed instrument, like a toothpick, match, or hairpin. Numerous instances are on record of injury to the drum membrane occurring from some one accidentally striking the arm of a person who is at the time engaged in picking his ear with a sharp instrument, which latter was by this means driven inward with force and suddenness.

applicator, place a few fresh crystals of the acid upon a piece of paper and hold in the left hand near the flame of the alcohol lamp. Using the right hand, hold the tip of the applicator in the flame until heated almost to the point of redness. Very quickly bring the heated tip of the applicator into contact with a crystal of the acid, which will adhere and fuse upon the instrument in the form of a little globule of most convenient size. Considerable practice will be necessary to prepare the chromic acid applicator satisfactorily.

Any foreign body that is hurled with sufficient force to enter the meatus may cause a direct rupture of the drum-head.   Children at play have been known to shoot paper wads, grains of corn, etc., into their playmates' ears by means of toy air-guns.   The membrana tympani of workmen may be wounded by pieces of stone or other material which fly off from the particular tools employed, as, for example, in the case of stone-cutters.   Another and rather frequent cause of direct injury to the membrana tympani is observed in the case of surf-bathers who permit the waves to strike the ear sidewise with considerable force.[1]

Those who perform high diving sometimes suffer an injury to the drum membrane from a similar cause, since the water enters the auditory canal with considerable force in case the head strikes the surface of the water sidewise.

It sometimes happens that rupture of the drum membrane will take place during treatment of the ear, even though this be conducted with great caution and skill.   Thus, if politzerization or catheter inflation of the tympanic cavity be performed, and too much air pressure be used, direct injury to the membrana tympani may be the result, the rupture taking place with a snap sufficiently loud to be audible a distance of several feet.   It is probable that when rupture occurs as the result of tympanic inflation that the membrane had been previously diseased and greatly weakened, and that it, therefore, gave way under much less air pressure than would be required to rupture the normal drum-head.   Of a somewhat similar nature is the rupture which occasionally results from the too vigorous suction upon the membrane by means of the Siegel otoscope—an accident which may happen when this instrument is employed for the purpose of giving massage to the membrana tympani and ossicles (see p. 174).

Blows upon the ear, as in boxing, and falls upon the head from a height or from a vehicle in rapid motion are among the most potent causes of severe injury to the drum membrane and middle ear (Fig. 133).   The injury thus resulting from such violent causes frequently extends beyond the ear, and may include extensive fractures at the base or other portions of the skull.   Fig. 305 represents a case of the latter,

---

[1] It is quite probable that a considerable number of deaths by drowning which occur during surf-bathing are due to injuries of this kind, and not to "cramps," as is commonly reported.   It is well known to all aurists that syringing the ears, even gently and with warm solutions, will in many individuals cause great giddiness or even total unconsciousness for a few seconds.   It is not unreasonable, therefore, to presume that the entrance into the ear of cold water with sufficient force to rupture the drum membrane might cause a more lasting unconsciousness, during which time the individual succumbs by drowning.

while Figs. 133 and 134 show the effect upon the drum membrane of severe falls upon the head, without a fracture of the skull itself.

Injuries to the membrana tympani from indirect violence occur principally as the result of the sudden condensation or rarefaction of the air in the external auditory meatus. Thus, any loud explosion, as of gun or cannon, when near the ear may bring about a rupture of the tympanic membrane.[1] In this instance the air is driven inward with such force and suddenness that the resistance. of this structure is overcome and it gives way before the violence of the increased air-pressure. Of a somewhat similar nature, though without the features of sudden compression of air incident to an explosion, is the effect of

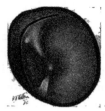

FIG. 133.—RUPTURE OF THE DRUM MEMBRANE WITH FRACTURE OF THE NECK OF THE MALLEUS IN A CHILD AGED NINE, THE RESULT OF FALLING DOWN A STAIRWAY.

Profuse hemorrhage at once occurred from the external auditory meatus, and facial paralysis developed in a few days on the affected side. There was also disturbance of taste on the same side, showing that the chorda tympani nerve had been injured. Recovery from the facial palsy was complete in a few months, showing that the injury to the nerve was probably due to an exudate or hemorrhage into the Fallopian canal.

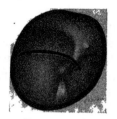

FIG. 134.—RUPTURE OF DRUM-HEAD AND FRACTURE OF HANDLE OF MALLEUS RESULTING FROM A FALL UPON THE HEAD FROM A RAPIDLY MOVING STREET-CAR.

Child aged eight years. Profuse hemorrhage immediately followed and child was unconscious for about twelve hours. Complete recovery followed in four weeks.

the air within a caisson upon the membrana tympani, occasionally causing its rupture.

It is a question of practical interest as to whether or not a severe injury or rupture of the normal drum-head can occur from such indirect causes as a loud explosion, or from an existence for a short time in a condensed atmosphere, as in a caisson or diver's bell. As a result of the examination of a considerable number of accidents to the membrana tympani from these causes, several authors have stated it as their opinion that the rupture under such circumstances was due to the fact of a pre-existing disease of the ear, usually in the nature of a

[1] During the war with Spain,, between the months of April and August, 1898, 10 cases of rupture of the membrana tympani, as the result of the firing of cannon, were reported among the crews of the North Atlantic Squadron, and 19 cases of this variety of injury to the membrana tympani occurred among the men of the Japanese crews in the battle of the Yalu during the recent Russo-Japanese war.

catarrhal inflammation of the middle ear accompanied by more or less occlusion of the Eustachian tube, and consequent rarefaction of the air within the tympanum.   Gruber (*Lehrbuch der Ohrenheilkunde*, p. 310) has experimentally shown that it is difficult to rupture the healthy drum membrane in the cadaver.   This author inserted the catheter into the Eustachian tube of a person recently dead, fastened it in position, and then suddenly injected 4 or 5 atmospheres—a pressure of from 60 to 75 pounds—into the middle ear and against the normal membrane.   He then reversed the experiment and injected equally high pressure against the drum membrane through the external auditory canal.   Such a high pressure thrown suddenly against the healthy drum membrane on either side was not sufficient to rupture it.

When injury occurs to the membrana tympani as the result of the penetration of some slender instrument, the particular quadrant which is perforated (see Fig. 187) depends in some measure upon the degree of suddenness and force with which the entrance is effected, and upon whether or not the entering end of the object is sharp or blunt.   It will be remembered that the drum membrane is normally placed at such an angle to the external auditory meatus that the posterosuperior quadrant lies nearer to the concha than does the anterosuperior quadrant.

If, therefore, the object is sharp pointed and is quickly thrust into the depths of the canal the posterosuperior portion will most likely be perforated, whereas, if the object be blunt pointed and is entered with comparative slowness, it may slip over the posterior portion of the slanting surface of the membrana tympani and penetrate one of the anterior quadrants.   Zaufal (*Archives für Ohrenheil.*, Vol. VIII.), in experiments on the cadaver, states that direct rupture of the drum membrane most usually occurs in the anterior half of the tympanic membrane, whereas Politzer (*Diseases of the Ear*, p. 242) and Dench (*Diseases of the Ear*, p. 292) state that when caused by the penetration of instruments the injury occurs in the posterosuperior quadrant.

Symptoms.—At the moment of the rupture of the membrane the individual experiences a sharp, lancinating pain in the ear which, while subsiding to some extent in a short time, continues as a feeling of more or less deep-seated pain and soreness.   Giddiness occurs at the instant of the injury, and is often of such severity that complete unconsciousness takes place for a short time.   Sometimes the dizziness persists for weeks or months and is accompanied by a tinnitus of varying degrees of intensity.   The degree of impairment of hearing that results from the injury depends upon the severity and nature of the wound and upon whether or not a suppurative inflammation is subsequently set up. Immediately following a severe wound of the drum membrane there is usually profuse bleeding from the external auditory meatus, and this is shortly followed in some cases by a discharge of serum, which after a few days becomes infected and assumes a purulent character. Should a fracture of the base of the skull complicate the aural injury, the subsequent discharge of bloody serum may be one of the notable symptoms of that occurrence. After suppuration is once established the subsequent symptoms of the case may differ in no important particular from those occurring in acute or chronic suppurative otitis media.

Otoscopic appearances of the drum membrane after a rupture or other injury vary according to the extent and cause of the injury, and also as to the time which has elapsed between the injury and the examination of the case. If the membrane has been penetrated by some slender, sharp instrument, and the wound is examined immediately afterward, a puncture-point will most likely be seen in the postero-superior quadrant, the site being marked by a small drop of blood. When of a severe nature, the bleeding from the meatus may be so profuse as to preclude an exact inspection of the drum membrane for several days, as was the case in each of the patients from which the drawings for Figs. 133 and 134 were made. In Fig. 133 the bleeding was so severe that it was necessary to tampon the meatus with sterile gauze for several days, after which the oozing of bloody serum interfered with accurately determining the extent of the wound until twelve days from the date of the accident. At this time the appearance was as shown in the figure.

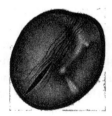

FIG. 135.—SLIT-LIKE RUP-
TURE OF DRUM-HEAD RE-
SULTING FROM A BOX UPON
THE EAR.

When due to indirect causes the injury to the drum-membrane occurs most frequently in the postero-inferior quadrant, and the rent, when viewed through the speculum, appears as a gaping slit (Fig. 135) through which the mucous membrane of the middle ear can sometimes be seen, provided the examination be made early. Later, if the wound be not large and the gaping therefore not extensive, nothing more is visible than a linear, blackish blood-clot, which has sealed the wound and furnished a most efficient natural dressing.

In all injuries to the ear, and especially to the membrana tympani and middle ear, it is important that the examining surgeon make a complete record at the time of the first examination of the results of the hearing tests, the history of the accident, and the exact appearance of the tympanic membrane when viewed through the speculum. Such a record is particularly important in all cases where there is a probability of subsequent suit for damages, at which time the attending surgeon will certainly be called to testify concerning the extent and probable permanency of any alleged defect resulting from the injury. When fortified by the record of a most careful and accurate examination of an injured ear, made at the time of the injury, the testimony of the surgeon becomes competent and most reliable evidence, upon which the court and jury must largely rely.

Treatment.—Many of the lesser injuries to the membrana tympani require little or no treatment. If seen early and the wound is found to be trivial, and especially if it is already sealed by a blood-clot, the best results are secured by non-interference with the injured part, since nothing more is required than the insertion of a sterile strip of gauze or a pledget of antiseptic cotton into the external auditory canal. When the wound is large and has been produced by direct violence, infection of the middle ear from the external auditory meatus is almost certain to follow. Hence it is wise to attempt the sterilization of the external auditory canal in the hope that a middle-ear infection may be avoided. Disinfection of the auditory canal is best and most safely accomplished by rubbing both the hairy and deeper integumentary surfaces with a cotton-tipped probe that has been dipped into either hydrogen peroxid or alcohol and boric acid solution. Under no circumstances should the external auditory meatus be syringed previously to the time when suppuration is already established as the result of the injury, for if syringing is practised previously to this time, infective material will almost certainly be carried from the meatus into the middle ear, where it will cause destruction of parts that might otherwise heal without undergoing the suppurative stage of inflammation. If the edges of the wound in the membrane are moist, it is permissible, after the application of the antiseptic to the meatal walls as just described, to insufflate a small quantity of some mild antiseptic or drying powder, like boric acid, in sufficient amount to form a delicate coating over the drum membrane and adjoining meatal walls. Following this, if any moisture is visible, superheated dry air may be injected into the meatus, after which the dressing is completed by the insertion of a strip of sterile gauze to the bottom of the auditory meatus, the gauze being left in place till healing occurs, unless infection has taken place and the dressing becomes soiled and foul smelling.

In case severe pain arises in the ear the same may be due to the collection of serum or blood in the tympanic cavity. This would, of course, happen only in cases where the perforation is small. An examination with the speculum would reveal a bulging and inflamed drum membrane which should be freely incised in order to provide the necessary drainage. In all cases in which suppuration is ultimately established as a result of the injury the subsequent treatment should be conducted upon the same plan which is advocated in the chapter on Acute Suppurative Otitis Media, from which the disease in question differs in no essential respect (see Chapter XXIII.).

CHAPTER XXI

ACUTE TUBOTYMPANIC CATARRH

Causation.—Catarrhal affections of the Eustachian tube and middle ear are of frequent occurrence, particularly during the cold and changeable seasons of the year and in damp climates. All the causes that are productive of colds in the head may be considered causative agents of Eustachian and tympanic catarrh. This affection is, therefore, very frequently observed to accompany or complicate a coryza or nasopharyngitis. The milder types of the exanthemata produce conditions in the throat that are causative of catarrhal affections of the tube and middle ear, whereas the more severe cases of scarlet fever or measles are more likely to be complicated by an actual inflammation and suppuration of the tympanic cavity. The accidental injection of fluids into the Eustachian orifice during the treatment of a nasopharyngitis may also be responsible for the disease under consideration, although such an accident is most often followed by the more severe affection, namely, an acute otitis media, either of the catarrhal or purulent variety.

The most common of the predisposing causes of this disease is the presence in the nasopharynx of adenoid growths, and it is entirely probable that it is in this particular ailment that adenoids prove most harmful to the individual. This is especially true since, occurring as they so frequently do in children, the causative relation between the adenoid and the accompanying deafness is not suspected early, or if at all suspected is not dealt with until structural changes within the ear of an incurable nature have already been established. A complete understanding by the student of the anatomy and physiology of the Eustachian tube and middle ear will make clear the necessity of having the nasopharynx free from all obstruction or inflammation. The presence of adenoids predisposes the individual to frequent or even continuous colds in the head, and to the production of congestion and oversecretion of mucus which blocks the Eustachian tubal orifices, and thus prevents the necessary entrance of air into the middle ear. Moreover, with the nasopharynx occluded by these growths, covered as they are by ropy mucus, a suction and rarefaction of the air in this space is produced by each act of swallowing. Then, too, the growth of numerous pathogenic bacteria in the nasopharynx is favored by the presence of the adenoids, and hence infection may arise in the middle ear as the result of the oft-repeated and forcible efforts of the individual to clear the obstructed nasal passages, during which efforts bacteria-laden mucus may be blown through the Eustachian tube into the middle ear.

Pathology.—In acute tubotympanic catarrh the inflammation may be limited to the Eustachian tube alone or it may spread to the middle ear. A catarrhal inflammation takes place with formation of serous or mucous secretion. The obstruction of the Eustachian tube when the inflammation is limited to the tube is generally followed by a serous transudation in the tympanic cavity due to rarefaction of the tympanic air. This rarefaction of the air is brought about by absorption of the air by the lining mucous membrane of the middle ear. Whether the inflammatory or mechanical obstruction is at the mouth of the Eustachian tube, a limited portion, or along the whole tube, the function of the tube (the wind-pipe of the middle ear) is destroyed and this results in a lessened air pressure in the middle ear. The equilibrium or balance of the drum membrane is destroyed because the outward atmospheric pressure is greater than the inner atmospheric pressure and the drum and malleus are pushed inward. This causes the short process to appear more prominent and causes the malleus to appear foreshortened. The head of the malleus is pushed toward the external attic wall. Meanwhile the whole middle-ear cavity becomes hyperemic and if the obstruction in the tube is not removed a transudate is formed. Also, as often happens in children with adenoid growth, the drum membrane becomes atrophied. This atrophy is brought about by the continual tension of the drum membrane which causes a lessened blood supply to the mucous membrane lining.

Symptoms.—The symptoms vary during the different stages of the disease. Thus, at the onset, when the affection consists of nothing more than a closure of the cartilaginous portion of the Eustachian tube, followed by the absorption into the blood of the air remaining in the middle ear, the membrana tympani is no longer supported by air pressure on its tympanic surface, and therefore the normal air column on the outside of the drum-head presses it inward with a force approximating 15 pounds to the square inch. The resulting symptoms are, therefore, largely of a physical nature. The hearing, which had been previously good, is suddenly very greatly diminished, and a tinnitus aurium of greater or less intensity is established. In cases where the onset is sudden and of marked severity vertigo may be a prominent symptom.

Since no active inflammation is present except perhaps in a portion of the Eustachian tube, but slight or even no pain is present. The patient complains rather of a soreness, which, if he is requested to locate, he will attempt to do so by pointing to almost every quarter of his neck and throat. A decided stuffiness in the ears is the chief complaint of many, who say that there is a feeling in the ears as though a foreign body occluded both external auditory meati, and hence persons so affected have an irresistible desire to be poking into the auditory canals with their fingers in their efforts to relieve this very uncomfortable feeling. Sometimes the suction produced by the sudden withdrawal of the finger from the external auditory canal will to some extent replace the sunken drum membrane and give the patient a very temporary relief—a result which will encourage him to repeat the procedure. The appearance of the drum membrane when viewed by means of an ear speculum and reflected light is usually one of great retraction (Fig. 136). The folds of the membrane are more distinct, the short process is more prominent, and, because the membrane is more tightly stretched over it, this process of the malleus looks whiter than normal. Since the handle of the malleus is driven inward, and hence away from the examiner, it appears more distant and much shorter than normal. The new position of the manubrium divides the membrana tympani into unequal parts, the antero-inferior portion appearing unusually broad while the posterosuperior seems greatly narrowed (Fig. 136).

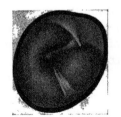

FIG. 136.—RETRACTION OF DRUM MEMBRANE.
Note the length of the light reflex, the shortening of the malleus handle, and the widened area of the antero-inferior quadrant.

Both the color and lustre of the membrane remain normal, but the light reflex is usually removed somewhat from its normal position; it is at times broken or multiple and may be altogether absent. The close proximity of the membrana tympani to the inner wall of the tympanic cavity occasionally permits the penetration of the reflected light through the membrane to such an extent that the color of the mucous membrane of the tympanic cavity is imparted to the tympanic membrane, in which case the color of the latter will be deceptive and may appear reddened or pinkish.

The appearance of the drum membrane after inflation of the tympanic cavity by means of the catheter or by politzerization is completely changed, the normal position of all the parts being at once restored unless, as sometimes happens, an exudate has already taken place into the tympanic cavity.

In the second stage of the disease, after the congestion has extended to the mucous lining of the middle ear, and exudation has taken place, all the symptoms previously enumerated, the impaired hearing, tinnitus, and stuffy feeling in the ear, continue, but in a somewhat lessened degree. In the more active forms of the tubotympanic congestion the attic of the middle ear may be involved, in which case pain in the ear of a varying degree of severity may be added. After the exudate has taken place and has partly filled the tympanic cavity, the patient may state that during the time the head is held in certain positions he hears badly, whereas, in other positions the hearing is relatively good. Thus, when sitting upright only slight impairment of function may be experienced, whereas, the moment the patient lies upon the back or holds the head toward the opposite side, great impairment immediately takes place. These marked changes occur chiefly in cases where the tympanic cavity, as above stated, is only partially filled with serous fluid, and hence the change in hearing results from the changed position of the fluid. Thus, when the patient is erect the round and oval windows are not covered by the contained fluid and the hearing is comparatively good, whereas, in the recumbent position, the exudate occupies these situations and the hearing is relatively bad. It is because of the movement of the fluid within the tympanum that the patient may also state that he sometimes feels as though a liquid were moving in the ear whenever the position of the head is changed. As patients sometimes express it, they "feel something slushing about in the head."

Autophonia, or a resonance of the patient's own voice in the affected ear, is a symptom in many cases, and when present in its worst form constitutes one of the most annoying features of the disease. The patient describes the sound of his voice as resembling that heard " when talking in a barrel." This sensation is so distressing to many individuals that they prefer to sit silent throughout the illness and are greatly annoyed when compelled to enter into even a short conversation. Gruber states that autophonia is most frequently an annoying symptom in mild cases of tubotympanic congestion, and in those cases in which there is present only a small amount of exudate in the middle ear. This symptom is also worse in those who are affected by the disease in one ear only. In most individuals who are afflicted with several of the accompanying symptoms of this form of aural catarrh, namely, impaired hearing, tinnitus aurium, vertigo, pressure in the head and autophonia, there quickly develops an unwarranted apprehension of permanent injury to the function, and of a subsequent life spent in social isolation. Children who suffer from this disease and who have in addition large nasopharyngeal adenoids, acquire a characteristic and expressionless countenance, which, together with the open mouth and lack of attention because of the poor hearing, constitutes that condition which Guye, of Amsterdam, has called aprosexia (see Fig. 117).

The appearance of the drum membrane during the second stage and after an exudate has taken place into the cavity of the middle ear varies somewhat according to the amount, character, and color of the exudate, the degree of transparency of the tympanic membrane, and finally, the amount of congestion within the middle ear, and the consequent color of the mucous lining which may be seen through the translucent membrane by reflected light. In the first place, the degree of retraction of the drum membrane is not usually so great as in the first stage, but the short process and handle of the malleus continue to stand out prominently. A comparison of the color of the upper with the

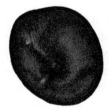
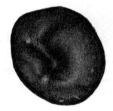

FIG. 137.—EXUDATE IN THE INFERIOR PORTION OF TYMPANIC CAVITY.
Note slightly crescentic line marking level of fluid. Viewed through speculum, patient's head erect.

FIG. 138.—SHOWING THE CHANGED RELATIONS OF THE EXUDATE WHEN THE HEAD OF THE PATIENT IS TILTED FORWARD TOWARD THE HORIZONTAL PLANE.
Same ear as shown in Fig. 137.

lower quadrant of the drum membrane will often show a decided difference in this stage, for whereas the upper portion of the membrane may retain its normal pearly-gray or slightly pinkish appearance, the lowermost portion looks slightly yellowish or straw colored, for the reason that the yellowish exudate within the tympanic cavity shows through the translucent membrana tympani. The level of this liquid in the drum cavity is indicated on the drum membrane by a distinct line, the color of which may be dark gray, white, or black. The direction of this line is, in the main, horizontal from before backward, but may be slightly crescentic (Fig. 137), concavoconvex, or inverted V shaped. If the contained fluid is thin and serous, and the patient's head be moved into different positions (Fig. 238) during the examination, the line may be seen to change its relation to the tympanic structures at each change in the position of the patient (Fig. 138). Should the exudate consist of a thick, ropy mucus, the above-mentioned changes may not occur at all, or if they take place they do so very slowly because of the greater density of the exudate. When the exudate is sufficient in quantity to fill the tympanic cavity, no line will, of course, mark its level and hence one cannot be seen. In this case the whole or at least some portion of the drum membrane will be found bulging to some degree, and a slightly yellowish and characteristic color will be observed over a greater or less area of the drum membrane unless the latter is from some cause opaque.

If during the examination of a drum membrane, beyond which there is a collection of exudate in the tympanic cavity, the tympanum should be inflated by means of the catheter or by the Politzer method,

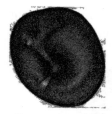

FIG. 139.—SHOWING AIR BUBBLES IN THE EXUDATE AFTER CATHETER INFLATION OF THE TYMPANIC CAVITY.

bubbles of air will be seen to arise from the antero-inferior quadrant near the tympanic ring—the tympanic orifice of the Eustachian tube—and finally to become lost above the surface-line of the fluid. In case this fluid is of a syrupy consistency the air-bubbles will be entangled in it, will rise very slowly, therefore, or they may stand quiescent in the fluid for a considerable length of time. During this experiment the catheter is inserted into the pharyngeal mouth of the Eustachian tube in the usual way, after which the instrument is held in place, and the inflation is performed by an assistant, while the examiner watches the effect of the entrance of air into the tympanic cavity, upon both the contained fluid and the membrana tympani (Fig. 139).

Mouth-breathing, due to an obstructed nose or nasopharynx, is a symptom which is observed in the majority of all cases of tubotympanitis occurring in children and young adults. An examination of the nasopharynx will usually reveal the presence of adenoids. In older persons the postrhinoscopic mirror will usually enable the examiner to make out a chronic nasopharyngitis, which may be seen to involve the lips of the Eustachian tube, the entrance to which is often blocked by tenacious mucus. Frequent head colds accompanied by nasal stoppage, blowing of the nose, and hawking and spitting are symptoms almost constantly present.

Diagnosis.—The diagnosis is made from the symptoms narrated by the patient, from the presence of an exudate in the tympanic cavity, and from the abnormal position of the membrana tympani. A physical examination of the fundus of the ear and also of the nose and nasopharynx is in every case essential to a correct diagnosis. Acute closure of the Eustachian tube may be strongly suspected from the symptoms alone, but the malposition of the membrane and the subsequent presence of an exudate within the tympanic cavity must each be actually seen before it can be said with certainty that a tubotympanic catarrh is present. The line marking the surface of the effusion into the drum cavity (see Fig. 139) is not often as well marked as the figures here given would indicate, and in many instances such a line is with difficulty distinguished by the examiner. The color of the exudate is usually of a light straw, or even deeper yellow color, and is therefore in strong contrast to the normal color of that portion of the membrane above the level of the fluid. A difference in the color of the upper and lower portions may not be noted by the examiner, for the reason that the whole tympanic membrane may be so thickened or congested as to entirely obscure the parts beyond. When this is the case the diagnosis as to the presence of fluid can be made from the character of the auscultatory sounds, which may be heard during catheter inflation, should the examiner connect the ear of the patient with his own, by means of the auscultatory tube (Fig. 113). The sounds heard, if fluid be present in the drum cavity, are bubbling or snapping, according to whether the fluid in the ear through which the air passes is thin or is mucoid and syrupy. If the fluid completely fills the drum cavity; if the drum membrane is opaque and the fluid cannot for this reason be seen; if the drum membrane is bulging at some point, for these reasons an incision of the membrana is justifiable for diagnostic purposes, and the outflow of serum or thick mucus which follows furnishes definite information concerning the nature of the tympanic affection.

Prognosis.—The prognosis depends much upon the early recognition of the exact nature of the aural affection and upon the promptness with which proper treatment is instituted for its relief. It is in this particular disease that procrastination as to treatment, especially in the case of children, is not only tolerated, but is also often desired on the part of those who have the care of these little unfortunates. The old and widely quoted advice, "to let the child alone and it will outgrow its aural ailment," has wrought incalculable mischief in this class of aural diseases, because when allowed to go untreated the child usually grows into and not out of the disease; and what is most unfortunate concerning this subsequent unfavorable progress of the aural affection is, that if left to itself, by the time the child has reached an age to think and act for himself in the matter, the aural disease has often reached a stage that is absolutely incurable.

When the patient is in good health otherwise and his environment

16

is in no way faulty, a rapid return to the normal condition of the ear
may be anticipated as a result of early treatment.   In cachectic individuals, who must continue to live under unhygienic circumstances, and
who are exposed a great deal to dampness and cold, the prognosis is
not so good.   In neglected cases the exudate, with its accompanying
symptoms of deafness, tinnitus, etc., may continue for months and
years, the retained secretion may finally organize, and bands of connective tissue may form as a result, these latter causing ankylosis of the
ossicles and permanent immobility of the membrana tympani.

Treatment.—In the first stage, while the affection consists merely
of a closure of the Eustachian tube together with the consequent displacement of the drum membrane inwardly, the treatment consists in
restoring the patency of the tube to the normal and of removing the
local predisposing cause of the disease.

The Eustachian tube may be opened and the tympanic cavity inflated by means of the Eustachian catheter or by the Politzer method.
It may in a general way be said that the catheter should be employed
in a majority of all adult cases in whom the nose or nasopharynx is not
greatly inflamed or exquisitely tender, whereas inflation by the Politzer
bag is particularly suited for use in young children and in adults where
the nose and nasopharynx are acutely inflamed and oversensitive to
the use of instruments.   Inflation, when successfully performed by
either method, will immediately improve the hearing to a very marked
degree, provided it was normal previously to the time of the present
affection.   When much swelling of the mucous lining of the Eustachian
tube is present as a result of the extension of the neighboring nasopharyngitis, it is sometimes difficult to inflate the tympanic cavity by any
method.   In such instances the catheter is preferable, but before attempting its introduction the nose and nasopharynx should be prepared
by thoroughly spraying the same with normal salt solution, and afterward applying a 4 per cent. solution of cocain to the inferior meatus,
to the lateral wall of the nasopharynx, and to the mouth of the Eustachian
tube.   The nasopharynx and nasal chambers are often found covered
with tenacious mucus, and the nasopharyngeal mouth of the tube is
commonly found to be filled with a similar secretion.   Any attempt,
therefore, to inflate the ear before this secretion is removed from the nose
and tubal orifice would most likely result in failure to accomplish the
desired end.   Only a small amount of cocain is necessary to sufficiently
anesthetize the oversensitive membranes and to render the introduction
of the catheter painless, provided it is applied only to the path the
instrument will traverse during its correct introduction.   The use of

cocain should be avoided after the first treatment in all cases who have nostrils sufficiently open to permit the ready passage of the instrument, provided the nasal mucous membrane is not hyperesthetic. The first few blasts of air through the catheter after it is properly placed should not be with force, since the sudden opening of the tube and replacement of the drum membrane may cause an unpleasant dizziness or even fainting on the part of the patient. With the auscultation tube in place, so that the operator may at all times judge the effect of the inflation upon the Eustachian tube and tympanic cavity, the air blasts are given with increasing force until the cavum tympani is entered and its normal air pressure is restored.

The greatly improved hearing which immediately results from the successful performance of this procedure will not likely prove permanent, the rule being that within a few hours after the inflation diminution begins, and by the end of one or two days the patient again hears almost if not quite as badly as before the treatment. It will, therefore, be necessary to repeat the operation in the worst cases at first daily, later every other day, and finally, once a week, as the necessity for the inflation disappears, while the hearing gradually improves, and at the end of two or three weeks becomes normal. After the first few inflations, when the patient is known to be improving satisfactorily, a good rule to follow is to request the patient to return for treatment only when he is convinced that the hearing power is again decreasing.

Proper local treatment of the nasopharynx is scarcely less important than the inflation of the drum cavity. The author considers the judicious management, either surgically or otherwise, of all inflammatory affections or new growths which may be found in this region, of such great importance in this and several other aural affections, that a separate chapter bearing on the subject has been prepared, and to which the careful attention of the student is here referred (see Chapter XIX.). At present all that need be said in reference to this treatment is that a successful result, both as to the cure of the present aural ailment and the prevention of future attacks of a similar or increasingly severe nature, will depend in great measure upon the skill and judgment with which the nasopharyngeal and nasal treatment is carried out.

If the affection is seen early and the above measures of inflation and nasopharyngeal treatment are carried out as directed, a large percentage of all cases of tubal catarrh will be cured before coming to the second stage or that of tubotympanic catarrh with exudate into the cavity of the middle ear. Should, however, the disease reach the tympanic cavity, into which an exudate takes place, the treatment, in addition to that already given, will consist largely of an effort to remove the exudate and to prevent its re-formation. Two methods of removing the exudate are in use: First, with the catheter introduced into the Eustachian tube in the usual way, the patient's head is held forward and somewhat toward the side opposite that which contains the fluid, when by means of air blasts driven through the catheter, first with a very moderate force, and later with a pressure of 15 or 20 pounds if necessary, the air current, aided by the position of the head, causes the secretion in the middle ear to flow out through the Eustachian tube into the nasopharynx and sometimes to trickle forward through the nose. If the tympanic exudate has by this means been removed, this fact may be known to the surgeon by an inspection of the drum membrane immediately after the performance, when the line denoting the previous level of the exudate will have been lowered or completely obliterated, and the yellowish color previously imparted by the contained fluid will have diminished or completely disappeared. This degree of success will justify a repetition of the catheter method of removal of the tympanic fluid every second or third day if there is a tendency to its reaccumulation. While this part of the treatment is being carried out the cleansing and appropriate local applications should be made to the nasopharynx. After ten days' trial of this means, if the exudate is not thereby removed, or if at the first examination of the case the tympanic cavity appears to be filled with the exudate to the extent of bulging in some portion of the drum membrane, the best procedure is to at once incise the drum membrane and remove the secretion through the external auditory canal.

Incision of the tympanic membrane, or paracentesis, which is performed for the purpose of entering the drum cavity from without and of evacuating secretions which are retained within, is employed as a curative and diagnostic measure in this and several other catarrhal and inflammatory aural affections. A complete description of the procedure and method of its performance is therefore given here, and reference will be made to it as may be subsequently required for the proper understanding of other sections of the work.

Incision of the drum membrane should always be preceded by a careful sterilization of the external auditory meatus, including the dermoid surface of the membrane itself. To accomplish this, a warm solution of mercuric bichlorid (1:4000) is sufficient when used for syringing the canal, after which a stronger solution of this drug may be rubbed into the roots of the hairs of the outer portion of the meatus and into the skin of the deeper portion. Hydrogen peroxid or the alcohol and boric acid solution are also effective for this purpose. Since it is frequently desirable to inflate the middle ear, either by the Politzer method or through the catheter after the drum membrane is incised, it is also necessary to spray the nose and nasopharynx thoroughly as a part of the preparation for the incision.

The question of the administration of an anesthetic arises in many cases, for when the membrana tympani is inflamed, and the patient has already passed one or more sleepless nights and is therefore exhausted by the continued and severe suffering, any additional or unnecessary pain should, if possible, be avoided. A thorough paracentesis, when performed during the height of a middle-ear inflammation, is exquisitely painful for a few seconds, and in highly nervous or sensitive individuals is regarded as a severe measure under all conditions. Therefore, while this operation can be performed upon a certain few without serious complaint, in the vast majority of patients requiring it the operator should either benumb the parts by the application of remedies locally to the drum membrane or he should administer a general anesthetic to the patient.

Of the many local anesthetics that have been suggested to prevent the pain during paracentesis and other operations on the drum membrane, the following, suggested by Gray, of Great Britain,[1] has proven serviceable

R. Cocain cryst.,	gr. xii–xxiv ;
Anilin oil,	3j ;
Absolute alcohol,	3j.—M.

After cleansing and drying the external auditory meatus the patient lies upon a cot with the affected ear uppermost, and the canal is filled with the warm anilin-cocain solution which is allowed to remain for ten or fifteen minutes, at the end of which time the membrana tympani is usually sufficiently anesthetized to permit of almost painless operating. This preparation should not be used without caution in any case in which a large perforation exists in the drum membrane, for the reason that should the tympanic cavity be filled with the solution toxic symptoms may rapidly develop, as in cases reported by Dupuy (*Laryngoscope*, Oct., 1901), Gray (*Lancet*, Mar., 1901), and St. Clair Thomson (*Lancet*, Apr., 1901).

A 5 to 10 per cent. solution of phenol in glycerin produces, when applied to the drum membrane, one of the most satisfactory methods of local anesthesia. The preparation should be used exactly as in the case of the anilin-cocain solution, but it requires more time to produce

[1] *Brit. Med. Journal*, April, 1900.

its full effect. Many combinations of cocain have been suggested as efficient local anesthetics in aural surgery, but most of them are unworthy of trial, for the reason that cocain will not be absorbed through the dermoid layer of the drum-head. The author has experimentally tested the membrana tympani and found it to be exquisitely sensitive after having been bathed for an hour in a saturated watery solution of cocain. No drug or combination of drugs has yet been discovered which will safely and completely anesthetize the inflamed drum membrane, and hence more or less pain will be experienced by the patient after the best of those suggested has been properly used. The preparation, when used in this way, very greatly lessens the pain, but does not usually completely prevent it.

In case of a child or of a very nervous and oversensitive adult the choice of a general anesthetic is frequently necessary. Because of the very short duration of the operation chloroform is preferable where not contra-indicated. In the case of older children and adults the administration of nitrous oxid is an ideal method of securing general anesthesia, since it is both rapid and safe, and the patient is almost immediately afterward conscious and free from the troublesome nausea which often follows the use of chloroform or ether. A further recommendation for the use of nitrous oxid is that the patient sits upright during the operation and the normal position of the quadrants of the membrana tympani are not altered from those most commonly seen by the operator.

The parts having been sterilized and the anesthetic provided for, the incision is made by means of a slender, sharp-pointed knife which may have either a straight or an angular handle (Fig. 141). This instrument should, of course, have been freshly sterilized, and must have its point and cutting edge in perfect condition. A dull-pointed knife is unfit for use and will cause very much unnecessary pain when employed in cases where only a local anesthetic has been used or perhaps no anesthetic at all. Under local anesthesia, or when nitrous oxid gas is used as a general anesthetic, the patient sits upright in a chair and the head is supported firmly between the hands of an assistant. The largest speculum is introduced into the canal which will give a good view of the drum membrane, and this latter structure is then clearly illuminated by means of reflected light from the head-mirror. The knife used for making the incision is slowly advanced into the external auditory meatus until its point is near the membrana tympani, when it is suddenly thrust through, and a cut is made upward or downward for the required distance before the blade is withdrawn (Fig. 142). Should the patient be in the recumbent position, the operator has only to remember the changed position of the landmarks from that in which he is accustomed to seeing them, and to operate accordingly.

The particular portion or quadrant of the drum membrane which should be incised in any given case and also the length of the incision depends upon the character of the disease which requires the operation, and upon whether or not there is fluid in the tympanic cavity in sufficient quantity to cause bulging of some part of the membrane. Thus, in

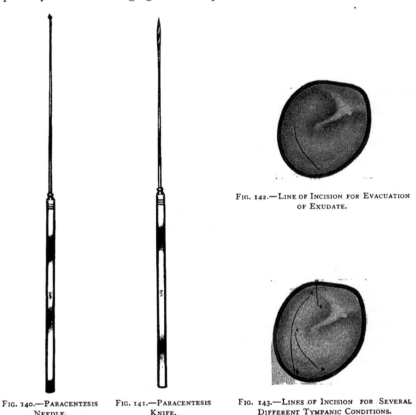

FIG. 142.—LINE OF INCISION FOR EVACUATION OF EXUDATE.

FIG. 140.—PARACENTESIS NEEDLE.

FIG. 141.—PARACENTESIS KNIFE.

FIG. 143.—LINES OF INCISION FOR SEVERAL DIFFERENT TYMPANIC CONDITIONS.

severe inflammation of the tympanic attic, where it is desirable to secure free depletion of the mucous lining of that region, it is necessary to make the incision in one of the superior quadrants, whereas if the disease be confined to the atrium the incision should be made in one of the inferior quadrants. However, whatever may be the causative disease, if the result has been an effusion of serum, an oversecretion of mucus, or a collection of pus which causes a decided bulging of some portion of the tympanic membrane, then the incision should be made so as to divide the swollen area and to include its highest point, as shown in Fig. 142.

The extent of the incision is a matter of judgment in each individual case, and must be governed by the severity of the disease, the pathologic condition which is present in the tympanic cavity, and the particular end that is desired to be accomplished. Since large incisions heal as rapidly as small ones, and since the efficiency of a paracentesis usually depends upon the freedom with which it is made, it is better to err on the side of making the cut too long rather than too short. A mere puncture of the membrana with the paracentesis needle (Fig. 140) or with the point of the knife is not sufficient. When the atrium is filled with fluid the knife may be entered at a point posterior to the short process of the malleus, just below the posterior fold and near the tympanic ring, and with the cutting edge turned downward be carried parallel to the ring to the inferior pole of the membrane (Fig. 143, A B). Or in case the attic is affected and its mucous lining is violently inflamed, the edge of the knife may be turned upward, and the cut be made as far as the upper pole of the ring and then carried outward through the skin of the posterosuperior wall of the external meatus (Fig. 143, E F). The depth to which the point of the knife should be carried varies also according to the nature of the disease within the tympanum. When the incision is made to evacuate fluid which is the result of a tubotympanic congestion it is not essential to incise the mucous lining of the inner tympanic wall at the same time that the drum membrane is divided; whereas, if there is in addition to a collection of fluid an intense engorgement of this membrane, and depletion of the latter is desired, then the knife should be entered deeply enough to include both the tympanic membrane and the mucous covering of the inner tympanic wall.

The recuperative power of the drum membrane is nearly always very active and not infrequently surprising in this respect. Hence when injured by a clean cut, and the wound is kept free from subsequent infection, a union of the severed parts takes place within one or two days, or just as soon as the exudate, or disease, within the tympanic cavity will permit. After a free incision of the membrana tympani, therefore, the danger is that the wound will heal too soon rather than not at all.

After a free incision of the drum membrane in case of the accumulation of exudate during the course of a tubotympanic congestion, a small amount may pour through the opening into the external auditory meatus immediately, provided the contained fluid be of a serous nature, but if it is thick and tenacious, only a bead of the exudate may protrude through the gaping incision, and none will subsequently be found in

the external meatus.   In either case it will be necessary to employ inflation for the purpose of completely dislodging the exudate and of
clearing the tympanic cavity.   Catheterization or politzerization should,
therefore, be immediately performed after the paracentesis and should
be repeated until all the exudate is driven through the opening into the
auditory canal.   It is sometimes impossible, even by vigorous inflation, to
dislodge all of the mucus, in which case resort may be had to Siegel's
otoscope (Fig. 97), which, when employed for this purpose, should be
used as a suction apparatus, by which means the remaining exudate
can be effectively dislodged and sucked into the auditory meatus.   It
has been proposed by some authors to wash the exudate out of the
tympanic cavity by means of an antiseptic fluid injected through the
catheter by way of the Eustachian tube, allowing it then to flow out
through the incision in the drum membrane into the auditory canal.
This procedure, as well as that of syringing the external auditory meatus,
has been proved to be harmful and should, therefore, not be practised.
The exudate usually reaccumulates, and the inflation of the middle ear
and suction with Siegel's apparatus will, therefore, need repeating, .at
first every day, then every other day, and finally only when the exudate
returns in quantity sufficient to impair the hearing.   At the same time
that these treatments are given the nasopharynx must receive attention,
and all inflammation or growths that are present should be skillfully
managed.   The general health of the individual may also be such as to
require the administration of tonics, the regulation of the diet, or a
change of environment to one that is less productive of frequent cold-
taking.

CHAPTER XXII

ACUTE CATARRHAL OTITIS MEDIA

THIS disease is, as the name indicates, an actual inflammation of the mucous lining of the tympanic cavity. Confusion as to the exact meaning of the terms used in the description of the acute diseases of the middle ear is apt to arise unless the student bears constantly in mind the pathology of each. In the preceding chapter a description of the acute congestive middle-ear affections was given, and it should now be recalled that the symptoms and objective signs accompanying them were not those which would indicate diseases of an inflammatory nature. While otitis media of the catarrhal variety is sometimes the result of a preceding tubotympanic congestion, it is usually an independent affection, behaves differently throughout its course, is in every way a more severe disease, and one that is dependent upon a more active form of infection of the cavity by one or more varieties of pathogenic bacteria.

Causation.—All the causes that have been enumerated as productive of tubotympanic catarrh are also active as etiologic factors in this disease. Thus, colds in the head, nasopharyngitis, and indeed the presence of all varieties of inflammation or new growths in the nose or nasopharyngeal space, may be considered as predisposing causes. Stoppage of the nose or throat by growths or inflammatory swelling of the mucous membrane in this locality is productive of middle-ear complication, first, because these conditions of the upper air tract favor the growth of bacteria in a neighborhood immediately adjoining the middle ear; second, the presence of such growths or inflammations favors an extension of venous congestion in the Eustachian tube and the mucous lining of the middle ear, and third, the obstruction of the pharynx and nostrils, together with the presence of the ropy secretion, requires that the individual blow his nose with undue force in order to clear the respiratory spaces; and this force is often great enough to blow some of the infected mucus through the Eustachian tube into the middle ear, the inevitable result of which is that the disease under consideration is at once set up. Faulty methods of using the nasal douche, either by the physician or the patient himself, is sometimes responsible for the disease. Patients who accidentally become strangled while gargling the throat, or from accidentally getting water into the mouth while bathing, may in their sudden and violent efforts to expel the fluid force some of it through the Eustachian tube into the middle ear. Watery solutions of all kinds, if forced from any reason to enter the tympanic cavity, invariably set up an otitis media, and the physician should, therefore, bear in mind certain rules concerning the proper method of nasal douching when personally employing this plan of nasal cleansing. Explicit directions should always be given for the methods of employment of the nasal douche should the patient be directed to use this as a method of home treatment. (See chapter on Nasal Treatment of Ear Diseases, p. 202.) The milder forms of measles, scarlet fever, la grippe, and other infectious diseases which nearly always affect the throat at the same time, are also frequent causes of acute catarrhal otitis media, the latter disease following as a complication, and is brought about in exactly the same manner that the pathogenic bacteria are caused to enter the drum cavity—namely, as a result of the entrance of pathogenic bacteria into the tympanum. The more violent varieties of the infectious diseases are usually followed by acute purulent otitis media, which will be described in the next chapter.

Pathology.—In acute catarrhal otitis media there is a general hyperemia of the middle-ear mucous membrane. The mucous membrane is swollen through enlargement of its vessels, serous and round-cell infiltration takes place, and there may be more or less exudate either serous, mucous, or seromucous lying on the surface of the mucous membrane. The air spaces are lessened through the swelling of the mucous membrane, the stapes may be hidden in the vestibular window, or the niche to the cochlear window may be occluded. The catarrhal secretion is a combination of inflammatory exudate and transudate. If the exudate is serous, it is clear and thin; if mucoid, it is thick and even tough, so that it can be drawn out by forceps. This disease is a combination of a tubotympanic catarrh and an inflammation not intense enough to cause necrosis of the middle-ear tissue, as in acute suppurative otitis media.

Symptoms.—Deep-seated pain in the ear is one of the earliest as well as the most pronounced symptom. When the inflammation has reached its height the pain is of a lancinating, tearing, and altogether unbearable nature. During the day, when the patient may endeavor to interest himself in his business affairs, less complaint is made, but during the night, and especially if the recumbent position is assumed, the suffering is greatly increased, sleep is impossible, and the patient frequently walks the floor, holds his head between his hands, and cries aloud. There are usually intervals in which the pain is less severe, but upon swallowing, coughing, or belching a lancinating pain shoots to the ear and the paroxysm of intense suffering is again renewed. Attempts to blow the nose forcibly will also bring on a sharp pain which seems to the patient to shoot from the nasopharynx into the depths of the ear. While in the beginning the pain usually centers in the middle ear, it sometimes radiates over the temporal region, to the teeth, or it may even simulate a trigeminal neuralgia.

Pain, or at least a feeling of soreness, is present in the space between the tip of the mastoid process and the ramus of the lower jaw—the external site of the pain corresponding to the position and direction of the Eustachian tube within. Pressure over this area frequently elicits considerable tenderness. Except in very severe cases, when the mastoid antrum and cells are simultaneously infected, little or no tenderness and no swelling can be detected over the mastoid region. The auricle can be freely moved and the external canal may be straightened by the examiner preparatory to the insertion of the aural speculum, without causing the patient the slightest increase of pain.

The hearing is greatly impaired. Beginning with a feeling of stuffiness in the ear, as the inflammation develops and the exudate takes place, the function becomes rapidly affected until within a few hours the degree of deafness is usually quite marked. Tinnitus aurium and high-pitched cracking sounds due to the passage of air through the inflamed Eustachian tube into the fluid of the middle ear are also symptoms, but complaint concerning these will scarcely be made while the pain in the ear is at its height. After a rupture of the drum membrane has taken place and subsidence of the aural pain has occurred, the chief complaint of the patient is frequently of the subjective head noises. These noises are due to the increased tension of the labyrinthine fluids produced partly by the presence of the exudate within the middle ear, and partly by the intratympanic vascular distention which complicates the changes in the middle ear.

The temperature is normal or but slightly elevated in the uncomplicated cases occurring in adults. If the otitis media is the result of an infectious general disease, like scarlatina or measles, the temperature may reach 103° F. or even higher. Should mastoiditis set up or should any of the intracranial complications arise, the temperature will be affected according to the particular complication that supervenes. (For symptoms of these complications see Chaps. XXXII.–XXXVIII.)

Rupture of the drum-head occurs at some period of the disease in the vast majority of all cases. After the suffering has continued with more or less intensity for from one to three days, the drum membrane gives way and a discharge of a seromucous fluid takes place into the auditory canal. Rarely a rupture may take place within twelve hours after the beginning of the disease, but the perforation may also occur as late as three days after the onset of the severe pain; or a rupture may not occur at all. In the latter instance the collection of exudate within the tympanum may escape through the Eustachian tube, or it may remain for an indefinite period, to be finally absorbed, to become organized, and form connective-tissue adhesions between the membrana tympani and some portion of the inner wall of the tympanum, or the ossicles may become first imbedded and finally ankylosed by the deposit of new tissue about them.

The general appearance of the patient is usually one that indicates great suffering. After one or more sleepless nights, during which the pain has been severe and perhaps incessant, the strongest individual may show evidence of great prostration, and even those having great fortitude will exhibit signs of the greatest cowardice toward further pain. After rupture of the drum membrane takes place the pain is usually much lessened, the patient falls into a long sleep, the appetite, which was previously lost, quickly returns, and the patient speedily enters upon the stage of convalescence. In some cases, however, the pain continues after the rupture takes place, and this fact is usually evidence that the opening through the drum membrane is too small, and that the drainage from the tympanic cavity is, therefore, insufficient.

The appearance of the drum membrane, as seen at the physical examination of the ear, varies with the stage of the disease at which the examination is made. During the first few hours after the onset of the inflammation a redness will be visible along the handle of the malleus, which, if observed later, will be found to have spread over the greater portion or even the whole of the membrane, and to have become a uniform, cherry-red color. At this latter period the individual injected vessels cannot be seen. The landmarks, with the possible exception of the short process of the malleus, will be found to have disappeared, and the whole fundus presents an inflammatory state in which it is not always easy to make out the ending of the walls of the external auditory meatus and the beginning of the membrana tympani. Very soon the exudate takes place into the tympanic cavity, and this is shown during the otoscopic examination by the bulging of some portion of the drum membrane which it causes. The greatest bulging is most frequently seen in the upper and posterior portion, although the whole membrane often bulges to a less degree, and either of the lower quadrants may be most greatly affected in this respect. Since in the purulent variety of acute otitis media the bulging is usually more limited in extent, and is most usually seen in the extreme uppermost portion of the membrane, the position of the point of greatest bulging becomes a feature in the differential diagnosis of the two diseases. Occasionally the postero-superior segment is bulged outward in the form of a sac, the lowermost portion of which is filled with exudate. Instances have been recorded in which such a protruding pouch has been observed to fill the postero-superior portion of the external auditory meatus, and even to appear as a polypoid-like mass at the orifice of the auditory meatus (Fig. 144).

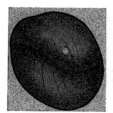

FIG. 144.—SAGGING OF SHRAPNELL'S MEMBRANE DUE TO THE PRESENCE OF AN INFLAMMATORY EXUDATE.

After spontaneous perforation of the drum membrane has taken place, the external auditory meatus is found, upon inspection, to contain more or less serous, seromucous, or serosanguineous discharge, which, if untreated, or only badly treated, will very rapidly become mucopurulent or purulent. The presence of a mucous or sero-mucous discharge is evidence of the occurrence of a perforation in the drum membrane, and the physical examination should be partially directed to the discovery of its location and extent. Occurring as the result of an acute catarrhal otitis media such a rupture is most frequently found in the lower half of the membrane, either in the postero-inferior quadrant just below the umbo, or in the antero-inferior quadrant over the site of the tympanic entrance of the Eustachian tube. It is not always an easy matter to locate a small perforation during the height of the inflammation when every surrounding tissue is infiltrated, and the normally small area of the fundus is thereby still more greatly encroached upon. If the exudate is small in quantity, it may be seen pouring through the perforation or a small bead of the material may be seen protruding through the opening, at which point a pulsation synchronous with the heart-beat may be observed. If the secretion is profuse and pours through the rupture in an amount sufficient to fill the external auditory canal it may be absorbed by the insertion of a cylinder of sterile cotton into the bottom of the external auditory meatus, or it may be washed away by syringing, after which, if the examination of the drum membrane is made immediately, the location of the perforation may often be made out. If the examination of the drum membrane is continued, while at the same time the patient performs the Valsalva inflation, or while an assistant performs inflation by the Politzer or catheter method, the observer will note the exit of air-bubbles at the point of rupture. He will also often be able to hear at the instant the inflation is performed a hissing sound due to the escape of air through the opening in the tympanic membrane.

It is of vastly more importance to determine the size of the perforation rather than its location, for the reason that the subsequent treatment will depend in no small measure upon whether or not the opening is sufficiently large to provide ample drainage to the inflamed cavities of the middle ear.

The diagnosis should be readily made when the examiner considers the symptoms in connection with the physical examination of the membrana tympani itself. The chief points upon which the diagnosis will be based are: the acute pain in the ear with accompanying deafness and tinnitus, in a case where examination of the fundus of the ear shows a uniformly reddened and infiltrated drum membrane which is also bulging and perhaps perforated. This disease must be distinguished from acute tubotympanic catarrh and from the acute suppurative diseases of the middle ear. The differential diagnosis is given in a comprehensive form at the end of the next chapter (see p. 277).

Prognosis.—The ultimate result of acute catarrhal otitis media is nearly always favorable in persons who were previously in good health, and whose environment is subsequently good. This is especially true of cases that are seen early and are skilfully treated until all the diseased parts have resumed their normal condition. When the disease follows an infectious fever or is the result of a tuberculous affection, the prognosis is not so good, and the discharge is apt to become first purulent and then ultimately chronic. In anemic, underfed, and poorly housed individuals the discharge may also become chronic. Children who are affected with adenoids and adults who suffer from chronic nasopharyngitis or from obstructive nasal growths are subject to recurrences of the aural inflammation during the damp and changeable seasons of the year. In such instances the pathologic condition of the nose and nasopharynx acts as a continued menace to the ear, and each attack of the tympanic inflammation predisposes the patient to another, until after a period of years the structures of the ear are hopelessly damaged. Mastoiditis rarely occurs in this disease, but when it complicates the tympanic ailment the dangers incident to this affection are added to the original disease. Intracranial extension with resulting meningitis, brain abscess, or infective thrombosis of the lateral sinus is still more rarely met with, and when one of these complications does take place it is the result of transmission of the infective material from the middle ear or mastoid to the cranial cavity through the medium of the blood or lymph streams, and not, as is the case in chronic suppurative otitis, through open channels that have been provided by the necrosis of the intervening osseous structures.

Treatment.—Since the patient is most usually seen for the first time after the pain has become severe, the relief of the suffering becomes the first and most urgent duty. This is most speedily and effectively accomplished by the administration of morphin hypodermically, if the patient be an adult, or, in the case of a child, an appropriate-sized dose of deodorized tincture of opium given per orum. It is safest to give paregoric to infants. Whatever form of anodyne is prescribed should be given in a sufficiently large dose to completely relieve the pain and to secure the much-needed rest for the patient. The continued administration of opiates is objectionable, and therefore just as soon as the patient is once relieved, active means of combating or aborting the inflammation should be instituted. If the individual is robust or plethoric, the administration of saline draughts should be begun at once and repeated until several large watery stools are produced. Local depletion is an effectual means of relieving the pain and of lessening the intratympanic congestion, provided it be practised early and before the exudate has taken place into the tympanic cavity. (See p. 125 for a description of the methods and benefits to be derived from local depletion.) In adults not fewer than three natural leeches should be applied, and if the artificial leech is used, from 2 to 4 ounces of blood should be withdrawn from the postauricular region.

When the inflammation of the tympanic mucous membrane is of a milder nature and the accompanying pain less severe, sufficient relief may often be obtained by the use of local applications which are made directly to the drum membrane and supplemented by the employment of dry heat applied continuously to the affected side of the head. Among the most useful remedies to be applied directly to the drum membrane for the relief of the pain may be mentioned the phenol-glycerin solution, in the proportion of 10 per cent. of the former and 90 per cent. of the latter. This can be most effectually applied to the affected part by twisting a cone of cotton on the end of a small applicator (Fig. 204), saturating the cotton in the solution of phenol-glycerin, and then holding the same over a flame until it is heated to the greatest degree of toleration when tested upon the back of the hand. After thus properly preparing and heating the medicated cotton cone, it is quickly removed from the applicator, seized between the jaws of the slender aural dressing-forceps, and before it has time to cool is quickly inserted to the bottom of the external auditory meatus where it is allowed to remain with the large end of the cone of glycerinated cotton resting directly against the outer surface of the drum membrane, while the caudal end projects slightly from the meatus, so that it may be easily removed at any time by the attendant or by the patient himself. If this cotton cone is prepared so as to fit the meatus snugly, if it is previously heated to the proper degree, and is then accurately inserted against the drum membrane, it acts beneficially in two ways: first, from the direct and continuous application of the heat, and from the action of the anesthetic qualities of the carbolic acid, the pain is relieved; and second, the presence of the glycerin in contact with the inflamed surface causes a transudate of serum in the direction of the auditory canal which is sometimes notably efficient in unloading the congested blood-vessels of the drum membrane and in lessening the quantity of the exudate within the tympanic cavity. This glycerinated tampon may be left in the auditory canal for several hours, provided there is no return of the acute pain. Immediately after its insertion dry heat in the form of the hot-water bottle or Japanese stove should be made over the external surface of that side of the head. The author has observed but slight relief from the instillation into the external auditory canal of such fluids as laudanum and sweet oil, which preparation is so commonly used by the laity for the relief of earache; nor has any appreciable benefit been obtained from the instillation of solutions of cocain even when of considerable strength. Any non-irritating solution if instilled warm into an aching ear will give some degree of relief, and the reputation which many ear solutions have acquired for the relief of earache is due to the fact that they are always instilled while warm rather than to any anesthetic or anodyne property of the drugs which they contain. Plain unmedicated water, when instilled after it has been heated to the proper temperature, will usually prove equally as efficient for the relief of aural pain as any of the more complicated and expensive combination of drugs which form the basis of ear-drops. The insertion of a Richards' aural bougie into the external auditory meatus has been helpful, particularly in the case of earache in very young children.[1]

[1] The formula for this bougie is as follows :

R.	Acidi carbolici,	ℳ vij;
	Extract opii fl.,	ℳ vj;
	Cocaini,	grs. iij;
.	Atropin sulphate,	grs. iij;
	Aquæ,	ℳ lij;
	Gelatini,	grs. xviij;
	Glycerini,	grs. clviij.—M.

To make 42 bougies. At the moment the bougie is to be used it is dipped into water as hot as the hand will bear. This renders it elastic, easy of insertion, and adds the

Should the foregoing measures fail to relieve the pain and abort the inflammation, and should it be found upon examination of the drum membrane that an exudate has taken place into the tympanic cavity, incision of the drum membrane should be performed at once. In case the bulging is greatest over the posterior portion of the membrane, the knife should be inserted just below the posterior fold, near the tympanic margin, and should then be carried downward parallel with the tympanic ring to its postero-inferior portion (see Fig. 143, A B). Since the exudate within the tympanic cavity is·usually thin, under pressure it immediately pours through the slit thus made in the membrana, and often in sufficient quantity to appear at the concha almost before the withdrawal of the

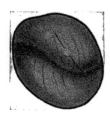

FIG. 145.—SHOWING LINE OF INCISION IN SAGGING SHRAPNELL'S MEMBRANE.

paracentesis knife. The bulging may occur in any quadrant, and wherever located, the incision must be made in such direction and position as to include it, and consequently to be most favorable to free drainage (Fig. 145). When the incision is performed early, and therefore during the height of the inflammation of the tympanic mucous lining, more favorable results will be obtained if the point of the knife is pushed inward to a sufficient depth to include the mucous membrane of the inner tympanic wall in the cut. A free hemorrhage will take place as the result of this incision of the mucous membrane, and as a consequence the congested parts are depleted, the tension of the vessels is relieved, and the swelling of the mucous membrane is greatly reduced.

The turbid seromucous discharge which follows the incision contains pathogenic bacteria of a low grade of virulence, and hence if the drum cavity is not subsequently infected from the auditory meatus through the incised wound in the membrane or from the nasopharynx through the Eustachian tube, the case will progress speedily toward recovery. The first duty of the physician following a paracentesis is, therefore, to provide as much as possible against the occurrence of such an infection from without. It is presumed, of course, that the external auditory meatus has been thoroughly sterilized before the drum membrane is incised, and it only remains to keep it in this state during the subsequent period of discharge and the healing of the wound. To valuable quality of heat in a form available for local application. The bougie should be inserted deeply into the auditory canal, where it dissolves and allows the several ingredients of which it is composed to come into direct contact with the membrana tympani. A pledget of cotton should be inserted into the meatus to retain the bougie, and the hot-water bottle should then be applied over the auricle and affected side of the head.

do this effectively is not so simple a measure as might at first be supposed, for unless the subsequent dressings be made in a perfectly aseptic dressing room it is easy to carry an infection to the middle ear upon either the gauze or instruments that are afterward used.   However, if the instruments, operator's hands, and the external auditory meatus of the patient are sterile, and reasonable care be taken not to handle the patient's head or objects in the treatment room, like chairs, etc., unnecessarily, it is possible to make a satisfactory aural dressing in the treatment room of the surgeon.

The author always prefers to begin the after-treatment following an incision of the drum membrane by the insertion of a sterile gauze wick to the bottom of the auditory canal, and so placing the innermost end of such a strip that it lies in direct contact with the incision in the membrane (Fig. 146).   Folds of the wick are then placed loosely over

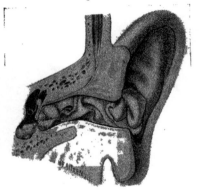

each other until the whole auditory meatus is full and a few coils are left lying loosely in the concha. Under no circumstances is it permissible to pack the auditory meatus tightly with the gauze, but the surgeon must always be sure that he has inserted the distal end of the wick deeply enough to lie in actual contact with the drum membrane, since otherwise the gauze will not serve the desired purpose of capillary suction of the exudate from the tympanic cavity, but would, on the contrary, act rather as an obstruction to the exit of the secretion, even after it

FIG. 146.—METHOD OF DRY PACKING IN THE TREATMENT OF SUPPURATIVE MIDDLE-EAR AFFECTIONS.

The distal end of the gauze strip lies in direct contact with the perforation in the membrana tympani, in which position it absorbs the pus as rapidly as formed.

has exuded into the external auditory canal (Fig. 147).   When the discharge is profuse, such a gauze wick is frequently saturated with the secretion in a very short time.   It is essential, however, to the carrying out of the antiseptic technic that no one but the surgeon or his trained assistant should remove this gauze and reinsert another.   The wisest plan is, therefore, to provide a thick pad of gauze which is placed over the outer ear and bound to it with a roller bandage, to take up the discharge as fast as it may appear at the outer end of the gauze wick, since in this way only can the infection of the wick itself be provided against and the necessity of frequent change of the dressing be obviated.

Hence, at the first and at each subsequent dressing, which is at the outset made daily, after the insertion of the wick into the auditory canal as above directed, a quantity of loose sterile gauze as large as can be conveniently accommodated in the closed hand is placed over the external ear and held in place by a roller bandage (Fig. 255). At each daily dressing of the ear the nose and nasopharynx should be given such treatment as may be indicated by any local congestion or inflammation that is present in these localities.

Until convalescence is well established the patient is safer and will make more rapid improvement if he remains indoors, or if while feverish and in pain he keeps his bed. The diet should be limited and of such character and quantity as would be indicated during the continuance

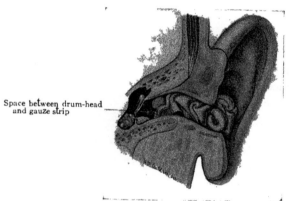

Space between drum-head
and gauze strip

FIG. 147.—FAULTY METHOD OF DRY PACKING THE EAR.

Note that the gauze strip only partially fills the external auditory meatus, and that pus can collect in the space between the gauze and membrana tympani. Compare the position of the distal end of the gauze strip in this illustration with that in Fig. 146, in which the gauze is properly placed.

of any inflammation. The presence of constipation must be remedied by the administration of salines, but if the patient is anemic and considerable prostration is present, the extract of cascara sagrada is preferable as a laxative. In this class of cases ferruginous tonics are also most helpful when given in connection with the local treatment.

After a persistence in the above treatment for four or five days by means of the gauze wick, if the aural discharge shows no indication of lessening, or if it should become more profuse and purulent in character, it may be deemed wise to abandon this method and to substitute therefor the plan of syringing the ear. The frequency with which a discharging ear should be syringed depends upon the amount of the secretion, which, when very free, may require cleansing every two or three hours, whereas, only once or twice a day may suffice if the discharge is scanty.

When the discharge has lessened to the degree that it no longer appears at the external orifice of the auditory meatus, the syringing should be withheld entirely, since persistence in its use after that time will often favor an exacerbation of the inflammation within the middle ear. When quite scanty, therefore, the discharge is best managed by wiping it away with a small pledget of cotton wound upon the end of the aural applicator, after which the meatal walls, and especially the outer or hair-growing parts of the external auditory meatus, should be sterilized by rubbing them with the boric acid and alcohol solution. Following any of the methods of cleansing the ear the whole auditory canal should be finally left dry, and as a finishing dressing a small quantity of powdered boric acid or boric acid mixed with zinc oxid should be blown into the canal and a thin coating everywhere deposited upon its walls and upon the dermoid surface of the drum membrane. The mistake must not be made of insufflating a large quantity of any kind of powder into an ear that is discharging, for the reason that the powder blocks the incision or perforation in the membrana tympani, and thus hinders rather than facilitates the drainage from the middle ear.

When the case is not seen by the surgeon until spontaneous perforation of the drum membrane has already taken place, and the opening through the tympanic membrane is seen to be ample to provide free drainage, the same methods of treatment may be instituted that have here been advocated as proper subsequent to an incision. But if the perforation is found to be small and the patient continues to suffer almost if not quite as much as before the rupture took place, then the opening should be enlarged by a free incision with the knife, exactly as if no perforation had ever occurred. It sometimes happens that even after a very free incision of the membrane that union of the lips of the wound takes place before the discharge subsides, in which case the good effects of the paracentesis which occurred immediately afterward are followed by a recurrence of the former pain and other symptoms which characterized the onset of the original attack of the catarrhal otitis media. Under such circumstances a second and equally free incision of the drum-head should be made.

During the height of the inflammation it is not wise to inflate the middle ear by any method. To do so usually increases the pain already present or causes a recurrence of that which is subsiding. As the acute inflammation abates, however, and when the pain and other accompanying symptoms of the acute catarrhal otitis have in great measure disappeared, inflation is to be advocated, and if the air is carefully injected through the catheter or by means of the Politzer bag the restoration of the inflamed middle-ear tissues to the normal is thereby hastened. During the course of this disease when left entirely to nature, the drum membrane is forced into an abnormal position, in which case the tympanic membrane is retracted or it may be bulged outward by the accumulations of exudate within the tympanic cavity. The tendency is often toward the retention in the cavum tympani, even after the most thorough paracentesis, of a portion of the exudate, which may ultimately organize and bind both drum membrane and ossicles into either of the above abnormal situations. The best means of avoiding this occurrence is the early and complete evacuation of the tympanic exudate as already stated, and then following this by the immediate replacement of the membrana by means of the air douche, or inflation by means of the Eustachian catheter. The employment of the catheter is usually preferable in adults provided skill is used during its introduction, for the reason that the amount of force with which the air is caused to enter the tympanic cavity can by this means be regulated more accurately, and moreover since very often only one ear is affected, it is undesirable to inflate both, as would happen when the Politzer method is employed. At first the inflation should be performed daily, but as the hearing distance increases and the drum membrane is seen on examination to be regaining its normal position and color, the inflation may be made only every second or third day, and finally, only rarely or not at all.

In case the ailment shows a tendency to become subacute or chronic, as indicated by its behavior subsequently to the incision of the membrane, notably by undue continuance of the discharge and delayed healing . of the perforation, stimulating vapors are sometimes more helpful than simple air, if injected through the catheter, the method of their employment being exactly similar to that already described.

Should the exudate within the middle ear become infected from without, either after spontaneous rupture or an incision of the drum membrane, the discharge becomes quickly purulent, tissue necrosis may take place, and the disease finally becomes chronic. The treatment for this latter disease is given in Chapter XXVII., to which reference is now made.

CHAPTER XXIII

ACUTE SUPPURATIVE OTITIS MEDIA

THIS disease is characterized by a group of symptoms that is more severe in every way than that which accompanies the two preceding varieties of middle-ear affection. The inflammation is not only more violent, but the resulting destruction of tissue within the middle ear is correspondingly greater, and therefore the permanent impairment of function is also greater. It is chiefly because of the extensive damage resulting from tissue necrosis of the middle ear during the progress of this disease that it is regarded by otologists as the most serious of all the acute aural affections. Chronic suppurative otitis media follows the acute variety in a very considerable proportion of cases, and especially in those in which treatment has been neglected.

Causation.—All the causes that were enumerated in the chapters on Acute Catarrhal Otitis Media and Acute Tubotympanic Congestion are also among the etiologic factors productive of the acute suppurative form. The chief difference between the two former diseases and the one under consideration lies in the violence of the causative disease. Thus a mild attack of nasopharyngitis, tonsillitis, or measles may be productive of nothing more than a tubotympanic catarrh, whereas in the same individual, if the pathogenic bacteria which are causative of the primary disease are of a more virulent nature, any secondary affection of the middle ear will usually be of a catarrhal or suppurative variety. Hence otitis media suppurativa is comparatively rare as a complication of the mild inflammatory affections of the throat or of the mild varieties of the acute infectious diseases, whereas it is quite common as a sequence of these affections when occurring in a severe form.

Of the general diseases which most frequently cause suppuration of the tympanic cavity, those of a specific infectious character stand first. The affections of this class which are most clearly responsible for the aural complications are, in the order of frequency in which the tympanic suppuration results, scarlatina, measles, epidemic influenza, and diphtheria. The disastrous effects of these diseases upon the organ of hearing are so frequently witnessed and occupy such an important place in otology that a complete discussion of each in its causative relation to aural diseases becomes essential to the student of this subject.

Scarlatina is probably the greatest enemy of the ear. In the worst forms of this disease, occurring during certain epidemics, and in damp, cold weather, the tympanic cavity is involved in an inflammatory or suppurative process in as many as one-third of all cases, and is the most frequent complication of scarlatina. Both the severity and frequency of the aural complication of scarlatina depends upon the character of the angina which accompanies the general disease. Thus, if the throat involvement which accompanies the exanthem is of only an erythematous type the ear is seldom implicated, and should extension to the tympanic cavity take place, its character is more apt to be catarrhal than suppurative. When, however, the angina which accompanies the scarlatina is more intense or is of the membranous variety, a suppurative otitis media is an almost constant complication, is of a violent nature, and mastoid extension is frequently met with. The direct and exciting cause of the aural suppuration in scarlet fever is the presence in the pharynx and nasopharynx of large numbers of pathogenic bacteria, in the worst cases, chiefly of the streptococcus, which finds its way directly into the tympanum through the Eustachian tube. This migration of the infective bacteria is favored in the case of infants and young children by the fact that in early life the Eustachian tube is shorter and more patent than in the adult, whereas in the latter the bacteria are often driven through the Eustachian tube by the powerful efforts the patient makes in blowing his partially or perhaps wholly occluded nose.

Measles, next to scarlet fever, must be regarded as the most frequent cause of acute otitis media. Both Tobietz and Bezold have ascertained by the collective post-mortem examination of 38 cases of death resulting from measles, during the early stages, that the inflammation had traveled to the tympanum and that there was already present in this cavity a mucopurulent or purulent exudate. In the early stage of measles the tympanic involvement is due, therefore, to the presence of the inflammation which is characteristic of this exanthem, and not to a secondary infection which results from the migration of pathogenic bacteria from the rhinopharynx. Later in the disease, however, streptococci and staphylococci, which are present in the nasopharyngeal space, find their way into the cavum tympani, and an active suppuration is quickly developed as a result.

Diphtheria causes a suppurative otitis media, in many instances at least, by an active extension of the diphtheritic membrane from the vault of the pharynx, through the Eustachian tube into the middle ear.

After the rupture of the drum membrane has occurred a bacteriologic examination of the aural discharge shows the presence of the bacillus of diphtheria associated with streptococci and staphylococci. Paralysis of the palatal muscles frequently occurs either during the progress of the diphtheria or as a sequel, and the impairment of function resulting to the muscles which act to open the Eustachian tube often produces a greater or less degree of deafness, and this temporary loss of muscular function no doubt furnishes a predisposing cause of the spread of the membrane to the tympanic cavity with resulting suppuration.

Epidemic influenza, as is now well known, exists in two well-defined types: that which affects principally the nervous system and that which involves chiefly the mucous membrane. The latter variety of la grippe is almost wholly responsible for middle-ear inflammation in so far as the latter is due to the former disease. In the catarrhal variety of la grippe the mucous membrane of the nose, pharynx, and nasopharynx becomes intensely inflamed, and from these central spaces the inflammatory process frequently spreads to one or more adjoining sinuses, as, for example, to the antrum of Highmore through the ostium maxillaire or to the tympanic cavity by way of the Eustachian tube. It has not as yet been determined whether or not the influenza bacillus is the sole cause of the inflammation of the upper respiratory tract, and of the accompanying suppuration which so frequently occurs in the middle ear or one of the accessory sinuses of the nose. In the severe forms of otitis media due to la grippe, streptococci, staphylococci, and pnuemococci are frequently found in the discharge from the ear. These bacilli have no doubt found entrance into the tympanum in an exactly similar manner to that already described in scarlet fever and measles, and have, as in those diseases, furnished the exciting cause of the otitis.

The presence of adenoids and enlarged tonsils in any individual who is attacked by one of the above infectious or contagious diseases adds greatly to the probability of an extension of the inflammatory process to the middle ear (see Chapter XX., p. 203).

An acute suppurative otitis media may be secondary to a traumatic injury to the drum membrane, following which an infection of the tympanic cavity takes place from the external auditory meatus, through the perforation. A tubotympanic catarrh in which spontaneous rupture of the drum membrane has taken place, or in which a paracentesis of the drum membrane has been made, may be followed by secondary infection of the tympanic cavity, and a purulent inflammation be thereby established in this cavity which was previously so mildly infected as to be comparatively but little diseased. Following a spontaneous rupture or an incision of the drum membrane in any case of non-infected middle-ear disease, a careless or indifferent mode of after-treatment on the part of the physician may quickly lead to infection of the drum cavity and to the establishment of the acute suppurative variety of the disease.

The most potent predisposing factor in the causation of this, as of the other acute middle-ear affections, is an inflamed nasopharynx or one that is occluded by growths, notably adenoids. The presence of this hypertrophy is productive of a retarded venous circulation of the Eustachian tube and middle ear, and of the secretion of a large amount of pathologic mucus. Nasopharyngeal obstruction furnishes both an ideal location and the most favorable conditions for the harboring and culture of these pathogenic micro-organisms which determine the character and severity of the different forms of inflammation which may occur within the middle ear.

Pathology.—The mucous membrane of the middle ear is more or less swollen, the subepithelial layer contains serous and round-cell infiltration, with more or less hemorrhage into the tissue. The infiltration spreads, according to the intensity and extent of the process, to the promontory, tegmen, and membrana tympani. The mucous membrane is bathed in pus or blood and pus mixed with bacteria. The process may involve the whole middle ear or only parts. By softening through necrosis, according to the intensity of the inflammation, the drum membrane gives way (see chapter on Bacteriology).

Symptoms.—The early symptoms of acute suppurative otitis media are much the same as in the catarrhal variety, the chief difference being the greater severity of those attending the suppurative disease. Thus, the pain is more severe and tearing, the temperature is higher, and the prostration of the patient is greater in the latter form. The temperature is nearly always slightly elevated, and may reach 102°, 103°, or even 104° F., and the pulse is correspondingly increased. After a continuance of the pain and fever for from one to three days the drum membrane ruptures and a yellowish discharge appears in the external auditory meatus. After the perforation takes place the pain completely subsides or is greatly modified, the patient sinks into the first sleep he has been permitted to enjoy since the onset of the pain, and both he and his friends are apt to believe that speedy recovery is assured. However, if the perforation is inadequate to provide perfect drainage or if it is badly located for this purpose, the pain very quickly returns and the suffering becomes almost if not quite as great as before. Tinnitus aurium and vertigo are usually present, but the intensity of the pain so obscures these symptoms that the individual makes no complaint in this respect until the pain has disappeared and the convalescent stage is entered upon; or in some cases not until the disease has become subacute or chronic.

When an acute suppurative otitis media results from an infective scarlatinal angina, it may come on at any time during the course of the disease, as early as the fifth day and as late as the thirty-fifth, from the onset of the scarlet fever. The most frequent period of the occurrence of the aural complication is the eighth to the tenth day of the primary disease. Either one or both ears may be involved, but if both are affected in the same case, usually an interval of from one to several days intervenes between the appearance of the discharge.

The symptoms of otitis media when occurring as a complication of scarlatina vary somewhat according to the stage of the general disease in which the otitis commences, and upon the severity of the fever and other symptoms present in the primary affection at the time. Thus, if the otitis occurs early, and therefore when the fever is high and the prostration of the patient very great, the symptoms denoting the onset of the aural complication may be so masked as to be completely overlooked until the discharge makes its appearance at the auditory meatus. Masking of the symptoms of otitis in infants and young children is common, and unless objective means of diagnosing the presence of the complication are frequently employed during the progress of the scarlet fever, the presence of the otitis will usually be entirely unrecognized at a period sufficiently early to enable the attending surgeon to institute the most effective treatment. Should the otitis occur during convalescence from the scarlet fever, and after the temperature has perhaps for several days been normal, the temperature will again suddenly rise and severe pain in the ear will be complained of by the patient. Immediately after rupture of the drum membrane or after a free incision has been made and the pent-up exudate of the tympanic cavity is set free, both the pain and fever usually subside.

Occurring as a complication of measles the otitis may develop early or late. When it appears early, and especially in the milder cases of measles, the tympanic complication is usually a catarrhal and not a suppurative otitis media, and is at this stage the result of the extension of the characteristic inflammation of measles from the throat to the middle ear. When, however, the tympanic complication occurs after the first week of the measles, it is then due to a streptococcic or staphylococcic infection of the middle ear, and suppuration, rupture of the drum-head, and subsequent aural discharge are the inevitable results.

The discharge is usually profuse at first, and in those severe cases where the destruction of tissue has been considerable it may continue so for many days, weeks, or even indefinitely. It is not offensive in odor and does not become so unless there is retention in some portion of the suppurating tract, or in the external auditory meatus after it has been discharged through the perforated membrane. In some instances the amount of the discharge is so great that it is at once recognized as impossible that all of it could be formed in so small a cavity as the middle ear alone. Politzer has stated that suppuration of the tympanic cavity is frequently accompanied by the presence of pus in the mastoid antrum, even when no symptom whatever of mastoiditis is present. Hence, it is always probable in cases of very profuse aural discharge that a portion of the pus is furnished by the cavity of the mastoid.

In case the mastoid antrum is involved and the drainage from it is poor, or in case the mastoid cells are infected and filled with suppurative products, and perfect drainage is therefore a physical impossibility, pain speedily develops in the mastoid region as the result of pus retention and subsequent intramastoid pressure. The onset of a complicating mastoiditis is, therefore, usually indicated by pain behind the ear, worse at night, and increased by pressure over certain areas of most frequent mastoid tenderness (see p. 281, Fig. 151). Any of the intracranial complications may follow an acute suppurative otitis media, and the possibility of such an occurrence should always be borne in mind, because the early symptoms of brain, meningeal, or sinus involvement are often obscure unless studied from day to day in their minutest detail. (For symptoms of Intracranial Complications see Chaps. XXXI.–XXXV.)

When acute suppurative otitis media results from a tuberculous deposit in the middle ear the disease runs its course up to the period of perforation of the tympanic membrane and subsequent discharge, without the development of any symptoms pointing to an aural affection. But little or no pain precedes the rupture of the membrana and no change in the temperature precedes or accompanies it. On the other hand, when occurring as a complication of a zymotic or other disease, the pain in the ear is intense, the temperature rises several degrees, and frequently symptoms of meningitis are developed. Enlargement of the cervical lymphatics is a symptom of some cases of acute suppurative otitis media, in which case the neck is stiff and painful upon pressure or when the patient moves or turns the head. If the whole chain of glands is infected and swollen the disease might be mistaken for the "sausage-like infiltration," which is said to accompany thrombosis of the lateral sinus and jugular vein, whereas if only the uppermost glands of the cervical chain are involved, the condition may somewhat resemble mumps.

The appearance of the drum membrane as seen by reflected light is not characteristic of this disease, for the infiltration and inflammatory discoloration and bulging may very closely resemble that which occurs during the acute catarrhal otitis or even a myringitis, in which latter the tympanic cavity is only rarely involved in the inflammatory process. However, the inflammation of the drum-head during an acute suppurative otitis media is oftenest seen to be more intense over Shrapnell's membrane and over the upper portion of the membrana vibrans than is the case in the other diseases just mentioned; and moreover in the latter disease the subsequent bulging of the parts from the pressure of the intratympanic exudate most often takes place in the upper quadrants of the membrana tympani. The membrane is always intensely and uniformly reddened, the landmarks are all obliterated with the possible exception of the short process, and in from twenty-four to forty-eight hours from the onset more or less bulging can usually be made out. Within from one to several days the pressure of the intratympanic fluid stretches the membrana at some point, weakens or impairs the circulation over some area, and as a result the membrane is ulcerated and finally gives way, allowing the pus to flow freely into the auditory canal. Previous to the occurrence of the rupture the height of the bulging area usually appears as a somewhat whitened or yellowish patch in the midst of the intensely reddened field (Fig. 148). After the rupture the pus is seen filling the auditory canal, and when this is mopped away by sterile cotton pledgets the point of rupture is often visible, a drop of pus is seen filling the opening, and this pulsates synchronously with the heart-beat.

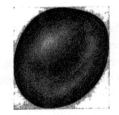

FIG. 148.—BULGING DRUM-HEAD WITH BEGINNING NE-CROSIS AT THE POINT OF GREAT-EST PRESSURE.

The shape of the perforation which has occurred spontaneously is slit-like at first and may run in any direction. After it has persisted for a time granulation takes place at the extremities of this slit, while dilatation occurs at the center, with the result that the opening usually takes on a circular form (see Fig. 194). In those cases complicating the infectious diseases in which the aural affection is violent, the greater portion of the membrana vibrans is sometimes quickly destroyed, leaving only a narrow margin at the annulus tympanicus. Should this have happened the inner tympanic wall will be seen through the large opening, but on account of the infiltrated and inflamed condition of the tympanic mucous membrane it may be mistaken for the drum membrane itself, and the true condition of the latter may therefore pass unrecognized. At the same time the membrana tympani is destroyed the ossicles, and especially the incus, may also suffer necrosis and be swept away together with other necrotic middle-ear structures. The handle of the malleus may still be recognized in its usual position, projecting like a peninsula downward and backward to the center of the field (see Fig. 191).

A small perforation always heals rapidly in otherwise healthy individuals, and will usually close permanently just as soon as the formation and discharge of pus has ceased. Indeed, in many instances the tendency of the opening is to close too rapidly, thereby blocking the discharge and bringing about the necessity for subsequent enlargement by a second incision. During the healing of the larger perforation, exuberant granulations often spring from the edges of the rupture, from a necrotic ossicle, or from a carious spot on some portion of one of the tympanic walls; and these when present can be seen, or at least felt, with the probe during the physical examination of the condition of the drum membrane. As the inflammation in the middle ear subsides and the perforation in the membrane heals, the inflammatory redness and thickness of the tympanic membrane are likewise seen to subside from day to day; and as the normal color and texture return, the landmarks reappear—first the short process of the malleus, then the manubrium, umbo, color, and light reflex, in the order mentioned. When the inflammation has almost disappeared, radiating injected vessels are sometimes seen coursing over the membrane. The very large openings which result from the loss of the greater portion of the drumhead remain permanently (see Fig. 197).

Diagnosis.—The diagnosis will usually not be difficult if the physician takes into account the history and symptoms of the case, the presence of an infection in the throat, or the coexistence of some one of the zymotic diseases in connection with the information he is able to obtain by an exacting physical examination of the drum membrane and middle ear. This affection is likely to be mistaken only for a myringitis, for acute catarrhal otitis media, or for a furunculosis of the external auditory canal. The differential diagnosis of these affections is given more concisely on p. 277, to which the reader is referred.

Early diagnosis of the tympanic complication of the specific infectious diseases is of the first importance for the reason that the best results from treatment of the same are only possible when such treatment is instituted at the very onset of the aural disease. It should be the rule, therefore, in any case of scarlet fever, measles, la grippe, or diphtheria to inspect the tympanic membrane of the patient from day to day; for, as has already been stated, aural complication in all these diseases is frequent, and the severity of the constitutional disease frequently so completely masks the tympanic·complication that the latter will often pass unrecognized unless the drum membrane is inspected daily by means of reflected light. Such an inspection in children is not always easy, and the interpretation of the appearances of the drum membrane is likely to be erroneous unless the patient is properly placed or held in position for such an examination, unless a good source of light is provided, and unless the examiner remembers that in an examination of the drum-head in the case of infants and the very young he must pull the auricle downward and backward, and not upward and backward, as should be the rule in adults (see Fig. 82).

The violence of the scarlatinal infection upon the tympanic structures is sometimes both rapid and extensive. Mastoiditis is frequently the result of an extension of the suppuration into the mastoid antrum and mastoid cells. Cases of necrosis of the labyrinth have been reported by Bezold, Pye, and many others. The necrotic extension of the disease within the temporal bone has, in a few instances, implicated the large blood-vessels in the immediate vicinity of the ear, resulting in a fatal hemorrhage. Hays and Hassler have each reported a case in which the carotid artery was eroded with an ensuing fatal hemorrhage. Baader narrates an instance of a child three years old suffering from scarlatinal otitis, in which death occurred from extension of the disease into the mastoid and with subsequent erosion of the sigmoid sinus. Huber, Kennedy, West, and Moller have collectively reported 6 cases of fatal bleeding as a result of the necrotic invasion of the carotid artery or lateral sinus subsequent to a scarlatinal involvement of the tympanic cavity.

Prognosis.—The termination of acute suppurative otitis media depends much upon the violence of the attack and upon the promptness and efficiency with which treatment is instituted. In those cases in which the onset is sudden and unusually severe from the first, extensive necrosis of both the soft and osseous structures of the tympanic cavity takes place so quickly that it is often impossible to successfully combat the destruction, and the result is a permanent loss of tissue and·a corresponding loss of function. When death takes place as a result of this disease, it usually does so from some intracranial complication which is set up because of the transportation of pathogenic bacteria into the cranial cavity, either through the blood or lymph currents or as the result of necrosis of the bone in the direction of the brain, and the direct admission of the septic fluid into the skull cavity. Such a complication may arise during the acute stage of the aural suppuration or it may occur at any subsequent period of the patient's life, should the acute disease become chronic.

The milder and more common forms of the affection, if permitted to continue untreated, will terminate differently, the difference depending greatly upon the patient's constitution, habitation, and mode of life. The tubercular case becomes quickly chronic and usually incurable. In the poorly nourished and badly housed individual who must perhaps resume his occupation in unfavorable weather and before the tympanic inflammation is cured, the disease will almost inevitably continue indefinitely, and finally become a chronic suppurative otitis. In children whose upper respiratory tract is obstructed by adenoids, recurrence of the suppurative inflammation of the middle ear is the rule, and ultimately more or less destruction of the drum membrane, or serious and permanent impairment of its function, as well as that of the middle ear, may be expected.

Early and well directed treatment influences the termination of this disease very greatly. When the patient is seen before serious necrosis of tissue has occurred, and a free outlet for the suppurative products is promptly provided and maintained, it may in all the milder cases be predicted with confidence that the inflammation will promptly subside, the discharge cease, the perforation heal, and that the hearing will be restored to normal or almost normal. In the very violent cases, however, the best directed and most vigorous treatment, even at the onset, will often be insufficient to prevent great loss of tissue and consequently a much impaired hearing. In these latter cases the question is often one of saving the life of the patient as well as of preserving the hearing apparatus, and the vigorous application of the known medical and surgical principles of modern otology in both these directions has proven to be one of the modern surgical triumphs.

Treatment.—Owing to the rapidity with which the purulent variety of otitis media often develops, and the widespread destruction of tissue that frequently follows, no time should be lost in meeting the earliest symptoms, combating the inflammation, and providing efficient drainage for the discharge. General depletion through the administration of salines, and local depletion by means of leeches about the ear, are more urgently needed here than in the catarrhal variety. These measures, when used in connection with heat applied locally to the ear, are often efficient in alleviating the pain; but since several hours may be required to affect the relief by this means, it is usually advisable in the beginning to administer a hypodermic injection of morphin to assist and prolong the effect. Owing to the fact, however, that under the continued use of morphin great destruction of tissue, or intracranial complication may occur and yet be unsuspected because of the apparent comfort of the patient, it is unsafe to repeat the remedy until the patient has been allowed to recover from its influence, and the physician has been given an opportunity to judge the condition of the case when free from the masking effect of the anodyne. The same local applications which were advocated for the relief of pain in acute catarrhal otitis (see p. 256) may also be applied to the inflamed drum membrane in this disease, but are not often efficient in relieving the suffering of the patient. Abortion of the disease by the foregoing procedures, even when applied at the earliest possible moment, is seldom to be expected, but modification of the severity of the inflammation and a certain degree of relief from the suffering is frequently accomplished.

Incision of the drum membrane is early indicated in a majority of all cases. When after the early employment of local and general depletion, of heat and anesthetic medicines to the membrana, the pain continues unabated or but little relieved, this fact is evidence of an inflammatory pressure within the tympanum which is due to engorgement of the lining membrane, or to the pressure of an exudate that has already taken place within this cavity. If paracentesis is not promptly performed, spontaneous rupture will sooner or later take place; but during the period of waiting for a spontaneous rupture the patient's suffering is not only intense, but pressure necrosis of the tympanic structures is meanwhile taking place, and the process if unchecked may spread to the mastoid antrum, mastoid cells, or even to the intracranial structures. If, therefore, the symptoms indicate that the middle-ear infection is of a violent nature, and the aural examination shows inflammation and infiltration of the drum membrane, a free incision should be made at once, even if only a few hours have elapsed since the onset of the disease. Experience has shown that early and free incision of the drum-head in these cases lessens the duration of the disease, shortens the period of suffering, and is the most reliable means of preventing mastoid or other complications.[1]

[1] Concerning the relation between an early incision of the drum membrane and the closure of the perforation, Körner states that as a result of paracentesis on the first day of the disease, closure of the perforation occurred on the seventh day; on the second day in 13 cases, closure occurred on the ninth day; on the third day in 8 cases, perforation closed on the fourteenth day; on the fourth day in 9 cases, perforation closed in fifteen days; on the fifth day in 13 cases, perforation closed on the sixteenth day;

18

The incision in the membrana should always be of sufficient extent to give free vent to the suppurative products of the middle ear. A mere puncture of the membrane with a "paracentesis needle" (see Fig. 142) is a procedure too trivial to merit consideration and is mentioned merely that it may be condemned. When the incision is undertaken before bulging of the membrane has occurred, the cut should be made by first penetrating this structure in the posterosuperior quadrant at a point opposite the short process of the hammer, and with the edge of the knife turned upward the blade is pushed inward until the point penetrates the mucous membrane covering the internal wall of the tympanic cavity, after which the instrument is carried upward in such manner that both the membrana tympani and mucous membrane are severed as far as the tympanic ring; and it is even better if the incision is then carried through the skin of the adjacent meatus for a short distance toward the concha, as the knife is withdrawn (see Fig. 143, E, F). When performed thus early a discharge of pus should not be expected to follow immediately, for the reason that it has not yet formed; but a free

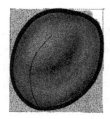

hemorrhage should be secured as a result of the incision, and this is of benefit for the reason that the engorged blood-vessels are thereby unloaded, the swelling of the mucous membrane is reduced, and the previous acute pain is greatly relieved because of the lessened tension within the blood-vessels.

FIG. 149.—SHOWING LINE OF INCISION.

Should the patient be seen at a later period, after pus has already accumulated in the middle-ear cavity, and when bulging of some portion of the drum membrane is apparent on examination (see Fig. 148), the incision is made so as to include the summit of the bulging, and is then extended to the lowermost portion of the tympanic cavity (Fig. 149).

The treatment subsequent to the incision depends somewhat upon the stage of the disease at which the opening is made. Following an incision during the first few hours of the inflammation, when no pus is yet present, and when depletion has been the primary object, it is not proper to irrigate the canal with any sort of solution; for if the external auditory canal had been properly sterilized before the paracentesis was made, better results will follow the insertion of a sterile gauze wick to the bottom of the canal (Fig. 146), and then applying the roller bandage

when paracentesis was done on the sixth day in 4 cases, healing of drum membrane took place on the twenty-fourth day; when the incision was performed on the seventh day the average time of closure in 20 cases was twenty-six days.

as previously described for the treatment of acute catarrhal otitis media (see p. 259, Fig. 146). If, however, pus is present in quantity at the time of the incision, better results will be secured by frequent irrigation of the auditory canal with one of the milder antiseptic ear solutions, after the plan already pointed out.

During the progress of the disease subsequent to spontaneous rupture or incision of the membrana, the latter structure should be frequently examined by means of the aural speculum and reflected light, when the amount of infiltration of the parts and the color of the drum membrane should be carefully noted. The size of the perforation should also be observed, and if found to be closing too rapidly, at the same time that pain and fever returns, a secondary incision should be performed at once. It sometimes happens, owing to the anatomical arrangement of the mucous folds found in the attic, or to the formation of adhesions that wall off one portion of the tympanic cavity from another, that a pocket of pus will form independently of the main tympanic cavity, and, therefore, a good opening may be seen through the membrana, whereas fever and pain will continue as a result of the retention of pus in the unopened pocket. In such case a careful examination will be sufficient to detect the bulging area, which should be freely incised and drained.

Those suffering from this disease should usually remain in doors and, during the height of the inflammation, in bed. During the height of the inflammation of the middle-ear tract the mucous membrane is hypersensitive to the temperature changes to which the patient is exposed should he be allowed to be up and around, a fact which is frequently demonstrated by exacerbations of the disease which follow even the most trivial exposure. Stuffy, overheated, and poorly ventilated quarters are to be avoided, whereas an equable temperature and a well-ventilated room are conducive to the best results. The patient should lie, after perforation or rupture of the drum membrane, upon the affected side and with the face somewhat downward, since this position favors the most perfect drainage. Systemic medication and local treatment of the nose and throat are always helpful and often most essential, and should be carried out after the plans detailed in another section of the work. The treatment of mastoiditis, which frequently accompanies or follows this disease, is also given in Chapter XXV.

In case the disease is first seen at a later stage, or should failure to cure have resulted from employment of the above measures, the use of astringents in the middle ear often prove beneficial and arrest the progress of the ailment before it has become chronic. The most efficient of this class of remedies is silver nitrate, but in order to secure the best results from its use certain rules must be followed. In the first place the irrigating solutions that have been previously used must be washed away with distilled water and the auditory canal afterward dried; catheter inflation of the middle ear should be performed and the fluid contents of whatever nature should be blown through the perforation into the external auditory canal, and mopped away by means of cotton cylinders. Silver solution should not be used stronger than 5 gr. to the ounce in the beginning. The patient lies upon a cot with the diseased ear uppermost, a few drops of the silver lotion are dropped into the canal, and the auricle is then retracted and the canal straightened by lifting the pinna upward and backward with one hand, while with the other the tragus is pressed into the concha repeatedly, so as to force the drops through the perforation into the tympanic cavity. By means of this manipulation the lotion is driven into all the recesses of the middle ear and quickly penetrates through the Eustachian tube into the nasopharynx. When the perforation in the drum membrane is quite small the employment of this procedure is unsuccessful and the opening should be enlarged by an incision. The silver solution may also be carried into the cavum tympani by means of a properly constructed aural pipette, the end of which is passed through the perforation, after which 2 or 3 drops of the solution are expressed. After the introduction of the silver by either of these methods, any excess of the solution should be syringed out of the canal, normal salt solution being used for this purpose. This not only neutralizes the further action of the silver but also prevents the discoloration of the visible portions of the ear, a most objectionable feature of silver preparations unless some such preventive measures as are here mentioned are employed. In cases where the discharge has been kept up by the presence of superficial ulceration of the soft parts, the use of this antiseptic and astringent frequently brings about a speedy cure. On the other hand, if deep-seated destruction of the soft tissues has occurred, and the ossicles or bony walls of the tympanic cavity are exposed, carious or necrotic, great benefit need scarcely be expected from this remedy, and the disease becomes chronic unless rational operative measures are instituted for the removal of the diseased areas.

Since efficient treatment of the acute tympanic affections depends in such large measure upon a correct diagnosis of the particular variety of the disease which may be present in any case, the following table of the leading symptoms present in each may prove helpful in a study of the subject.

DIFFERENTIAL DIAGNOSIS OF ACUTE TUBOTYMPANIC CATARRH, ACUTE CATARRHAL OTITIS MEDIA, AND ACUTE SUPPURATIVE OTITIS MEDIA

	Acute Tubotympanic Catarrh	Acute Catarrhal Otitis Media	Acute Suppurative Otitis Media
Pain.	Absent in the ear; usually amounts only to a sense of soreness in throat, as of foreign body. More or less pain along course of Eustachian tube.	Severe in depths of the ear, radiating over side of head. Worse on lying down. Pain increased by blowing nose or cough.ng.	Very severe, of lancinating, tearing variety. Increased by recumbent position, by coughing, sneezing, blowing of the nose, etc.
Fever.	Absent, unless the tubotympanic catarrh is secondary to some other ailment, as a mild form of measles, which primary disease gives rise to the fever.	Temperature usually elevated, 100°-101° F. in infants and young children.	Ranges from 102° to 104° F., the height of temperature depending much upon the presence of some general disease, as measles, scarlet fever, or la grippe.
Deafness.	Moderate. Patient complains of great deafness, however, largely because of the suddenness of onset.	Very considerable in affected ear.	Very great in affected ear. Patient very deaf when both ears are involved.
Prostration of patient.	None.	Usually moderate. Sometimes considerable.	Often very great.
Tinnitus, vertigo, etc.	Present and often severe.	Head noises not a prominent symptom except in later stages, after the pain and fever have subsided. Vertigo and nausea rare.	If present in beginning are so masked by severe pain that they are not mentioned. Sometimes present during convalescence.
Drum membrane.	Greatly retracted in first stage, less so in second stage. Inflammation absent, vessels along handle of malleus sometimes injected. After exudation into the tympanic cavity has occurred, a dark, or sometimes a light line may be seen crossing membrane, and indicating level of fluid. All landmarks present.	Little or not at all retracted at onset, later is bulging over some quadrant. Injected at first, and later a diffuse uniform redness covers whole membrane. Landmarks usually all obliterated with possible exception of short process of the malleus.	Intensely reddened, especially in upper portion; swollen, bulging, opaque. Landmarks all obliterated. Drum membrane may be largely destroyed during first two or three days.
Perforation.	Drum membrane seldom ruptured.	Drum membrane usually perforated after from one to three days.	Always present after first two or three days.
Discharge.	None except after paracentesis.	Thin seromucous discharge immediately after rupture or paracentesis. May later become purulent from infection.	Sanguinopurulent at moment of perforation, purulent later. Usually very profuse.
Tympanic cavity.	Rarefied in first stage. In second stage frequently contains a yellowish serum, or ropy mucoid exudate, which is visible through non-inflamed membrana tympani.	Contains seromucous exudate, which bulges membrane, but is not visible through inflamed membrane.	Contains pus. Mucous membrane greatly swollen, with necrotic areas in worst cases. Incus and hammer sometimes carious.
Tympanic inflation.	Not painful. Immediate and marked improvement results to hearing.	Painful. Little or no improvement in hearing, except in later stages.	Painful, and should seldom be performed during height of inflammation.
History.	Usually accompanies or follows a cold in the head or a nasopharyngitis. May result from mild attacks of exanthemata or tonsillitis.	Accompanies or follows the exanthemata of moderate severity, and the acute tonsillar and nasopharyngeal inflammations.	Follows or accompanies the more violent forms of the exanthemata, la grippe, ulcerative tonsillitis, diphtheria, etc.
Mastoid complication.	Never occurs.	Seldom occurs.	Frequently occurs.

CHAPTER XXIV

ACUTE MASTOIDITIS

ACUTE inflammation of the osseous structures of the mastoid process may take place at any time during the progress of an acute otitis media, especially of the suppurative variety. During certain epidemics of the exanthematous diseases and of la grippe the mastoid complication has been known to occur with great frequency. Extension of an acute suppurative inflammation of the middle ear to the mastoid antrum and the adjoining cellular labyrinth of the mastoid process, is in all cases an occurrence of more or less gravity, adds very much to the suffering of the patient, and greatly decreases both the immediate and remote chances of recovery. The affection, therefore, presents one of the most important of the several diseases which arise in the temporal bone, and which have a common origin in an existing suppurative process within the tympanic cavity.

Causation.—Acute mastoiditis is in nearly every instance secondary to a previous infection and suppuration of the tympanic cavity. It has been estimated that not over 1 per cent. of all the cases of this disease originate in the mastoid antrum itself, and of this small number nearly all cases of primary mastoiditis are due to traumatism. Certain general diseases, and local nose and throat affections, are primarily responsible for acute mastoiditis. Among the former may be mentioned scarlatina, measles, diphtheria, and la grippe; while among the latter, quinsy and the different varieties of tonsillitis may be cited. In general it may be stated that the more violently severe the middle-ear infection, the more likely is a mastoid inflammation to follow as a complication.

Inefficient drainage of a suppurative middle ear must be counted among the most potent determining causes of mastoiditis. When the provision for the outflow of pus is inadequate, either because the rupture through the drum membrane is too small or because the incision was not sufficiently extensive, pus is retained in the tympanic cavity under more or less pressure, and some of it must inevitably find its way into the mastoid antrum where a secondary focus of infection is established. In view of the fact that the cavities of the mastoid antrum and middle ear lie in such open communication with each other (Fig. 150), it is quite

278

probable that in all cases of tympanic suppuration in which the drainage is not entirely free, that pus from the middle ear finds its way into the mastoid antrum, and that as a result mastoiditis is quickly established unless the tympanic drainage is speedily improved.

The greatly lowered vitality of the patient who suffers from a severe attack of aural suppuration is without question a factor in the establishment of a mastoiditis, for when an individual has undergone great pain as the result of some general disease, in which a middle-ear suppuration has also taken place, the mucous lining of the mastoid antrum is undoubtedly less resisting to the invasion of pathogenic bacteria than is the case when the tympanic inflammation results from some local affection of the throat, in which less pain and constitutional disturbance is manifest.

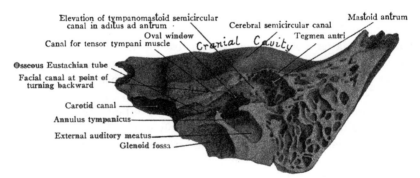

FIG. 150.—SECTION OF TEMPORAL BONE IN PLANE OF MASTOID ANTRUM. ADITUS, TYMPANUM, AND EUSTACHIAN TUBE, SHOWING DIRECT CONNECTION OF ALL THESE SPACES.

Diagnosis.—The diagnosis of acute mastoiditis must be determined by the physical condition of the patient; by the manifestation of the presence of underlying disease as indicated by external changes in the tissues over the mastoid and around the external ear; by the physical changes that have taken place at the bottom of the auditory canal, and in the drum membrane and middle ear, as shown by actual inspection of these parts by means of reflected light and the use of instruments when necessary.

1. *The Physical Condition of the Patient.*—In most instances of acute mastoiditis it will be found that the middle-ear suppuration which is responsible for the mastoid complication has been of more than the average violence, and that, unless the mastoiditis developed soon after the beginning of the middle-ear involvement, the patient is more greatly prostrated than would have been the case had the sole disease been nothing more than a simple aural inflammation. In cases where the

extension of the inflammation to the mastoid occurs several days after the beginning of the tympanic disease, it is usually found that the discharge from the ear has at no time since its appearance shown any tendency to lessen, or if it has done so, that there was at once set up, as a result of the pus retention, a decided increase of pain in the ear and over the temporal region. Anemia, due to the continued and severe pain, with the consequent loss of sleep and disturbed digestion, is often so marked as to be suggestive of a more serious affection than a simple otitis media. The temperature may vary greatly in different cases and during the different stages of the same case. When the mastoiditis comes on during the continuance of the general disease which is responsible for the middle-ear suppuration, the temperature may reach 103° F. or even 105° F. In such instance, however, the high temperature is due largely to the causative general disease, as, for instance, measles, scarlatina, or la grippe, and not so much to the complicating mastoiditis. Should this latter complication arise subsequently to the subsidence of the general disease, as is often the case, the temperature may be but little or not at all elevated. Mastoiditis in which considerable destruction of tissue has resulted is sometimes observed in cases in which the temperature remains normal. In the case of infants or very young children the temperature may be considerably elevated at the beginning of the mastoid complication, whereas subsequently there may be a normal or even subnormal temperature, even though a large postaural abscess is present.

2. *The External Manifestations Over the Mastoid Region.*—Swelling of the soft tissues over the mastoid region occurs only after the pus which has collected in the mastoid cells has ruptured through the exterior bony walls, or after an inflammation and infiltration of the soft structures which cover the bony cortex has taken place as a result of the transportation of septic material from the infected interior, through the vascular channels, to these superficial structures. A postauricular tumefaction should, therefore, not be expected to occur as a result of mastoiditis until the suppuration has existed in the mastoid process for several days. Such a swelling does not occur at all in many cases even though the mastoiditis continues into the chronic form. The author has repeatedly found both the mastoid cells and antrum filled with pus at the time of the mastoid operation, when not the slightest external swelling had previously existed to indicate its presence. Swelling above and behind the auricle sometimes occurs as a complication of either a circumscribed or diffuse external otitis. As has already been pointed out in the chapters on these subjects, either a boil or a general

inflammation of the external auditory canal will, when severe, often be accompanied by a tumefaction behind the auricle which is sufficient to cause protrusion of the ear and to give a deformed appearance to the individual's head. To the casual observer this condition looks identical to that produced by the postaural swelling which sometimes takes place during a mastoiditis (see Fig. 181), but the examiner can usually differentiate the one from the other if he will only remember that manipulation of the auricle is accompanied by very severe pain in case the swelling is due to an inflammation which is located in the external auditory canal, whereas if it be due to an underlying suppuration of

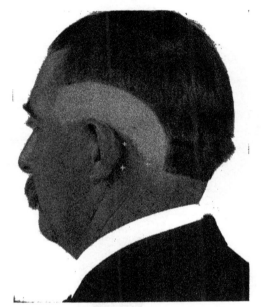

FIG. 151.—POINTS OF MASTOID TENDERNESS IN ACUTE MASTOIDITIS.
The uppermost X is over the site of the mastoid antrum, the lower one is over the mastoid tip, and the posterior one is over the point of exit of the mastoid vein. The hair of the whole head is clipped close and the mastoid region is closely shaved preparatory to the mastoid operation.

the bone, as is the case in mastoiditis, the auricle can be retracted or otherwise handled without causing the slightest suffering to the patient.

Mastoid tenderness is almost constantly present, but except in the more severe cases, and where there is an accompanying periosteal inflammation over the mastoid process, this tenderness is usually confined to three small postauricular areas. The first and most common point of tenderness can be covered by the ball of the finger and lies directly over the site of the mastoid antrum. As will be seen by the external markings which indicate the position of this cavity, and as

shown upon the surface of the skull by the suprameatal triangle
(see Fig. 165), this area lies just behind the attachment of the auricle
and slightly above the posterosuperior border of the external meatus.
The second area of greatest tenderness is over, and sometimes beneath,
the tip of the mastoid process (Fig. 151). The third point of tenderness
lies over the exit of the mastoid vein (Fig. 151). In that type of mastoid
process in which the mastoid cells are large, and consequently lie near
the surface (Fig. 152), the amount of pain resulting from deep pressure
over the mastoid tip, especially during the height of the suppurative

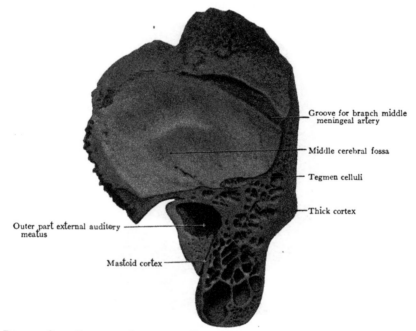

Groove for branch middle
meningeal artery

Middle cerebral fossa

Tegmen celluli

Thick cortex

Outer part external auditory
meatus

Mastoid cortex

FIG. 152.—OUTER PORTION OF A SECTION OF THE TEMPORAL BONE ON A PLANE EXTERNAL TO THE TYMPANIC
CAVITY AND MASTOID ANTRUM.
Specimen shows large cells at the mastoid tip. Bezold's abscess is favored by this type of mastoid.

period, is usually very considerable. On the contrary, if the bony cortex
is thick, and the mastoid cells are but slightly developed (Fig. 153), the
tenderness on pressure may be correspondingly less marked. In testing
any of the above situations for tenderness, the pressure of the examining
finger should be firm and prolonged for a few seconds. Rude manipulation in the examination of the mastoid is apt to be painful, even when
the underlying structures are entirely normal, and some individuals
are so unduly sensitive to pressure exerted over this region that the
rule should be followed in all instances of suspected mastoiditis to make

exactly similar pressure over the mastoid of the healthy side, for by exercising this precaution the examiner is able to determine whether or not the pain elicited by the examination of the presumably diseased mastoid is or is not normal. In testing the sensibility of the mastoid tip it is essential to hook the finger around the lower end of this projection and into the digastric fossa as much as possible, in order that the desired pressure may be exerted in an upward direction and against the large cellular space that often fills the point of the apophysis (see Fig. 152). By carefully executing this procedure exquisite tenderness is

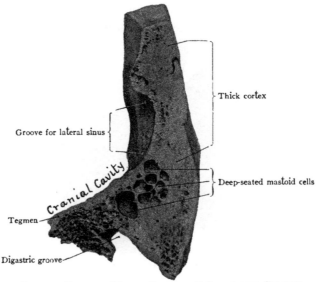

Thick cortex

Groove for lateral sinus

Cranial Cavity

Deep-seated mastoid cells

Tegmen

Digastric groove

FIG. 153.—SECTION OF MASTOID POSTERIOR TO STYLOMASTOID FORAMEN.
Note the thick cortex and the comparatively thin tegmen. Compare this drawing with Fig. 152.

sometimes discovered that would otherwise have been entirely overlooked.

3. *Changes that Have Taken Place at the Inner End of the Auditory Canal, in the Membrana Tympani, and in the Middle Ear Itself, which May be Determined Only by a Thorough Examination of the Depths of the Ear.*—The upper and posterior portion of the inner end of the external auditory meatus lies in close relation to the adjoining cellular structure of the mastoid process. It follows, therefore, that when the adjacent cells of this process are distended by inflammatory exudate or pus that sagging of this portion of the canal wall will take place (Fig. 154). Such a swelling of the inner end of the meatal wall is not constantly present in acute mastoiditis but in the author's cases has been

observed in a majority of instances. Numerous authors have spoken of this sagging, when present, as a pathognomonic symptom of mastoiditis.

A perforation in the tympanic membrane will most likely be present in one of the superior quadrants, and in the acute cases of mastoiditis the rupture is usually small and therefore provides inefficient drainage for the rather considerable suppurating area beyond. When the bead of pus which fills the opening is mopped away by means of a cotton-tipped applicator, another will be seen to take its place almost immediately, the discharge thus appearing much more profuse than in uncomplicated cases of otitis media purulenta. Politzer has called attention to a pulsating light reflex which may frequently be seen on the drop of pus which fills the perforation, and he believes that when

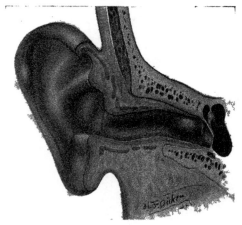

Fig. 154.—Sagging of the Posterosuperior Wall at the Inner End of the External Auditory Meatus, the Result of Mastoid Suppuration in the Adjacent Pneumatic Cells of the Mastoid. Compare location of the sagging with tumefaction of canal due to furuncle (see Fig. 74).

this pulsation continues to be present after the continuance of the discharge for a period of two weeks from the date of the rupture of the drum-head, that the same is indicative of a complicating mastoid abscess. The author has confirmed this belief in many instances, and attaches considerable importance, in a diagnostic way, to the presence of the pulsating reflex, especially if present in conjunction with other symptoms.

In those violent middle-ear suppurations which so often complicate scarlet fever, the middle ear, mastoid antrum, and mastoid cells are, no doubt, frequently involved simultaneously, as in such instances it is not uncommon to find that the drum membrane and ossicles have been entirely swept away, thus providing for ample drainage, but not before necrosis of the soft and bony tissues of the middle ear and mastoid have taken place.

Not all or even a majority of the above diagnostic points are found in every case of acute mastoid suppuration. Those upon which most reliance is usually placed are: tenderness upon pressure over the site of the antrum, mastoid tip, and exit of the mastoid vein, the presence of a profuse unchecked discharge, the pulsating light reflex at the point of rupture in the drum membrane, and the sagging of the posterosuperior meatal wall. In any case in which the discharge from the ear is profuse and persists beyond two weeks without perceptibly diminishing in quantity, when the pain is unduly severe, interfering with sleep at night, and when there is more fever and general prostration than should accompany an uncomplicated middle-ear suppuration, acute mastoiditis may, with reasonable certainty, be diagnosed even though postauricular swelling and tenderness are not present.

Prognosis.—The termination of acute mastoidits is nearly always favorable provided the present well-known and efficient means of treatment are applied sufficiently early. Left untreated, it is sometimes a fatal malady. Politzer has demonstrated that pus is present in the pneumatic spaces of the mastoid process in most cases of suppuration of the middle ear, and a study of the anatomic relation of the labyrinth of cavities—the middle ear, mastoid antrum, and mastoid cells—clearly shows the likelihood of such an occurrence in any case. The mere presence of pus in the mastoid cells does not, however, constitute a mastoiditis, for it is only when the parts are greatly inflamed and suppurating and the pus is retained under pressure that the disease under consideration may be said to be present. Many of the milder mastoid inflammations subside after the establishment of better drainage through the perforated drum membrane, the inflammatory deposits which have already taken place within the cellular structure of the mastoid being in time fully removed by absorption. If, however, the drainage from the cells into the mastoid antrum, from the antrum into the middle ear, and finally from this latter cavity through the perforated tympanic membrane is at any point seriously impeded, the pus retention may result in pressure necrosis, and consequent rupture of the pus through the bony walls may take place (a) outwardly upon the external surface of the mastoid, producing a subperiosteal abscess behind the auricle (Fig. 181); (b) through the tegmen tympani into the middle cranial fossa, causing a cerebral abscess (Fig. 155); (c) backward into the cerebellar space or lateral sinus with cerebellar abscess formation, or lateral sinus thrombosis (Fig. 155), and finally (d) rupture into the digastric fossa with escape of pus into the tissues of the neck, and giving rise to a Bezold's abscess (see Figs. 179 and 180). Infection of the cranial contents through a fistula caused by necrosis of the intervening tissues is rare in acute middle-ear suppuration. Rupture of the pus outward upon the mastoid surface or into the digastric fossa is much more common.

The lymphatic and venous communications between the structures of the temporal bone and cranium are intimate, and septic material is sometimes carried to the brain and its coverings through these channels, the result being a localized or general meningitis, a cerebral or cerebellar abscess. Thrombosis of either the superior or inferior petrosal vein or of the sigmoid sinus may also result from the adjacent mastoid suppuration. While these intracranial complications are by no means rare, they do not follow the acute aural suppurations nearly so frequently as is the case in the chronic forms of mastoid disease.

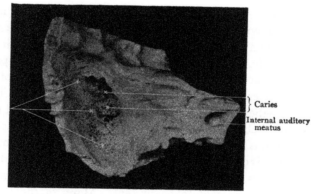

Axis of sinus groove

} Caries

Internal auditery meatus

FIG. 155.—CARIES OF SIGMOID SINUS GROOVE.
External cortex of antrum. Phlebitis of lateral and petrosal sinuses and jugular meningitis. (Warren Museum, Harvard Medical School. J. Orne Green Collection.)

A frequent termination of acute mastoiditis is the establishment of the chronic variety, which will be subsequently described.

Treatment.—The management of this disease is abortive and operative. If seen in the very beginning and it is intelligently treated by the physician, many of the milder acute mastoid inflammations are undoubtedly aborted or cured by means other than the mastoid operation. Free drainage through the middle ear and perforated drum membrane is absolutely essential to a subsidence of the inflammatory state of the mastoid antrum and cells. The first duty of the attendant is, therefore, to ascertain by a most careful examination of the fundus of the ear the location and size of the perforation in the tympanic membrane, and if this is not already sufficiently large or is not favorably situated, to immediately perform a free paracentesis. Following this procedure a sterile gauze wick is inserted directly against the drum membrane in order to more efficiently empty the tympanic cavity of its pent-up contents (see p. 259, Fig. 146).

It has in the past been a common practise to apply, in all cases of mastoiditis, an ice-bag (Fig. 156), to the postauricular region, leaving the same on constantly for a period of from one to several days. More recently dry heat applied by means of the hot-water bottle has had its advocates. Either cold or heat when continuously applied in this way for twenty-four or thirty-six hours will produce a sedative effect on the pain, and in the earliest stages of the ailment, no doubt, acts favorably upon the inflammatory process. The question as to which of the two, heat or cold, shall be applied in any given case, should be largely determined by the individual preference of the patient. Whichever one is used should not be kept on continuously for more than twenty-four hours, or at most thirty-six hours, for the reason that the benumbing effect which is produced will often so mask the necrotic progress of the disease within the bone that both the attending physician and the patient may believe that all is well, whereas the exactly opposite condition possibly prevails. Therefore after either of these measures has been applied continuously for a day, the same should be discontinued for one night, when if the pain returns in its former severity, the fact would be highly significant of an unfavorable progress. On the other hand, if the former

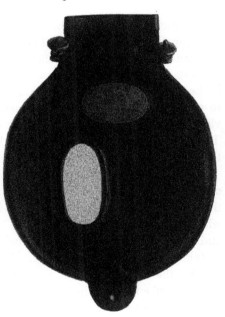

FIG. 156.—SPRAGUE'S AURAL ICE OR HOT-WATER BAG.

suffering does not return at all or only mildly, this fact, taken in connection with the coincident betterment of other conditions should be looked upon favorably, and the mastoid heat or cold may be again employed.

The use of morphin or other form of opiate is sometimes advisable and at times urgently demanded. The patient should not be kept under its continuous influence for the same reason that has just been given in the case of the prolonged applications of heat or cold. However, the author believes it advisable at the onset of acute mastoiditis, if the accompanying pain is severe, to administer a small hypodermic of morphin, which should not be repeated until sufficient time has elapsed for its full effects to have passed off, at which time the amount of mastoid pain can again be noted independent of the masking influence of an opiate or local application. Applications of iodin, the inunction of mercurials, or the use of blisters over the mastoid surface are not advisable, especially after the first few hours subsequent to the onset of the mastoiditis. The application of a blister should especially be condemned for the reason that it creates so much external soreness that subsequent examinations are interfered with, and the pain resulting from the blister will be so confused with that which is due to the mastoid inflammation that an intelligent estimate of the progress of the disease is subsequently impossible.

Mention need scarcely be made of the requirement that a patient suffering from mastoiditis shall remain indoors and preferably in bed. The suppurating middle ear should receive the same attention, as concerns its irrigation and other medication, that has already been outlined in the chapter on Acute Suppurative Otitis Media (see p. 272). Attention to the alimentary and digestive tracts, if the same has not been previously given, is early indicated in the complication under consideration. The bowels should be emptied by the administration of salines and the patient should be put upon a limited but nourishing diet.

In the event the patient fails to improve as a result of the application of the foregoing measures, or grows worse during the continuance of this treatment, the mastoid operation is indicated. The length of time which should be devoted to efforts directed to aborting the disease and rendering mastoid surgery unnecessary varies with each case or, certainly, with each type of case. In some the inflammatory invasion is from the onset so violent that the cellular structure of the mastoid may be broken down, the cortex perforated, and a subperiosteal abscess form within a week, whereas in the milder forms such an event may be delayed for months or may never take place, the mastoiditis continuing into the chronic form and the patient subsequently suffering only from the annoyance incident to a chronic discharging ear. In the fulminating variety of the disease it is unwise to delay operative measures longer than two or three days or at most a week after a thorough examination has demonstrated the extension of the disease to the mastoid process. The less violent cases may be treated for a week or ten days in the hope that subsidence of the inflammation may take place, and yet the author believes that both the present and future safety and comfort of the patient is usually best served by opening the mastoid and securing perfect drainage at an earlier date. The opinion held by some writers that one should wait for the appearance of redness and swelling behind the ear or for intracranial or other danger signals before resorting to surgical measures for relief, is entirely unwise, unsurgical, and unsafe, since, as has already been seen, a postauricular tumefaction usually denotes that perforation of the cortex has already taken place with escape of pus to the subperiosteal tissues, and intracranial disease would certainly point to a transfer of septic material directly through a rupture into the cranial cavity or indirectly by means of the vascular communication. An early mastoid operation in cases where it is clearly a justifiable procedure has the double advantage of checking further destruction, by the disease, of the middle-ear structures, and of preventing further and dangerous complications. The effect of this

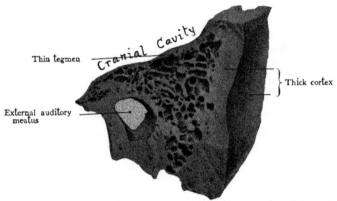

Fig. 157.—Section of Temporal Bone External to Tympanic Cavity and Mastoid Antrum. Showing marked contrast in the thickness of bone which separates the exterior of the skull from the cells and that which separates the cranial cavity from the cells.

operation in the way of arresting the tympanic suppuration and the consequent preservation of function in the affected ear, is in most cases so notable that the mastoid operation, if performed to secure these results alone, is often justifiable (see p. 308).

A study of the anatomic environs of the mastoid structures will show (Figs. 152 and 157) that the thickness of the bone covering these cells externally is as great and, in most cases much greater, than that which separates the cells from the middle-cranial fossa above, and from the sigmoid sinus posteriorly, and that, therefore, the pressure necrosis which occurs as a result of the pent-up pus within the mastoid cells is as apt· to take place brainward as outward. The sacrifice to life by operative procrastination in those clearly operative cases of mastoid suppuration must, even at the present time, be very considerable.

19

CHAPTER XXV

THE MASTOID OPERATION FOR ACUTE MASTOIDITIS

THE operation here described differs in so many important respects from the radical mastoid operation, which is performed for the cure of chronic mastoiditis, that the author believes a clearer understanding concerning the technic, and the extent and purpose of each procedure may be imparted by describing each one separately. What is said, therefore, in this chapter pertains only to the surgical methods applicable to acute mastoiditis, whereas the radical mastoid operation is discussed in another section of the work (see Chapter XXX.).

Preparation of the Patient.—On the evening preceding the operation, unless the bowels have already been thoroughly cleansed, sufficient saline should be given to secure one or more watery stools. The evening meal should consist of bouillon, milk, or other liquid food, and no breakfast whatever should be allowed on the morning of the operation. If pain is present of sufficient intensity to interfere with sleep during the previous night, the administration of morphin hypodermically is indicated, and its use in securing needed rest will add much to the patient's resisting powers, both at the time of the operation and during the subsequent treatment.

An examination of the heart, lungs, and urine ought to be made the previous day in order that the anesthetic to be given may be selected with intelligence. If the heart is sound, chloroform is preferable, for the reason that bleeding is much less profuse during its administration than is the case when ether is used. The hemorrhage itself is usually of little consequence, but as the wound deepens during the progress of the operation, the capillary oozing that takes place from every quarter during ether anesthesia often so obscures the operative field as to greatly delay the work or to render its progress somewhat hazardous. Especially is this true in those cases where the soft tissues around the ear are greatly congested and swollen at the time of the operation, and it is in just such instances that the use of chloroform, when not contraindicated, is most helpful. Chloroform should also be given if bronchitis is present or if the urine contains albumin or casts. If, however, the heart's action is irregular or feeble or if valvular lesions are present, ether is much safer, and the possibilities of annoyance from bleeding during its administration should not interfere with its employment.

The hair should be shaved from the head of the affected side for a distance of from 2½ to 3 inches around the attachment of the auricle (see Fig. 151). If the patient be a man, it is advisable to have the remaining hair of the head cut short with clippers. Women often object to extensive removal of the hair, but no such objection should be permitted to influence the operator to attempt so important a surgical procedure without first having provided a clean surgical field; and this can only be accomplished by clearing the hair from an area at least as far from the auricle as above designated. If the surgical necessity for this measure is fully explained to the patient all objection to this plan of preparation of the operative field is usually withdrawn. The remaining hair of the female head should be combed horizontally over the crown and tightly braided upon the opposite side, since this disposition of it has proven effective in keeping it well away from the wound during the operation and at subsequent treatments.

When shaved, the parts adjoining the auricular attachment are scrubbed with soap and water, the external auditory meatus is syringed with bichlorid solution (1:4000), a sterile gauze wick is inserted to the bottom, and a bichlorid gauze dressing is applied over all, and held in place by a roller bandage (Fig. 255). This dressing is not removed until the patient is anesthetized, when the parts are again scrubbed with tincture of green soap and water, then rubbed with ether, and this is in turn followed by an alcohol bath. A rubber cap or a wet sterile towel should cover the balance of the hairy scalp, and sterile towels are placed over the chest and about the neck.

. Operations upon the mastoid process for the relief and cure of acute mastoiditis should if possible be made in a well-appointed hospital. This is, however, frequently not possible, and in such instances careful antiseptic preparations should be made at the home of the patient. Excellent results are often obtained after the home operations, provided aseptic conditions are assured and a good light can be provided for the performance of the work.

Two assistants and a nurse are necessary. The first assistant constantly watches the progress of every step of the work; he removes the chips of bone the instant they are detached, and he keeps the wound free from blood by frequently mopping it dry with the gauze sponges. The second assistant retracts the flaps or attends to other duties that may be assigned. The nurse provides all needed supplies promptly, rinses the instruments as they may be soiled, and keeps them arranged in the particular order designated by the operator.

The Operation.—The initial incision (Fig. 158) is made from just below the center of the mastoid tip to a point slightly posterior to and above the upper attachment of the auricle. Throughout its course the cut follows the postauricular groove, parallel to it and at a distance of about ¼ inch behind it. The operator stands at the head of the table, the left forefinger outlines the mastoid tip, at which point the

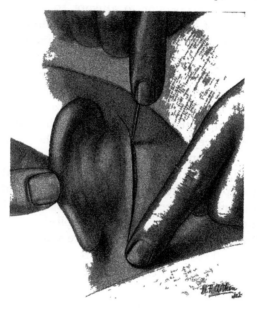

FIG. 158.—INCISION THROUGH SOFT TISSUES.
Showing second stroke of knife which severs the periosteum throughout the entire length of wound.

knife (shown in Fig. 159) is inserted, and the line of incision is quickly but deeply carried through its course to its upper termination. In adult cases firm pressure is made upon the knife, which is held with the blade almost perpendicular to the mastoid surface. In very young children cartilaginous and membranous areas still exist between the centers of ossification, and therefore the initial cut must be made with a lighter touch lest the knife enter the cranial cavity. The first stroke of the knife usually severs the tissues down to the periosteum and divides one or more blood-vessels which require clamping with artery forceps (Fig. 160). The wound is then dried, when a second cut, following the exact course of the first, will be sufficient to penetrate to the bone at every point. The periosteotome (Fig. 161) is then carefully inserted under the periosteum at the middle of the anterior flap, and the periosteum is separated from the bone in a forward direction until the posterior portion of the superior and posterior walls of the external auditory meatus are clearly exposed to view. In like manner the periosteum of the posterior flap is lifted

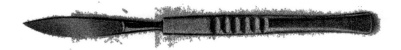

FIG. 159.—MASTOID KNIFE.

from the bone throughout the entire extent of the incision, with the exception of that portion which lies above the linea temporalis, which is covered by the temporal muscle. The greatest care should be exercised by the surgeon in separating the periosteum from the underlying bone, for if this is performed rudely or indifferently the periosteum may be torn, shredded, or be so much bruised that it may subsequently become

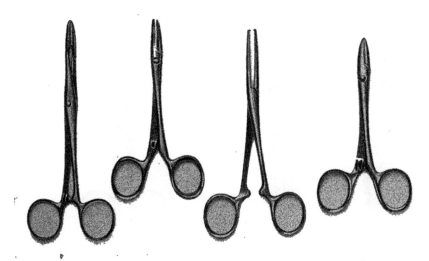

FIG. 160.—DIFFERENT SIZES AND SHAPES OF ARTERY FORCEPS USED IN MASTOID SURGERY.

inflamed or slough, and will therefore fail to adhere to and properly cover the exposed portion of the mastoid process during the healing of the wound. To the mastoid process are attached the sternomastoid, the splenius capitis, and longissimus capitis muscles, the fibers of which, together with their aponeurosis, must be separated to a greater or less extent by means of the blunt-pointed, curved scissors (Fig. 162), which are caused to hug the bone closely until the muscular attachments are free to the desired extent.   Suitable retractors are then placed in such position as to separate the flaps and expose the denuded mastoid process to its fullest extent (Fig. 163).

It is unwise in any case to attempt to perform the mastoid operation through a small incision of the soft tissues, for the reasons that the landmarks upon the surface of the skull cannot be seen sufficiently well, and that unnecessary difficulty is experienced in manipulating the instruments intelligently and safely within the narrow space thus provided.   Hence, if the incision just described proves insufficient in any instance, the operator should feel no hesitation in making a second one backward and at right angles from the center of the first for a distance of at least

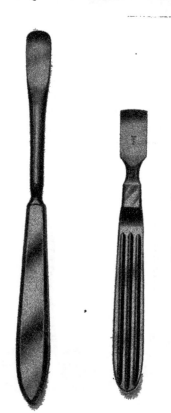

FIG. 161.—TYPES OF PERIOSTEAL ELEVATORS.

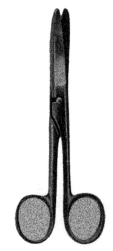

FIG. 162.—BLUNT-POINTED CURVED SCISSORS FOR DETACHING MUSCULAR ATTACHMENTS TO MASTOID PROCESS.

1 inch, after which the soft parts are lifted from the bone, and the posterosuperior, and postero-inferior flaps are turned respectively upward and backward, and downward and backward (see Fig. 240) in such a way as to greatly increase the area of denuded skull.   This second incision is especially indicated in those cases where there is great tumefaction of

the postaural tissues, which thus causes the bone to lie deeply, and hence increases the difficulties of operating through a small opening. The additional incision is also necessary when the disease in the underlying bone is extensive, and to do a complete operation requires a wide removal of the mastoid osseous structure. The author has never seen any unfavorable results follow this extensive exposure of the skull, and since the advantages arising from its employment in the items of safety to the

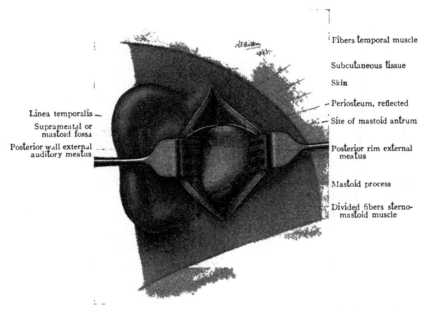

Fibers temporal muscle

Subcutaneous tissue

Skin

Periosteum, reflected

Site of mastoid antrum

Linea temporalis

Suprameatal or mastoid fossa

Posterior wall external auditory meatus

Posterior rim external meatus

Mastoid process

Divided fibers sternomastoid muscle

FIG. 163.—THE FIELD FOR THE MASTOID OPERATION (ACUTE) COMPLETELY EXPOSED, SHOWING ALL LAND-MARKS NECESSARY TO OBSERVE DURING THE OPERATION.

The muscular attachments to the tip of the mastoid process are shown cut away to a greater extent in this, and the subsequent illustrations, than is usually necessary. In all the drawings of the mastoid operations shown in this work the periosteum and other soft tissues are, for purposes of greater clearness, slightly exaggerated. Observe that the periosteum is not incised above the linea temporalis, and that the fibers of the temporal muscle are not divided.

patient and ease of operating are very considerable, he employs it in a constantly increasing number of his operations.

Although the hemorrhage incident to the operation is in no case severe unless the sigmoid sinus should be accidentally injured, yet in order to accomplish the successive steps of the procedure speedily, safely, and accurately, the blood must be frequently mopped from the wound by an assistant. For this purpose, several sizes of gauze sponges are most convenient, the largest being used during the skin incisions, and the smaller and still smaller ones substituted as the bony opening is deepened.

A moderately slender dressing-forceps is a most convenient instrument (Fig. 164) with which to use the mops rapidly and efficiently.

Inspection of the Landmarks upon the Mastoid Portion of the Temporal Bone which are Exposed by the Primary Incisions (as shown in

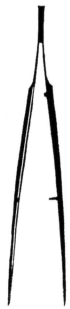

Fig. 163).—When the wound is thoroughly dried, certain landmarks which are usually present must be sought for and their position afterward borne in mind, because they form important guides to the safe and speedy entrance into the mastoid antrum. The posterior root of the zygoma continues backward above the superior margin of the external meatus, forming a ridge that can be seen, or at least felt with the examining finger, in almost every instance. This ridge (Fig. 165, 1, 2) indicates the lower boundary of the middle cranial fossa, and the removal of bone above it to any considerable extent will expose the contents of the cranial cavity. Therefore in the mastoid operation when performed for the relief of acute mastoid suppuration, the chiseling or other means used to remove the bony cortex should be carried on entirely below this ridge. In case the ridge cannot be made out, owing to its lack of development, the superior meatal margin must be taken as a guide, and an imaginary line drawn backward and slightly upward

FIG. 164.—DRESS-
ING-FORCEPS.

from it will serve the same useful purpose as the ridge itself.

The suprameatal triangle (Fig. 165, 3), lies just below the posterior zygomatic ridge and immediately behind the upper margin of the external auditory meatus. Since this triangle forms the outer wall of the mastoid antrum its importance as a guide to the exposure of this cavity is of first value. Macewen, who first described this triangle and established its surgical importance, gives the following description of its boundaries: "The base is formed by the posterior root of the zygoma running somewhat horizontally above; the portion of the descending plate of the squamous, which forms the arch of the osseous part of the external auditory meatus below, and a base line uniting the two, dropped from the former on a level with the posterior border of the external auditory meatus."[1] It will thus be seen that this triangle is not wholly bounded by visible landmarks, and many times no marks at all are present except the superoposterior meatal margin. However, when the flaps of overlying soft tissue are widely dissected, exposing the osseous surface of the mastoid

[1] *Dis. of Brain and Spinal Cord*, p. 9.

process extensively and the wound is free from blood, the experienced operator will at a glance map out the region of this triangle with sufficient accuracy for operative purposes, even though all the landmarks are poorly defined. The beginner will obtain a better knowledge of this triangle from a study of Fig. 165, which was made from a specimen on which these landmarks are clearly visible, than can be obtained from a study of the temporal bone itself, especially should the lines on its surface be but poorly developed.

Upon the surface of this triangle, and immediately posterior to the upper part of the postmeatal margin, are seen the suprameatal fossa

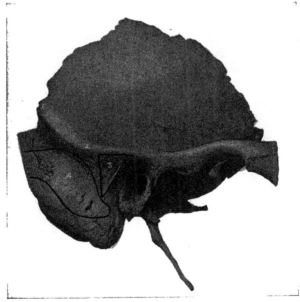

FIG. 165.—RIGHT TEMPORAL BONE ON WHICH THE LANDMARKS ARE VERY WELL DEVELOPED.
1, 2, linea temporalis; 3, suprameatal triangle; 4, course of sigmoid sinus. Note the unusal length of styloid process.

and spine (see Fig. 8). These external markings are not present in some cases, but in others are so well developed that the spine is quite prominent, and the fossa is sufficiently large to accommodate the ball of a small finger.

The mastoid process may be found broad or narrow. If broad, the fact is probably indicative of a normal situation of the sigmoid sinus, middle cranial fossa, and facial nerve; whereas a narrow, thin process is suggestive of a crowded condition of these important structures, and serves as a warning to the operator that unusual care must be observed in order to avoid wounding one or more of them during the operation.

Opening the Mastoid Antrum.—Since no mastoid operation can be considered good surgery in which the antrum has not been entered, and since when this cavity is once exposed it furnishes the best guide for the extension of the wound in any necessary direction, it should be the aim of the surgeon to open the antrum as the first step of the bone ablation. To accomplish the removal of the bony cortex, as well as the denser portions of the mastoid interior, the author recommends the employment of chisels and gouges as both efficient and rapid, since either of these instruments is safer than the various drills and burrs which are propelled by a dental engine. Several chisels and gouges of different sizes (see Figs. 167 to 172) should be at hand. These, as well as every other cutting tool that is to be used, should in every case be as

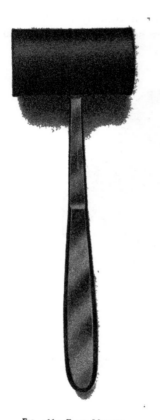

FIG. 166.—FIBER MALLET.

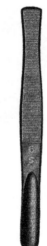

FIG. 167.—MASTOID GOUGE.

sharp as the grinder's art can provide, since dull instruments not only retard the progress of the operation, but also necessitate heavier strokes of the mallet (Fig. 166) in the cutting than should, for obvious reasons, be employed when operating on the cranium. The largest chisel or gouge (Fig. 167) is selected for removing the cortex. Its cutting edge is placed against the bone just posterior to the suprameatal fossa if this landmark is present, or about the center of the suprameatal triangle if this latter area be taken as the guide (Fig. 168).   The cutting operations must be conducted throughout with the chisel directed at all times toward the auditory meatus.   The reason for beginning the chiseling so near the posterior rim of the auditory meatus is that by this precaution only can the operator avoid wounding the sigmoid sinus, should this vessel run abnormally far forward, as shown in Fig. 182.   Thin slices of the bone are rapidly removed, the operator noting the nature of the underlying structure before making each cut, he being thus able to recognize the wall of the sigmoid sinus or the dura of the middle fossa should either be accidentally uncovered.   Frequent drying of the wound by means

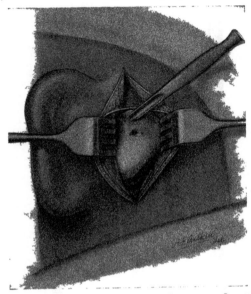

FIG. 168.—CASE OF RUPTURE THROUGH MASTOID CORTEX NEAR SITE OF ANTRUM.
Gouge shown in position of safety to begin removal of cortex.   The gouge may, if desired, be pointed in any other direction toward the auditory canal.   When the osseous structure surrounding the point of rupture is softened by the disease, the use of a sharp curet is often preferable to the gouge or chisel.

of the gauze sponges and the removal of the bony chips as rapidly as they are cut away are necessary to safe operating.   As the osseous cavity is by this means deepened, it becomes necessary to work with a smaller chisel (Figs. 169 to 172 and Fig. 242).   If the cellular structure of the bone is found sufficiently soft, either naturally or as a result of the mastoid disease, a stout, sharp curet or scoop (Fig. 243) can be used to good effect, and often the greater part of the osseous tissue between the cortex and antrum can by this means be rapidly and safely removed. The curet, like the chisel, should always be driven in the direction of the auditory meatus.   When the usual depth of the antrum is approached, a bent silver probe (see Fig. 200) or the explorer (Fig. 173) should be inserted into any cell that is opened, so that the antrum may be recognized at the earliest moment.   It often becomes necessary, as the wound deepens, to enlarge the cortical portion of the mastoid opening in order to give more freedom for the manipulation of the instruments. This can safely be done at any time after the cone-shaped opening is well begun, provided that the same care be given in the removal of each bony chip that has already been suggested.   It often happens that when

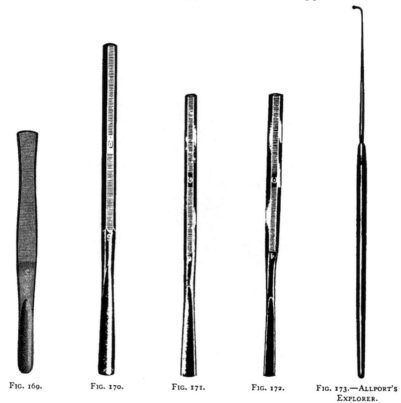

FIG. 169.   FIG. 170.   FIG. 171.   FIG. 172.   FIG. 173.—ALLPORT'S
                                                                    EXPLORER.

the superficial cells are reached the outer table of bone will overhang them in such manner that the bone forceps (see Fig. 269) can be used rapidly and safely in the removal of large superficial areas.

When the antrum is entered it may be readily recognized both by its situation and large size.   Its walls should be at once explored (Fig. 174) in all directions by means of the probe in order to determine the extent of overhanging bone that must subsequently be removed.   To accomplish this removal, the chisel, scoop, and forceps may be used, and the outer wall of the cavity cut away until the opening into the antrum thus provided is as large as any portion of the antrum itself.   To test this point the bent explorer is inserted to the bottom of the antrum at any portion, when if it can be withdrawn without meeting any overhanging ledge, it may be considered that a sufficient amount of bone has been removed.   The antrum is now temporarily packed with a strip of gauze to arrest the bleeding in this portion of the wound.

The mastoid cells are next attacked if the previous history of the case and the present inspection of this portion of the mastoid indicates that the disease has extended to the tip.   The broadest gouge is applied at the mastoid tip, and with the edge directed upward the cortex is rapidly removed by a few strokes of the mallet.   The outer portion and

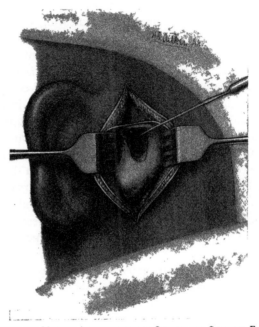

FIG. 174.—SHOWING THE MASTOID ANTRUM PARTIALLY OPENED, THE OPERATOR ENTERING THE CAVITY WITH THE EXPLORER FOR THE PURPOSE OF DETERMINING ITS SIZE AND THE EXTENT OF THE OVERHANGING OSSEOUS LEDGES WHICH MUST BE REMOVED

cellular interior of the tip of the apophysis should be entirely removed in many cases.   The cellular interior should be scooped and bitten away until the bottom of the entire wound in every direction is smooth and free from pockets or suspicious areas of diseased bone.   The ragged edges of the cortex at the mouth of the bony wound must also be smoothed, beveled, and honed with appropriate instruments until a strictly surgical margin is everywhere encountered.

The packing which was a few moments before placed into the mastoid antrum is now removed and since the pressure of the gauze has by this time arrested the bleeding, the walls of the cavity can be better inspected than before and any remaining portion of diseased membrane or roughened bone can be detected and removed. When the antrum has been thoroughly cleansed of disease, a small sharp curet, bent to an appropriate curve (Fig. 216, D), should be passed through the aditus ad antrum, by which means this channel is very gently cureted in an outward direction and a free communication between the antrum and the middle ear is thus established. Care must, of course, be exercised as to the distance to which this instrument is inserted into the aditus, since if it is passed too far in the direction of the tympanic cavity this latter space will be entered, injury to the ossicles or membrana tympani may result, and unnecessary damage to the hearing will follow.

The posterior root of the zygoma, which overhangs the antrum to a greater or less extent in many cases, sometimes contains several cells that are also apt to become infected in any case of mastoiditis (see Fig. 18). Before the mastoid operation can be considered completed, therefore, the operator should continue the removal of bone in this direction in order to determine if this adjacent portion of the zygoma is solid or pneumatic, and if the latter, whether or not the cells are infected and suppurating. If pus is found, the cortex must be bitten away with forceps, and the cellular tissue cureted out to the extent that this portion of the wound is left free from pockets and smooth in every direction. To accomplish this as thoroughly as good surgery demands requires that the primary incision of the soft parts be extended somewhat forward above the ear in order to give a sufficiently large exposure of the post-zygomatic region.

The entire wound is then irrigated with hot boric or saline solution for the purpose of removing any loose spicula or bony chips that have previously escaped attention. Following this procedure, the whole cavity is thoroughly dried with gauze mops, after which every portion of the bony cavity should be finally inspected to make sure that no diseased area or roughened surface is permitted to remain. A few moments spent at this stage of the operation in smoothing any irregular surface, or in removing some small area of suspicious looking bone, will unquestionably shorten the time required for healing, or even obviate the necessity for a second operation. Perhaps nowhere in surgery is judicious care as to detail in the respect just mentioned more amply rewarded by successful results than in the mastoid operation. When the osseous wound is completed it has the appearance shown in Fig. 175.

During this final inspection, or at any previous examination of the posterior or superior walls of the mastoid antrum, it may be discovered that a fistulous tract leads into the middle fossa of the skull above, or into the sigmoid groove posteriorly, exposing the dura of the cerebrum to infection in the one instance and the lateral sinus and cerebellum in the other. In case granulation tissue or plastic lymph is found covering the exposed sinus or dura, it is not wise to remove the same by curet-

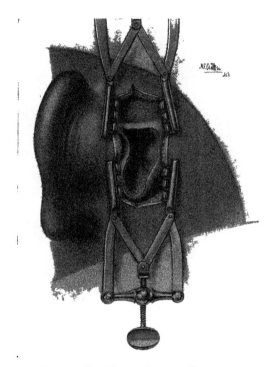

FIG. 175.—THE MASTOID OPERATION COMPLETED.

The bottom of the mastoid antrum is seen in the upper and anterior portion of the osseous wound. On the posterior wall the thin bony covering of the sigmoid sinus projects into the opening. The method of using Allport's retractors is shown. It should be remembered that the shape and extent of the osseous wound of no two mastoid operations are exactly the same. The above illustration shows only a completed operation in this particular case.

ment unless it is proposed to open the sinus immediately afterward, for the reason that such granulation tissue or plastic lymph forms nature's most effective barrier to the entrance of pathogenic bacteria from adjoining sources. This form of protection is quite analogous to that which is provided for the bowels during septic peritonitis. The abdominal surgeon formerly wiped this barrier away during abdominal operations with a resulting high mortality. Now he allows it to remain undisturbed, greatly to the betterment of his statistics. The otologist may wisely follow the safer practise of the gynecologist in this respect.

Packing the wound with gauze constitutes the next step.[1] Although every suppurative tissue of the mastoid has been thoroughly obliterated, suppuration within the middle ear continues, and now finding the easiest exit through the aditus ad antrum, it naturally enters the mastoid wound.

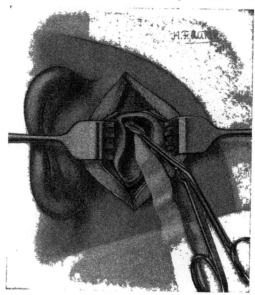

FIG. 176.—INSERTING THE GAUZE PACKING.
The distal end of the strip should be inserted to the bottom of the antrum and against the aditus ad antrum. Folds of the gauze are then loosely packed, one over the other, until the whole wound is loosely filled.

For the purpose of favoring the discharge of pus from the middle ear through the channel of the aditus, and thus preserving the function of the tympanic cavity, the strip of gauze packing is first inserted to the

[1] Instead of packing the wound with gauze, several operators, notably Blake, Reik, and Sprague, have advocated and practised the method of allowing the wound to fill with a blood-clot, which, through subsequent organization of the clot, brings about a much more speedy closure of the mastoid cavity. The blood-clot dressing, as this method has been called, would be ideal were it not for the fact that in the acute mastoid case the wound which is to be filled and healed by the clot is a septic one, and one which, because of the coincident suppuration in the tympanic cavity, cannot be rendered absolutely sterile. The blood-clot dressing therefore usually becomes speedily infected, breaks down and is discharged. Jack reports that of 60 cases treated at the Massachusetts Charitable Eye and Ear Infirmary by the blood-clot dressing that the clot broke down in 48 cases, and that uncomplicated healing occurred in only 4 of the 60 cases. By this method the accompanying aural discharge is not so favorably affected, and this constitutes another and a most excellent reason for using the gauze packing rather than the blood-clot dressing.

bottom of the antrum (Fig. 176) and against the antral mouth of the aditus.   Folds of the strip are packed over each other with moderate firmness until first the antrum and finally the entire mastoid excavation is filled with the gauze to the level of the skin flaps (Fig. 177).

A word concerning the gauze strip which is to be used for packing the mastoid wound will be of service to the beginner.   It should be somewhat firmly woven with selvage edge, 18 to 24 inches long and $\frac{3}{4}$ inch wide.   In simple mastoid cases the strip may be only plain sterile gauze, but if the mastoid has been the seat of a violent suppuration, or if the dura of the sigmoid sinus or middle cranial fossa has

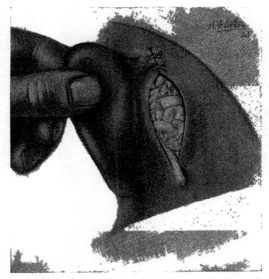

Fig. 177.—The Mastoid Wound Packed and the Flaps Sutured down to the Linea Temporalis.
The illustration gives an impression that the gauze is tightly crowded into the wound.   The packing should in reality always be lightly inserted.

been either accidentally or intentionally exposed or wounded during the operation, a 5 per cent. saturation of the gauze with iodoform should be used for the first dressing, but afterward borated gauze may be substituted.   Before inserting the strip into the cavity it should be scrutinized carefully to determine if its edges or ends (Fig. 178), carry any loose threads; and should this be the case, to remove them for the reason that if such be carried into the wound, they are apt to be caught in the granulations or upon the bony surface, where they are retained, and, escaping the subsequent attention of the surgeon, act as foreign bodies to delay or even prevent healing.

That portion of the wound through the soft tissues which lies above

20

the temporal ridge should not be packed. The periosteum of both the anterior and posterior flaps should be seized with tissue forceps, drawn out to a level with the skin, and two or three sutures of catgut should be so accurately passed through both integument and periosteum that a perfect coaptation of this portion of the flaps is obtained and a union by first intention will result (see Fig. 177).

The balance of the opening is left unsutured. Experience has taught that the broadly open wound is not only more easily and painlessly dressed, but that it is also much more certain to finally heal completely, for the reason that inspection of the progress of the healing is at

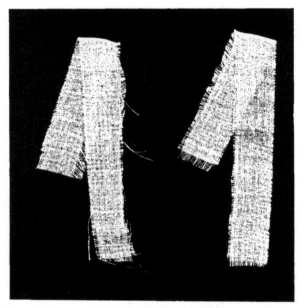

Fig. 178.—Fragments of Gauze representing Proper and Improper Preparation for Insertion into the Mastoid Wound.
The loose ravelings shown in one would be detached in the granulating wound and cause delay in healing.

all times easy, and therefore early measures can be taken to correct any questionable tendency to repair that may arise.

The gauze strip that was inserted into the external auditory meatus before the beginning of the operation is now removed and a fresh one is inserted to the bottom of the canal. It is essential to pack this with some firmness against the outer end of the posterior wall of the meatus for the reason that during the dissection of the anterior flap, during that part of the operation in which the flaps were formed, the skin and periosteum of this portion of the posterior meatal wall were separated from the underlying bone, and if the two are not now pressed together snugly, sagging of this wall may subsequently occur to such an extent as to lessen or obliterate the lumen of the external auditory canal.

After the mastoid wound has been completed and packed, it is the practise of some operators to incise the drum membrane freely before inserting the gauze wick into the external auditory meatus, as just described. Such an incision is always indicated in cases in which, for any reason, the mastoid antrum has not been entered during the mastoid operation. While no harm can result from the free incision of the drum membrane, such an incision is scarcely necessary, provided both antrum and aditus ad antrum have been as freely opened during the mastoid operation as has been advised by the author, because under such circumstances the subsequent formation of pus in the tympanic cavity will find a perfectly free outlet through the mastoid wound, and the discharge from the middle ear will, as already stated, rapidly cease.

Boric acid powder, because of its mildly antiseptic and detergent qualities, is dusted freely over the edges of the mastoid wound; loose gauze is placed liberally over and around the auricle, and the dressing is completed by an accurately applied roller bandage. Some caution is necessary in arranging the gauze behind and around the external ear, and in the application of the roller bandage, to avoid kinking the pinna to such an extent as to produce great discomfort or even unbearable pain until the first dressing is removed and the error is corrected. The completed dressing is shown in Fig. 255.

As a rule but little shock follows this operation. The subsequent pain is only occasionally severe enough to require the administration of an anodyne. Severe pain within the first twenty-four hours is sometimes due to a faulty dressing. After this time it will more likely arise as a result of infection of the skin flaps and the consequent swelling and tension upon the sutures. Soreness and stiffness of the muscles of the neck of the operated side is a natural consequence in those cases in which it has been necessary to partially or entirely separate the muscular attachments from the mastoid tip, but in most instances this symptom rapidly disappears.

The postoperative temperature seldom rises above 100° F. If it was high preceding the operation it usually falls almost immediately to the normal or near the normal. Any marked postoperative rise, coincident with an increase of pain, is commonly indicative of a stitch or flap infection, and usually subsides promptly after a change of the dressing and the correction of the fault.

The length of time the first dressing should be allowed to remain undisturbed varies with the symptoms which arise. If the temperature remains normal or is but little elevated, if the pain is slight or entirely absent, and if the gauze coverings remain dry and free from odor, a change of dressing is not indicated earlier than the fifth or sixth day after the operation.   Should the patient complain of pain in the wound during the first twenty-four hours an anodyne in the form of codein or morphin hypodermically may be given.   Persistence of the pain for a longer period would dictate the removal of the outer coverings and an inspection of the condition of the auricle, skin flaps, and sutures.   Saturation of the dressings with exudate or blood, with the result of rendering them foul smelling or uncomfortably stiff, is an indication for earlier change. During this time the patient himself is treated surgically and is kept quiet in bed on a restricted diet.   The bowels should be moved on the third or fourth day.   If the previous prostration of the patient has been marked, extra care must be exercised in the selection of a most nourishing diet, in addition to which, benefit is often obtained from the early administration of elixir of iron, quinin, and strychnin, or some other equally efficient tonic.

The first change of dressing is painful unless the physician is gentle in every manipulation.   In the typic case that has continued without change of the dressing for five or six days the gauze in the depth of the bony wound will have become so saturated with exudate as to be somewhat slippery and therefore easy of removal.   If taken out at an earlier date the folds of gauze are often somewhat adherent to the structures against which they have lain, and their withdrawal requires more effort, and consequently causes more pain.   When all are removed the wound usually appears dry and granulations are seen springing from almost every point.   The good effects of the mastoid operation on the suppurating middle ear may be judged from the fact that the gauze wick which was inserted into the external meatus at the time of the operation, when withdrawn at the first dressing is often found moist only at the inner end, and may be dry throughout, thus demonstrating the fact that the discharge from the middle ear has either ceased or that it has found exit through the mastoid wound.   The greatest improvement in this respect is often noted in cases where, previous to the mastoid operation, the discharge had been so profuse that a similar gauze wick when inserted into the meatus would have been saturated with pus in an hour.   It is seldom necessary to irrigate the mastoid wound at the first dressing. Any collection of dried secretion or blood that may be found on the adjoining skin or edges of the flaps is best removed by gently rubbing the same with a pledget of cotton saturated with hydroyen peroxid, and held in the jaws of a dressing-forceps.   Any slight collection of exudate in any part of the mastoid opening should be absorbed by means of small gauze sponges applied directly to the suppurating area. Antiseptic powder may or may not be dusted into the wound, according to the preference of the surgeon or to the appearance of the granulating surface. If used, only a quantity sufficient to lightly cover the raw surfaces should be employed. A fresh gauze strip should then be inserted into the mastoid wound and a separate one into the auditory canal, exactly as at the primary dressing, and the roller bandage should be again applied.

Subsequent dressings must be made every twenty-four to forty-eight hours, depending largely upon the rapidity with which the gauze coverings are soiled. When the granulating process becomes active, the secretion may become correspondingly profuse, in which case irrigation is properly performed each time. For this latter purpose a saturated solution of boric acid or the normal salt solution is sufficient. It is not advisable to irrigate the external auditory meatus at any time subsequent to the mastoid operation, provided the discharge through this channel has ceased or is only slight.

On the occasion of each dressing it is essential that the surgeon should carefully scrutinize every portion of the healing surface in order that he may be able to detect at the earliest moment any area of bone that fails to be covered by healthy granulations, for it sometimes happens that, following an operation in which the destructive disease of the bone has been violent, additional death of osseous tissue may subsequently occur, even though at the time of the operation every suspicious area had been thoroughly removed. Should such an occurrence take place, granulations will fail to form over the necrosing areas or, having once formed, will soon become sufficiently luxuriant to conceal the area of dead bone. If extension of the necrotic process be recognized sufficiently early, and its surface be vigorously cureted at this time, healthy granulations may thus be stimulated and the part may be sufficiently covered to preserve its life. Should it not do so and should separation of the bone occur, the resulting sequestrum is felt with the probe under the semipolypoid mass of granulations and should be entirely removed.

The open wound must heal by filling in with granulations from the bottom and sides. The unsutured portion of the skin flaps should, therefore, be kept widely separated by means of the gauze packing. If the external portion of the wound is allowed to close too rapidly there will likely result a fistulous tract leading to a more or less diseased cavity within. It is from this cause that secondary operations are frequently necessary. The granulations when healthy are always small and firm.

Large and flabby granulations are pathologic and require removal by the curet or caustic. A bead of silver nitrate fused on the end of a probe (see Fig. 132) furnishes an excellent means of destroying the diseased granulations without risk of injury to adjacent healthy structures.

It will be seen that a successful termination of the operated cases depends in no small measure upon the amount of painstaking care the surgeon devotes to the after-treatment. It is always desirable, therefore, that the patient remain until well under the immediate observation of the operator or his trained assistant.

The length of time required for the complete healing of the wound varies greatly. Some cases are well within a month, while others require a much longer time. After a week, many times earlier, the patient may sit up in a chair and be permitted to walk about his room. After ten days or two weeks the average patient may leave the hospital, and subsequent attention may be given at the surgeon's office. Postaural deformity of any consequence results only in the worst cases—those in which, in order to do a successful operation, it becomes necessary to remove a large amount of bone, and also in that class where the patient is old or decrepit, and in which granulation takes place with such slowness that the skin covers the depression before the granulation tissue fills the cavity of the wound sufficiently to reach the skin level. The scar usually resulting from the operation for acute mastoiditis is so slight that it amounts to nothing more than the line indicating the union of the flaps, and this, because of its hidden position behind the auricle, is not commonly observed.

BEZOLD'S ABSCESS

The name has been given to a collection of pus in the tissues of the neck that has resulted from the rupture of a mastoid abscess into the digastric fossa (Fig. 179), from whence the pus finds its way down the neck. Reference to Figs. 152 and 252 will explain the ease with which Bezold's abscess may take place during a mastoid suppuration, provided the structure of the mastoid process is of the large cellular type. Bezold's abscess is quite likely to occur in any case in which a large cell exists at the tip of the process, especially when the cortex of this cell is exceedingly thin, as in the specimens shown in Figs. 152 and 232. It is entirely improbable that such an abscess ever occurs in cases of which Fig. 153 is a type. Since the purulent material is discharged from the mastoid process into the cellular tissues of the neck at a point beneath the deep cervical fascia, its natural tendency is to subsequently dissect its way downward along the cervical vessels, nerves, and muscles,

and in this way it has been known to reach the thorax.   In any case
of discharging ear that is complicated by mastoid inflammation, if a
hard and painful swelling should occur below the tip of the mastoid proc_
ess (Fig. 180), together perhaps with increased temperature and rigor,
infection of the cervical tissues in the manner just described should be
suspected.   Owing to the great depth of this accumulation of pus and
the tension of the intervening tissues, fluctuation is not present, at least
not as an early symptom.   In order to prevent the dangers resulting
from the migration and dissemination of the pus after it has broken
through the mastoid cortex the condition should be detected at the
earliest possible moment, in order that correct surgical measures may at
once be instituted for its removal.   Local applications in the form of

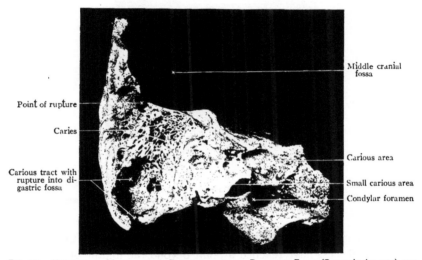

Point of rupture

Caries

Carious tract with
rupture into di-
gastric fossa

Middle cranial
fossa

Carious area

Small carious area

Condylar foramen

FIG. 179.—NECROSIS OF MASTOID WITH RUPTURE INTO THE DIGASTRIC FOSSA (BEZOLD'S ABSCESS) AND
ALSO INTO THE MIDDLE CRANIAL FOSSA.
This most interesting and instructive specimen shows the direct course of the necrosis from the mastoid
interior through the cellular structure which is completely broken down, to the digastric groove in one direction
and to the cranial cavity in the other.
(Specimen of J. Orne Greene, Warren Medical Museum, Harvard Medical School.)

liniments or poultices should have absolutely no place in the treatment.
That the abscess is present in any case is only proof that the mastoid
operation has been already too long delayed and that it is now urgently
indicated.   In such cases the deep abscess in the neck is operated on at the
same time and as a necessary part of the mastoid operation.   The mastoid
should be thoroughly opened and the tip completely removed, as has
been fully described above.   Following this a director or, preferably, the
finger of the operator, is inserted into the abscess cavity at the bottom
of the mastoid wound, and the tissues are by that means dissected along

the tract of the abscess, to its lowermost position in the neck. At this latter point the intervening structures between the skin and finger-tip should be freely incised, and a counteropening sufficiently large to permit free drainage be thus established. A strip of gauze is then inserted from above, through the passage made by the finger, and this is brought out through the lower opening, above which the entire cavity is filled with the gauze. If the pus is foul smelling and its range through the neck has been wide, after the counterincision is made through the

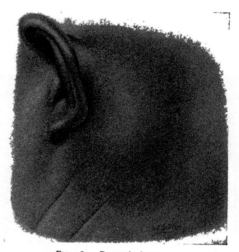

FIG. 180.—BEZOLD'S ABSCESS.
Compare the position of the auricle and of the tumefaction with that produced by rupture through the mastoid cortex over the site of the antrum, as shown in Fig. 181.

lowermost portion, it will be advisable to thoroughly irrigate the wound. Should the abscess have reached a point beyond the middle of the neck, or perhaps near the clavicle, its obliteration will be most certainly and safely accomplished by laying the tract open for a considerable distance, and then packing the open wound with gauze until healthy granulations are everywhere established and the wound is thus filled in from the bottom.

SUBPERIOSTEAL ABSCESS

Subperiosteal or postaural abscess occurs over the mastoid region as a symptom in a considerable number of all cases of acute mastoiditis (Fig. 181). While it is most commonly observed in the neglected cases, yet it is sometimes seen within a week after the beginning of a severe mastoid complication. In adults the occurrence of such an abscess is nearly always the result of a perforation of the bone caused by the rupture of the abscess externally and a leakage of pus through to the under surface of the periosteum (see point of rupture in Fig. 168), which latter is everywhere detached in the directions of least resistance. Since the attachment of the periosteum over the postauricular region becomes closer as it approaches the tip of the mastoid process, where the muscles are inserted, the pus in these cases finds an easier passage in an upward and backward direction; it usually collects posterior to and somewhat above the attachment of the auricle, which latter is thereby pushed outward and downward to the extent of giving a deformed appearance to that side of the head. This form of abscess is most frequently met with in infants and young children, in which cases the pus may escape from the interior to the surface of the

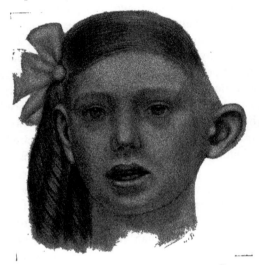

FIG. 181.—PROJECTION OF THE AURICLE IN MASTOIDITIS WITH POSTAURAL ABSCESS.
The collection of pus is above and behind the auricular attachment. Compare this condition with that produced by a rupture of pus into the digastric fossa (see Figs. 179 and 180). Note also the expression indicative of an adenoid which was a causative factor in the production of the aural and mastoid affection.

mastoid, through the squamomastoid suture (Fig. 9), which exists at this period of life, and hence in this class of patients it is not necessary to presuppose the presence of a bony perforation.

Since a subperiosteal abscess is only a symptom of the underlying osseous suppuration, the treatment of any case thus complicated differs but little from that afforded by the mastoid operation already described. When the periosteum has been separated from the bone for a period of several days the surface of the latter structure is sometimes found roughened and grayish in color over the denuded area. When this has occurred, it should be cureted in every quarter after the complete mastoid operation has been performed, and just previously to suturing the skin flaps. The periosteum itself is frequently found necrotic in places or covered on its under surface by unhealthy granulations, while the soft parts covering the periosteum itself are infiltrated with septic fluids. When so diseased, the flaps should be freely dissected from the bone, then turned outward to an extent that widely exposes the under surface of the periosteum, when, if found granular or necrotic, the curet or curved scissors, if necessary, is vigorously applied and the diseased areas are completely removed.

Dangers of the Mastoid Operation.—The dangers which may be encountered in the performance of the mastoid operation are injuries (*a*) to the facial nerve with resulting facial paralysis; (*b*) to the walls of the lateral sinus, causing severe hemorrhage; and (*c*) to the dura mater above the tegmen antri, with resulting exposure of the cranial contents to infection. In cases in which the anatomic relations of these structures are normal, injury to any of them is not probable, provided the operator possesses that almost perfect knowledge of the anatomy of the parts without which the operation should never be undertaken; provided the operative landmarks are kept in mind throughout the entire procedure, and also provided that the same exceeding care which should always characterize the work of the trained and experienced surgeon be exercised when removing the tissues adjoining the facial nerve, sigmoid sinus, or brain covering.

Abnormalities as to position of these important structures may be present in any case, and when this is true the possibility of injuring one of them is greatly increased even though the greatest care be exercised by the surgeon. The temporosphenoidal lobe of the cerebrum may be found on a lower level than the ridge of the posterior root of the zygoma, and the sigmoid sinus may run so near the posterior margin of the external auditory meatus that it will be injured even when the chiseling is performed within the most anterior portion of the suprameatal triangle (Fig. 182). It has already been stated that the width of the mastoid process and the angle which the auditory meatus forms with the surface of the skull furnish some information concerning the near or remote situation of the sigmoid sinus to the postmeatal margin; nevertheless, the careful operator prefers to avoid the risk of injury to so large a vessel by following the advice already given—namely, to make the initial opening into the bone at a point well forward in the suprameatal triangle, to at all times direct the cutting edge of the chisel toward the external meatus, and to always hold the chisel at such an obtuse angle to the surface of bone to be removed that it is possible to remove only thin chips of osseous tissue when the instrument is driven forward. When any cell or space of whatever nature is uncovered on either the upper or posterior wall or in the bottom of the wound, the same should be inspected at once by an examination with an exploring instrument in order to learn the exact nature of the cavity and thus to prepare the way for safely removing any additional portions of bone. In the acute mastoid operation it is scarcely possible to injure the facial nerve unless the operator invades the bone recklessly and without correct anatomic knowledge or experience as a guide. One exception should be made to this statement—namely, that the mastoid inflammation is occasionally of such violence as to cause the death of a considerable portion of the process *en masse.* In such instances the facial nerve

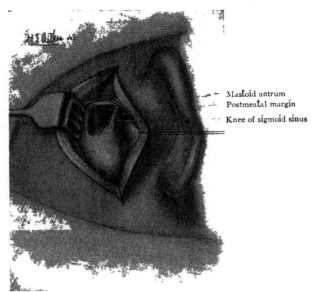

Mastoid antrum
Postmeatal margin
Knee of sigmoid sinus

FIG. 182.—CASE IN WHICH THE SIGMOID SINUS WAS FOUND ABNORMALLY FAR FORWARD.
In this instance the vessel lay immediately under the posterior and lower part of the suprameatal triangle, (Fig. 165, 3) and would have been opened but for the precaution of first chiseling away the anterior portion of the triangle. Note that the mastoid antrum is small and crowded far forward.

may be destroyed by the disease coincidentally with the death of the surrounding bone, but should its function continue for a time, and should the mastoid operation be then performed, the nerve would in all probability be unavoidably injured. The wall of the sigmoid sinus may be wounded by any of the instruments used in the performance of the mastoid operation, or a spicula of the overlying bone may be driven into it in the efforts of the operator to remove the diseased osseous tissue from the sigmoid groove. If only a puncture of the sinus is made, the bleeding from the vessel will be profuse, but not alarming, whereas if a large incision or tear of the sinus wall is made the resulting hemorrhage is severe, persistent, and dangerous unless prompt and efficient measures are at once instituted to arrest it. In case one of the more trivial wounds has been inflicted upon the walls of the vein the outpouring of blood is at once so considerable as to obscure the entire operative field and thus to stop further operating until the bleeding has been arrested. The end of a strip of gauze $\frac{1}{2}$ inch wide should be immediately placed over the site of the injury, and over this a strip is folded, forward and backward, until a half dozen layers have been superimposed upon the first, when the ball of the finger of an assistant should be placed firmly upon the top of the last fold, and continuous pressure be exerted until the flow of blood has ceased. If the mastoid operation were well under way before the injury to the sinus occurred, and a large mastoid opening therefore exists in the bone, it will be entirely possible to proceed with the operation in some other part of the field while waiting for the fibrinous sealing of the wounded vessel. After a few minutes, during which time the pressure has been constantly exerted upon the pressure pad which covers the puncture in the sinus, the gauze pad may be cautiously removed, when, if bleeding recurs, it must be immediately replaced. In most cases the hemorrhage will have stopped and the operation may proceed as though no accident had occurred, only the operator and assistants must use great care not to disturb the wounded vessel by rude manipulation or sponging in the immediate vicinity of the part.

Should the sigmoid sinus be extensively incised or torn during the mastoid operation, it becomes imperative to at once check the bleeding. This may be accomplished, provided the sinus wall has already been widely exposed by the removal of its osseous covering in the sigmoid groove, by quickly turning the incised edges of the vessel walls into the lumen of the vein, and then making firm pressure upon the same by means of a properly shaped pad of sterile gauze. Should this plan fail, it may become necessary to insert a strip of sterile or medicated gauze into each end of the injured vessel. If by either of these means the bleeding can be controlled, the operation should be continued until completed; but if it is found difficult to control, and the pad of gauze, which must be used as a hemostat, is sufficiently large to cover the field of operation, the procedure should be abandoned for a period of one or two days.

Injury to the sinus during the mastoid operation is always likely to be followed by sinus infection and sinus thrombosis. This result should be expected, since the wound of the vessel exposes its contents directly to the suppurating mastoid wound. Of course, if the mastoid process has been thoroughly opened and cleaned previously to the accidental wounding of the sinus the risk of infection will be lessened, but as a matter of fact it is difficult to render this class of wound sterile, and, moreover, the instrument which causes the wound is of necessity an infected one. When the bleeding has been controlled after such an accident, the exposed portion of the sinus wall should be covered with iodoform gauze while the operation is completed, and the entire wound is as completely sterilized as possible. A fresh strip of the iodoform gauze is then placed over the sinus so as to form a pressure pad on the site of the wound and the mastoid dressing is completed as described on p. 307. A separate dressing for the exposed sinus and for the balance of the mastoid wound should, if possible, be maintained at each subsequent dressing until a substantial layer of healthy granulation has covered and protected the sinus. In case an infection of the sinus takes place at any time, symptoms denoting this fact will quickly arise (see p. 418).

One of the surest means of guarding against the accidents and dangers that may occur during the performance of the mastoid operation is to provide, by the ample dimensions of the soft-tissue flaps, a wide field in which to operate; and another is to keep this field so thoroughly cleansed from blood that the operator may at all times clearly see the minutest details of the entire surgical area.

MASTOIDITIS IN INFANTS

Because of the frequency with which mastoiditis in infants and very young children is met, and also because of the differences that arise as to its cause and behavior, as compared with the same disease when occurring in older children and in adults, a discussion of the subject should be of great practical value to the student and practitioner.

The chief differences observable in this class of patients are unquestionably due to the developmental state of the temporal bone at birth and during the first two years of extra-uterine life. The facts that have already been stated concerning the development of the temporal bone have a bearing upon the cases which is of such practical nature that they cannot be ignored, because frequently neither an accurate diagnosis of mastoiditis can be made in the infant nor a satisfactory treatment instituted unless the surgeon is familiar with the rudimentary state of the temporal bone at this early period of life.

It is a clinical fact that subperiosteal mastoid abscess is most frequently seen in the infant and very young child, and this fact is readily accounted for by the persistence of the squamomastoid suture at this period of life (Fig. 9). The plate of the squamous portion of the temporal bone is also quite thin, sometimes paper thin, and the mastoid antrum lies directly under it without any intervening cellular tissue. In short, the antrum is very superficial, necrosis can take place outwardly with ease, and hence, in some cases at least, the very superficial situation of the antrum itself may account for the postaural abscess.

The *causation* of mastoid abscess in children is the same as in adults— namely, infection of the mastoid antrum through the channels of the Eustachian tube and middle ear. The frequency of the occurrence of acute mastoiditis in infants may at least be partially accounted for on the anatomic reasons that the Eustachian tube in the infant is proportionately much wider and shorter than in the adult, whereas the middle ear and mastoid antrum are almost as large as they ever become,— anatomic conditions favoring the admission of disease germs from the nasopharynx.

The *symptoms* are usually not so well marked as in adults. The first indication of the extension of the suppurative otitis to the region of the mastoid may be the occurrence of the postauricular swelling. It is a noteworthy fact that infants do not, as a rule, appear to suffer great pain during the establishment and progress of this disease. It is not at all uncommon to meet with cases in which the postaural abscess is already large, and yet the child shows few if any evidences of acute suffering. This may be accounted for, first, from the fact that the large spaces of the antrum and the large and comparatively short Eustachian tube permits, in addition to the perforated membrana tympani, a better drainage into the nasopharynx than is possible through the same channels in the adult; and, secondly, by the ease with which the pus finds its way outward through the squamomastoid fissure which lies inferior to the antrum and marks the boundary between the mastoid and squamous portions of the bone (Fig. 9). Sometimes, however, the temperature runs high, the pain is severe, exhaustion is evident, and pulmonary or meningeal symptoms, that lead to error in diagnosis and treatment, may develop.

Diagnosis.—Extension of the suppuration to the mastoid antrum in an infant should be suspected in any case that has been preceded by a middle-ear discharge, which does not promptly cease after the establishment of good drainage, and in which anemia, prostration, continued fever, or malnutrition become evidence of some complicating ailment. Mastoid tenderness is too uncertain to be helpful in many cases because an infant will usually cry or squirm if pressure be made anywhere on its body. Swelling behind and above the ear, when occurring in connection with an aural discharge, is the most certain external evidence of the mastoid complication. The sagging of the posterosuperior meatal wall at its junction with the tympanic ring, which is frequently present as an important diagnostic aid in adults, when occurring in those under three years of age will be seen upon the superior instead of the superoposterior wall of the canal, for the reason that there are as yet no cells developed in the mastoid process which can fill with pus and cause the bulging on the adjacent posterior wall. The mastoid antrum and attic lie almost wholly above the tympanic ring, and hence collections of pus within these spaces would affect chiefly the superior meatal wall. The treatment directed to the abortion of the disease differs in no essential respect from that already advised in the adult (see p. 286). The surgical treatment, however, must be greatly modified by reason of the anatomic differences that exist in the infantile bone.

The Mastoid Operation as Performed on Children under Two Years of Age.—Previous to this age there is commonly no development of the mastoid process, and consequently there are no cells to be opened and no mastoid tip to be removed. There is, however, present at birth the one large cell, the mastoid antrum, and it is with this single cavity that the operator must deal when operating on the infant or young child for mastoid abscess. To open this cell the primary incision should begin a little below Reid's base line (Fig. 269), and follow the post-auricular attachment at the usual distance to a point above and posterior to the superior attachment of the auricle. In making this incision down to the bone, the operator should not forget that the osseous tissues of the skull at this age are soft, that they may in addition be necrotic, and that, therefore, by undue pressure upon the knife it is easily possible to enter the cranial cavity. Instead of trying to make one incision that will extend entirely to the bone throughout the entire distance, it is much safer to cut through the skin, fascia, and periosteum by separate and careful strokes of the knife, the blade of which, while so used, should be held somewhat away from the perpendicular. The soft parts are then reflected in the usual way and the whole osseous field of operation is exposed to view. The suprameatal triangle (see Fig. 165, 3) should be sought for just as in the adult case, but the operator must remember that the position of this is changed from that already studied in the fully developed bone. The posterior ridge of the zygoma, forming the linea temporalis, lies on a higher plane in the infant and must be sought for at a greater distance above the superior margin of the tympanic ring. It is not well developed in every case and may be difficult or impossible to find, but, as in older persons, it forms the superior boundary of the triangle and indicates the uppermost line of safety in operating.

The postero-inferior border of the triangle is formed by the squamo-mastoid suture, which can, as a rule, be distinctly traced (see Fig. 9). The triangle is completed by the antero-inferior border which is formed by the postero-superior part of the tympanic ring (see Fig. 35). The posterior skin flap must be dissected from the skull for a sufficient distance in every case to expose the squamomastoid suture, because this marks the lower limit of safety in the operation.

It will thus be seen that in order to safely open the mastoid antrum of an infant it will be necessary to do so through a small triangle, which lies in a higher plane than the suprameatal triangle of the adult; and that this space lies more nearly above than behind the orifice of the external meatus. Any attempt to enter the antrum in the usual way would not only fail, but would also endanger the facial nerve which emerges from the bone as high up as the line drawn horizontally through the center of the external auditory meatus. The sigmoid sinus in infants was posterior to the above triangle in all the cases examined, and, therefore, if the operator keeps within this area when removing the bone he will run slight risk of injuring this vessel.

Since the antrum occupies a position under the above triangle, it is covered only by the very thin plate of the squamous portion of the temporal. Hence, to expose it requires but a few gentle strokes of the mallet upon the small sharp gouge, after which the overhanging ledges can be bitten away by a small bone-forceps. The interior of the cavity of the antrum is then cureted with thoroughness, but with the exercise of very gentle care. The after-treatment varies in no essential particular from that already advised in adult cases (see ·p. 307).

CHAPTER XXVI

CHRONIC PURULENT OTITIS MEDIA. CAUSATION, PATHOLOGY, SYMPTOMS, AND DIAGNOSIS

This disease, because of its frequency, variety, and dangerous complications, forms one of the largest, most interesting, and important chapters in otology. It is highly probable, however, that when the profession becomes more familiar with the modern principles of otologic practise and applies the same more vigorously in the acute stages of aural diseases than at present, the number of cases of chronic discharging ears, together with the numerous and serious complications of the same, will be greatly diminished.

Pathology.—In chronic suppurative diseases of the middle ear the suppurative inflammation attacks the mucous membrane of the tympanum, causing polypoid degeneration with the formation of polypi or cushions of granulomata. The inflammation may extend to the bone, especially in tuberculosis and syphilis. Acute suppurative otitis media blends into the chronic disease after eight weeks' duration. This rule is arbitrary, for there is no sharp division between acute and chronic suppurative diseases. Accompanying the granulomata caries takes place, sometimes necrosis or caries necrotica. Loss of the incus is common, especially its short process and head. The head of the malleus or its handle is often destroyed and such changes take place as are described under caries of the temporal bone (p. 550). The formation of cholesteatomata is not uncommon and the bone may become porous or it may become sclerotic, even ivory-like (see Fig. 241). Destruction of the drum membrane may be slight or entire (see Figs. 196 and 197). Fig. 183 shows a section of drum membrane which is very much thickened and opaque as a result of chronic aural suppuration. The mucous membrane epithelium is lacking on the right and the drum membrane thins down to scar tissue with a layer of mucous membrane and a dermal layer, that is, the membrana propria is wanting. In this figure the membrana propria is not clearly defined. The layer of mucous membrane is greatly thickened with areas of infiltration and enlarged blood-vessels. The elastic fibers are clearly shown

in each of the three layers of the drum membrane. A layer of desquamated epithelium nearly the thickness of the thickened drum is
adherent to the dermal layer. The discharge may be mucopurulent,
seropurulent, thin, and acrid, as in tuberculous diseases; very thick
and stringy when the Eustachian tube is involved. The discharge may
be very abundant or very slight, sometimes so slight as to form crusts
and deceive the patient, who believes the ear is not discharging. The
odor is sometimes offensive. Small particles of bone may be found in
the discharge. The disease may end in any of the so-called complications, such as brain abscess, meningitis, sinus thrombosis, extradural
abscess, or labyrinthine disease. In early childhood, even up to twelve
years of age, acquired deaf-mutism is common.

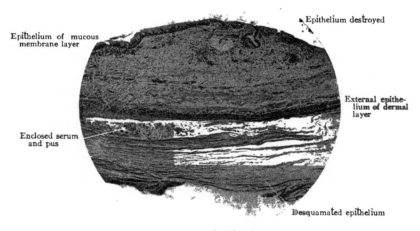

FIG. 183.—SECTION OF DRUM MEMBRANE; CASE OF CHRONIC OTITIS MEDIA SUPPURATIVA.
(Prepared by Dr. H. C. Low.)

Granulations are found in the middle ear and consist of newly
formed tissue composed of round cells richly supplied with blood-vessels.
These new growths develop under the influence of long-continued
inflammatory irritation. The superficial layers of the mucous membrane are destroyed and granulomata spring up, at first little papules
with raspberry-like appearance. These granulomata bleed easily when
touched. They may be covered with squamous, ciliated, or columnar
epithelium, according to where the granulomata are located, and their
internal structure may become differentiated. They are called polypi.
The term polyp indicates the shape of the new growth and does not
indicate the character of its tissue. Sometimes the polyp is covered

with flat epithelium in one part and with glandular-like epithelium in another part [1] (see Figs. 184 and 185).

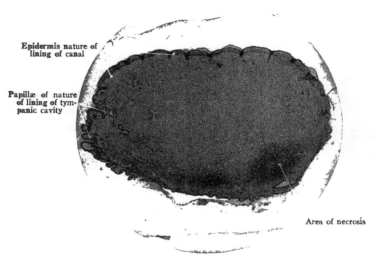

Epidermis nature of lining of canal

Papillæ of nature of lining of tympanic cavity

Area of necrosis

FIG. 184.—TRANSVERSE SECTION OF AURAL POLYP.
(Prepared by Dr. Wales.)

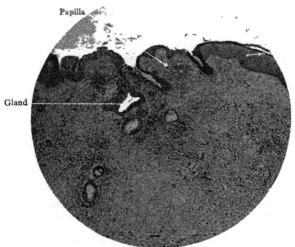

Papilla

Gland

FIG. 185.—TRANSVERSE SECTION OF AURAL POLYP SHOWING CHARACTER OF COVERING EPITHELIUM.
(From a preparation by Dr. Wales.)

Causation.—Chronic aural discharges, with the exception of the comparatively few cases that complicate tuberculosis or syphilis, are

[1] Goerke, *Archiv. f. Ohrenheilkunde*, Bd lii., Heft. 1 and 2, p. 63, 1901.

the sequelæ of a preceding acute tympanic inflammation. The violence of the acute affection has usually been so great that necrosis of the mucous membrane or osseous structures has taken place to such an extent that nature, even when assisted by rational treatment, is unable to repair the damage and consequently the disease has become chronic. Chronicity of the discharge will probably result if, during the acute

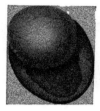

stage, the perforation in the drum membrane is too small to permit free drainage. Failure on the part of the physician to apply, during the acute stage and at the earliest possible moment, the well-established principles of treatment is also responsible for many chronic cases.

FIG. 185 a.—AURAL POLY-
PUS SPRINGING FROM ATTIC
AND PARTIALLY FILLING EX-
TERNAL MEATUS.

The presence of adenoids, nasal inflammation, and new growths in either the nose or naso-pharynx have the unquestioned tendency to pro-long an acute purulent otitis into the chronic form. Whatever may have been the cause of failure to arrest the suppurative disease in its incipiency, if it continues beyond a period of six to eight weeks it is, by common consent, said to be chronic.

Prognosis.—The points of most concern as to prognosis relate to the cessation of the discharge, the restoration of the impaired hearing, and the danger to the life of the individual. A trustworthy prognosis is impossible unless an examination has been made with sufficient accuracy to determine the location and extent of the middle-ear disease as well as the complications which may be present in a given case.

Crura of stapes   Long process of incus

Course of chorda tympani nerve

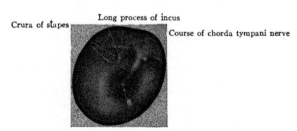

FIG. 186.—RIGHT DRUM MEMBRANE WITH TRANSPARENCY EXAGGERATED, SHOWING COURSE OF CHORDA TYMPANI NERVE AND THE RELATION OF THE OSSICLES AS SEEN THROUGH A SPECULUM.

In the milder forms, where the disease has become chronic from the neglect of aural cleanliness or from the presence of adenoids or nasal growths, and when there is no bone involvement, the discharge may be said to be always curable. Even where granulations or polypi are present or when one or more ossicles are necrosed, the discharge will cease after the complete removal of the offending parts. When the osseous tympanic walls are denuded of their covering membrane to any considerable extent, and particularly if the tegmen antri, tegmen tympani, or other distant and more inaccessible parts are affected, the prognosis as to cure of the discharge is bad, except as a result of the most skilful and well-directed mastoid surgery.

The fact is now generally recognized that grave danger to life attends the majority of all chronic suppurative ear diseases. It is becoming apparent that, excepting traumatic and systemic causes, nearly if not all suppurative and inflammatory affections within the cranial cavity have their origin in an infected condition of one or more of the air spaces which lie in close proximity to the base of the brain. Two of these spaces, the middle ear and mastoid antrum, lie in such intimate relation to the dura mater of the cerebrum and cerebellum that infection of these latter structures would seem an almost inevitable consequence of a prolonged suppuration within the former.

When the attic of the ear and the adjoining mastoid antrum are involved, and the osseous walls of these cavities are invaded by the destructive process, the dangers of intracranial extension are always grave. If cholesteatoma is present softening of the surrounding bone takes place from the pressure of the mass, thus exposing the brain and sigmoid sinus to almost certain infection unless the progress of the disease is promptly arrested by surgical interference.

The results of treatment for the restoration of the impaired hearing are usually unsatisfactory. The original disease has in most cases wrought irreparable damage. A drum membrane or ossicle that is once destroyed by the chronic suppurative process can never be restored to usefulness. Where the impairment of hearing is largely due to a thickened mucosa, to an imprisoned stapes, or to adhesions of some part of the drum membrane or long process of the malleus, appropriate treatment will often yield good results. When the tympanic membrane and ossicles have been swept away and the mucous membrane of the middle ear becomes ultimately "dermoid" and dry, the hearing power is often less acute than during the continuance of the discharge.

Symptoms.—A large percentage of cases of chronic aural discharge complains of nothing except the discharge itself, and this is quite often looked upon by the patient and his friends as a trivial annoyance which is scarcely worth the trouble required for treatment. Among the more careless or ignorant it is not unusual to find those who have had running ears for long periods, and yet have never thought it necessary to do more than to wipe away the pus when it appeared externally in the auditory meatus.

The amount of discharge varies in different cases from that so profuse as to fill the auditory meatus several times a day to a quantity so small that it seldom or never wets the whole auditory canal. When produced in such minute quantity the pus dries about the edges of the membranous perforation or upon the adjacent meatal walls into hard masses, in which condition it is easily mistaken for inspissated ear wax. This class of patient will state that formerly his ear discharged, but he is apt to believe that for a long time it has been absolutely free from any suppuration.

The pus may be mucopurulent and stringy, thin and sanious, or creamy and yellow, depending much upon the particular part of the middle ear most affected and upon the kind of tissue involved. Mucoid discharges are found in cases in which the lower portion of the drum cavity and Eustachian tube are the chief seats of the disease, while creamy pus usually originates in a diseased attic or mastoid antrum. A bloody discharge occasionally occurs in cases where granulations or polypi are present, since these growths are highly vascular and the vessels so thin walled that the bleeding may take place spontaneously. The occurrence of such a hemorrhage is indicative of no additional gravity, but becomes important from the fact that the patient is sufficiently alarmed by it to seek curative measures at once, whereas previously he had been entirely satisfied with nature's indefinite, uncertain, and, perhaps, dangerous course.

In the mildest cases and those that have received proper care in the way of cleansing, the pus may have little or no odor. In many cases, however, even after the most thorough cleansing possible, the penetrating odor of the purulent discharge persists and is often characteristic of chronic aural suppuration. Fetid odor is present in attic necrosis in connection with involvement of the ossicular chain, and especially in cases where cholesteatomatous masses are present in the tympanic cavity. Such odors, here as elsewhere, are due to retention and decomposition of the secretions or to decay of the soft or bony structures, and can, in most cases, be permanently arrested only by providing perfect drainage and after complete obliteration and removal of the diseased tissues. Chronic suppurative otitis media sometimes results in the destruction of the chorda tympani nerve, which traverses the upper anterior portion of the cavity of the middle ear (see Fig. 186; also Fig. 24). When this takes place the patient complains of a disturbance of taste on the lateral half of the tongue corresponding to the affected ear. Complaint is also occasionally made that there is present in the mouth a continual bad taste. This latter is due to the fact that some of the aural discharge finds its way into the nasopharynx and mouth through the patulous Eustachian tube. Severe stomach and intestinal disturbances have been known to follow when the patient swallows the pus, which thus finds its' way into the pharynx through the Eustachian tube.

Facial paralysis is also an occasional symptom, particularly when the aural suppuration is complicated by cholesteatoma, mastoiditis, or labyrinth necrosis. The facial palsy occurring in this connection may be the result of an extension of the inflammation and infection into the Fallopian canal, in which instance an inflammatory exudate takes place about the nerve sheath, and the pressure consequent upon the increased amount of fluid is sufficient to inhibit the function of the nerve. The facial nerve may be invaded by necrosis of the bone comprising the canal, a sequestrum may form, and the nerve trunk may, as a result, be exposed to direct infection from the middle ear. In such case the exposed portion of the nerve trunk may be completely destroyed; or, as a result of the exposure of the nerve from necrosis, granulations or polypi may spring up over the site of the diseased bone, the pressure from which may be great enough to impair the nerve or even to completely destroy it for a considerable distance.

The hearing power, even when there has been considerable destruction of the drum membrane, ossicles, and other tissues of the middle ear, often remains so good that the patient makes little or no complaint concerning it. Even when the tympanic membrane, hammer, and incus have been entirely swept away by the violence of the original disease, the patient may yet be able to hear the conversational voice quite well. Children who have suffered such destruction of the middle-ear structures as a result of measles, scarlet fever, or other violent diseases, are subsequently often able to attend school with remarkably slight inconvenience from the resulting deafness.

All chronic suppurative middle-ear cases, however, are not so fortunate in this respect, for in some, labyrinthine inflammation or even suppuration may be a complication from the first, in which instance the loss of hearing is always much greater and is sometimes complete. When very considerable impairment occurs in the very young, deaf-mutism is an inevitable consequence (see Chapter XLVIII.). Deafness is also more pronounced when in the course of the long-continued discharge the foot-plate of the stapes becomes imbedded and immovably fixed in the oval window by the formation of connective tissue over and about it. Connective-tissue deposits in the round window, adhesions of the handle of the malleus to the promontory, and ankylosis of the ossicular chain may occur singly or together during the progress of any case, and when present will greatly impair the hearing power of the individual.

Pain is not a prominent symptom of this disease. Patients are not uncommon who have had running ears for many years with absolutely no suffering since the onset of the ailment. When present in any case pain is indicative of imperfect drainage. Either the perforation that was formerly ample for the purpose has become too small from gradual closure, or else a granulation, polypus, or crust of dried secretion is blocking the opening and retaining the pus under pressure. When the suppurative process has extended to the mastoid antrum and cells a free outlet for the pus through the middle ear is frequently no longer possible, and this is often a cause of suffering, either as a result of the pent-up pus or of the periosteal inflammation and external swelling which is produced by the fluid in its effort to liberate itself through some part of the temporal bone.

Tinnitus aurium is present in many cases, but seldom with such intensity as that which accompanies chronic non-suppurative aural inflammation. The head noises are oftenest found, when coexistent with chronic suppuration, in those cases where physical examination reveals the presence of adhesions of the remnant of the drum membrane to the inner tympanic wall or of the long process of the malleus to the promontory. Tinnitus is also very apt to result from the imprisonment of the foot-plate of the stapes in the oval window, which occurs as a consequence of the connective tissue that is deposited about it during the long course of the disease. This symptom is also present in an exaggerated form in many patients in whom the aural discharge has ceased for weeks or months, but with resultant cicatrization and contraction of all the middle-ear tissues which were formerly inflamed and suppurating.

Dizziness becomes an annoying symptom in some cases. It may occur only at the time the ear is syringed or otherwise treated or it may be constantly present and so severe that the patient is unsafe when walking abroad alone. Where faintness occurs when the ear is irrigated, it is usually due to the presence of a large opening through the drum membrane which permits the fluid entering the ear to strike the oval window with considerable force. If the dizziness is constant and severe, labyrinthine involvement should be suspected.

The symptoms of the complicating ailments which may arise in the course of the disease, for example, mastoiditis and the various intracranial affections, are more properly discussed in chapters devoted to this subject (see p. 353, Chapter XXVIII.).

Diagnosis.—1. *Physical Examination.*—Preceding any examination of the drum-head in which there are suspected changes in its position, thickness, color, or, more particularly, if there is a probable loss of a large portion of the membrana (Fig. 191), the examiner will do well to recall the landmarks of the normal structure. For purposes of rendering intelligible the description of the pathologic condition that may be found, and in order that the results of the inspection may be properly recorded, the quadrants, their location and boundaries, should also be noted (Fig. 187).

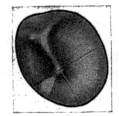

FIG. 187.—THE QUAD-RANTS OF THE DRUM-HEAD VIEWED THROUGH A SPECULUM.

In no branch of medicine or surgery is a painstaking and thorough examination into the exact state of the diseased parts more necessary to successful treatment than in chronic otitis media purulenta. Neither empiricism nor inference has a place among modern methods, as they pertain to the diagnosis of chronic discharging ears. Every feature of the disease as presented by each individual patient must be noted and given proper significance. In any case of chronic otorrhea the disease may have extended to the mastoid region. Indeed, such complication may have constituted the patient's sole reason for consulting the physician. However this may be, as a first step of the examination the region of the mastoid process should be inspected, and comparison made with the corresponding portions of the opposite side, in order to determine if there be present any tenderness, redness, swelling, or fistula leading into the mastoid antrum or cells. During this part of the examination the patient is placed with his back toward a good light from a window, in which position any malposition or tumefaction about the auricle will be readily noted. If there is much swelling behind the ear and over the mastoid or in the posterior wall of the external auditory meatus, the pinna will be pushed forward so as to stand most noticeably away from the head and will cause the latter to appear decidedly unbalanced (see Fig. 181). Pressure over the tip of the mastoid process at the point of exit of the mastoid vein and over the site of the mastoid antrum should not be neglected, because in disease of the underlying cavities these situations are most constantly sensitive to deep pressure (see Fig. 151). Should a mastoiditis have existed for a long time as a complication of the chronic discharge in the tympanic cavity, there is a possibility that the bony cortex and soft tissues covering the mastoid process may have ruptured, leaving a discharging fistula in the post-auricular area (Fig. 188). Such an occurrence may be best observed with the patient in the above position, which is also a favorable one for gently probing any such sinus in order to ascertain the depth and direction of the channel, and also to learn whether or not bony sequestra or necrotic areas lie in its tract. The condition of postaural fistula leading to deep foci of disease is one calling urgently for operative measures, and although the patient may make little or no complaint concerning it, experience has shown that there is the gravest danger of extension of the disease to the sigmoid sinus, where thrombosis may

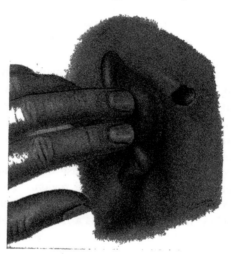

Fig. 188.—Postaural Fistula of Long Duration Resulting from Acute Mastoiditis. Chronic tympanic and mastoid suppuration were present at the time the drawing was made. A radical mastoid operation was performed.

be produced, to the meninges causing meningitis, or to the cerebral or cerebellar structures, where abscess may result.

The patient is next placed in the examining chair in proper position to use reflected artificial light. The external meatus is first inspected and the lumen of its canal noted. In cases where there has been a discharge covering a period of several years, or perhaps only a few months if the discharge has been irritating, the skin lining the meatus at times becomes greatly thickened, fissured, or eczematous, any one of which complications may have caused the patient more annoyance or suffering than the primary ailment. Accumulations of epithelia or of inspissated pus or cerumen are sometimes seen lying more deeply in the canal, all of which must be removed before an examination of the drum membrane or middle ear can be satisfactorily made. If a crust of dried secretion is found covering Shrapnell's membrane and the adjacent superoposterior wall of the external meatus (Fig. 189), the same possibly indicates a perforation of the membrane above the short process of the malleus (Fig. 199). Examination of the crust after it is removed will show its composition to be dried pus. Accumulations in this region are often pathognomonic of attic disease and in such instance the surgeon should be cautious not to state to the patient that the same is ear wax and that the condition is, therefore, a trivial one.

The external meatus, having been cleared of all obstruction by syringing or by the use of appropriate instruments used under the direction of the eye and a good reflected light, the examination of the membrana tympani and middle-ear cavities is begun. A proper-sized speculum is inserted and the canal straightened by traction. It cannot

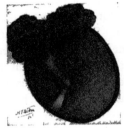

FIG. 189.—CRUST OF DRIED PUS COVERING PERFORATION IN SHRAPNELL'S MEMBRANE AND EXTENDING OUTWARD INTO AUDITORY CANAL.
Fig. 199 shows perforation in Shrapnell's membrane after crust has been removed.

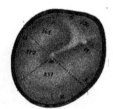

FIG. 190.—SHOWS THE RELATIVE FREQUENCY OF PERFORATION IN EACH QUADRANT OF THE DRUM-HEAD IN 1000 CASES, AS OBSERVED BY B. A. RANDALL.

be too often repeated that the patient's auricle must be lifted strongly upward and backward until the canal is straightened, for in this position only it is possible for the light to penetrate to the fundus in sufficient volume to fully illuminate the drum membrane. The observer will first note the presence or absence of the landmarks (see Fig. 96) and normal color, the disappearance or modification of which will bear a close relation to the amount of disease or destruction of the membrane. The membrana tympani may have become thickened, perforated, or otherwise pathologically altered in any portion of its structure. The whole membrane may have been swept away by the violence of the original ailment or only portions or all of a given quadrant may be found wanting. While any shape, size, or position [1] of the perforation may be present, certain types are seen in practise, the most common being the following:

[1] B. A. Randall, *Trans. Otol. Section*, *A. M. A.*, 1898, gives the tabulated result of a study of the location of 1000 consecutive cases of perforation of the drum-head. Fig. 190 graphically represents the position of the different groups of perforation by quadrants.

(*a*) The short process and all or portions of the handle of the malleus remain intact even when large portions of the surrounding drum membrane have been destroyed, the projecting handle with its remnant of

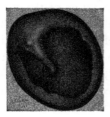

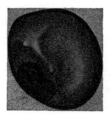

FIG. 191.—LOSS OF GREATER PORTION OF THE MEMBRANA TENSA.
The long process of the malleus remains intact.

FIG. 192.—PERFORATION IN ANTERO-INFERIOR QUADRANT, NEAR THE TYMPANIC ORIFICE OF THE EUSTACHIAN TUBE.

membrane attached, forming a kind of peninsula, which will be seen extending from above downward and backward in normal position (Fig.

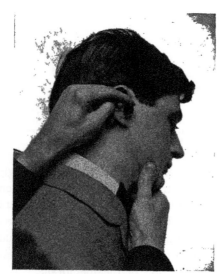

191). Sometimes in such instances the umbo is adherent to the promontory, in which case the condition is not so clearly made out by vision alone, and when such is the case the probe can be efficiently employed to determine this point.

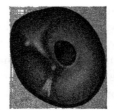

FIG. 193.—POSITION OF PATIENT'S HEAD WHILE INSPECTING THE ANTERIOR PORTION OF THE DRUM MEMBRANE.
The face is turned somewhat away from the examiner.

FIG. 194.—PERFORATION POSTERIOR TO THE UMBO.

(*b*) Perforation in the antero-inferior quadrant, near the site of entrance of the Eustachian tube, the shadow of the mouth of which is often visible if the opening into the drum cavity is sufficiently large (Fig. 192). A perforation of the membrane in this locality is best seen when the patient's face is turned slightly away from the examiner, who looks along the rays of light, which should penetrate the depths of the ear somewhat in the direction of the tip of the patient's nose (Fig. 193).

Perforations in this location have usually originated from some mild infective process which became chronic either because of inefficient treatment or from the existence of a catarrhal affection in the nose or nasopharynx. The presence of an adenoid is a great hindrance to the cure of any aural discharge, but is particularly influential in keeping alive the tubal and middle-ear inflammation with its mucopurulent secretion in cases of perforation in this quadrant. Very rarely are the osseous tissues carious or necrotic in this class of perforation.

(c) Perforation behind the handle of the malleus near its tip (Fig. 194). This class usually occurs in childhood and, like the preceding, is most likely the result of neglect, of the presence of nasopharyngeal inflammation, or of adenoids. It represents the least difficult class to

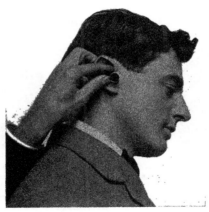

FIG. 195.—POSITION OF PATIENT'S HEAD DURING THE EXAMINATION OF THE CENTRAL PORTIONS OF THE DRUM-HEAD, INCLUDING THE HANDLE OF THE MALLEUS AND UMBO.
Head erect and face forward.

cure, since there are commonly few important changes in the middle ear itself and polypi seldom spring from the edges of the opening. The proper position of the patient's head for examining this portion of the drum membrane is shown in Fig. 195.

(d) A class in which the membranous rupture lies below the posterior fold and covers the site of the incudostapedial articulation (Fig. 196). Unlike the two preceding varieties, this one represents more deep-seated and violently destructive pathologic conditions within the drum cavity. Polypi frequently arise from within, grow through the perforation, and wholly or partially fill the auditory canal. Adhesions of the margins of the perforated membrane below and on each side to the adjacent mucous lining of the middle ear often occur, but the upper margins remain free, forming the mouth of a channel, the other extremity of which is usually high in the attic.   Necrosis of one or more ossicles or of some portion of the adjacent bony walls is common, and mastoid involvement is not an infrequent complication.

(*e*) Destruction of practically the whole membrana tensa. In such cases there is apt to remain a rim of thickened membrane along the whole line of attachment of the drum-head to the annulus tympanicus (Fig. 197). The membrana flaccida—Shrapnell's membrane—is usually present, but has become in most instances so much thickened, granular, or polypoid as to be wholly changed from the normal. Sometimes the short process and neck of the malleus, together with the stump of its handle, may be seen or felt with the probe imprisoned in the diseased tissues. The incus has usually suffered death, has already been discharged with the pus, or a remnant of the ossicle may be found lying dislocated and useless in some portion of the middle ear. If the

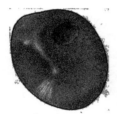

FIG. 196.—RUPTURE BELOW THE POSTERIOR FOLD OVER SITE OF INCUDOSTAPEDIAL ARTICULATION.

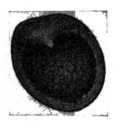

FIG. 197.—LOSS OF GREATER PORTION OF MEMBRANA TENSA.
Stump of malleus handle remains, membrana flaccida thickened. Tympanic mucous membrane granular.

head of the patient be tilted far to one side and away from the examiner (Fig. 198), the head and portions of the crura of the stapes may possibly be visible if not located too high, and are not imbedded in granulations or connective tissue.   In cases of comparatively short duration the mucous lining of the tympanic cavity presents an inflamed, thickened, and granular appearance.   In this condition it is not always easy to determine whether the drum membrane is present or totally wanting, since the entire appearance may very closely simulate that in which the intact drum membrane is so much thickened and inflamed that its landmarks are entirely obliterated.   Where the disease has been of long standing and the suppuration is very scant, the tympanic cavity is sometimes covered with a dermoid epithelium which has grown inward from the external meatus, a "dermatized" mucous membrane, that is far less sensitive to the touch and which serves none of the secretory functions of the normal lining; but for purposes of protection to the widely exposed cavity the new covering is vastly superior to a mucous membrane.

(*f*) From the standpoints of pathology, prognosis. and treatment, perforations through Shrapnell's membrane are the most important. These ruptures are of necessity small and are most often located immediately external to or just above the short process of the malleus (Fig. 199). Their external appearance usually gives no indication of the serious nature of the underlying disease, and they are entirely overlooked unless the examiner is both skilful and thorough. The small amount of pus discharged through this variety of perforation often dries as fast as it appears in the opening, and a crust thus forms about the edges of the perforation and its adjacent parts; this finally covers not only the

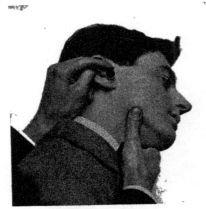

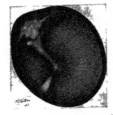

FIG. 198.—POSITION OF THE PATIENT'S HEAD FOR EXAMINING SHRAPNELL'S MEMBRANE.
The head is inclined away from the examiner, the face of the patient approaching somewhat the horizontal.

FIG. 199.—PERFORATION IN SHRAPNELL'S MEMBRANE, SHOWING DROP OF PUS IN OPENING.
Same case as that shown in Fig. 189.

perforation but also the whole of Shrapnell's membrane, and may then extend outwardly along the superoposterior wall of the external meatus (see Fig. 189). It is such a crust that is often mistaken for hardened ear wax and, as previously stated, the surgeon should be warned against the mistake of telling his patient that the condition is trivial. Upon the removal of this inspissated pus, and when the patient's head has been placed in a position away from the examiner and horizontally to one side, the perforation will be seen filled with purulent secretion (Fig. 199). Examination of the crust after its removal will also show its true composition. The condition is one distinctly indicative of attic and mastoid involvement. Necrosis of the head, neck, and, often, the short process of the malleus have usually taken place, and the osseous attic walls and mastoid antrum are frequently involved. The entire pathology is one to be dealt with surgically, since local applications and general medication have only a subsidiary place in the treatment.

Visual impressions are not always entirely reliable in aural diagnosis. Conditions are often present that would lead to error if sight alone were depended on. A delicate silver probe that may be bent to any suitable angle is a most valuable aid in diagnosis (Fig. 200). A polypus projecting through the membrane, and partially or wholly filling the canal (Fig. 201), can be moved about by the gentle use of such an instrument; the consistency of such a growth and the point of its attachment can be determined, and thus a positive diagnosis of the nature of the tumor can be made. Foreign bodies at the fundus of the meatus are apt to be mistaken for new growths unless the probe be delicately and intelligently used to aid the

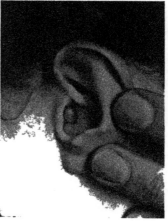

FIG. 200.—DELICATE SILVER AURAL PROBE.

FIG. 201.—AURAL POLYPUS PROJECTING INTO THE CONCHA. See microphotographs (Figs. 185 and 186) prepared from growth here shown.

examination. Necrosis of an ossicle or of any part of the bony walls of the drum cavity can be detected with certainty only by the dextrous use of this little instrument. During the examination it is often necessary to bend and rebend the probe until that particular angle is found that will enable the instrument to follow the diseased parts into the depths to which the latter have extended. Should the tip of the probe touch uncovered.bone, the grating sensation imparted to the hand of the examiner is unmistakable. The situation of any carious region should be noted and the probable tissue involved should be determined, in order that proper measures may be more ration_ally applied in the subsequent treatment. The region behind and above the short process of the malleus should always be most thoroughly inspected with the probe in any case in which the drum membrane is seen to be perforated near this landmark. It is a well-known pathologic fact that the largest number of chronic discharging ears follows acute suppuration in the attic, and when such discharges result from the violent infectious diseases of childhood, necrosis in this locality will almost certainly be found if sought for with sufficient persistence and skill. The head of the malleus is sometimes largely

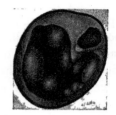

Fig. 202.—Loss of Greater Portion of Drum-head including Head and Most of Malleus Handle.
Aural polypi present. Ossiculectomy; curettage; recovery.

or wholly destroyed, the perforated drum membrane being covered by one or more polypi that spring from the necrotic tissues (Fig. 202).

The posterosuperior wall of the external meatus should also receive careful consideration in this examination, because if the suppuration in the middle ear is of long standing, and especially if the mastoid has been involved, there sometimes exists a perforation in this location which leads not only through the soft tissues of the external auditory canal but also penetrates deeply into the underlying osseous structures. The probe should be entered into the mouth of any such fistula and the direction and extent of the channel thus be ascertained. Sequestra or carious bone can in this way, even though they lie deeply in the mastoid process, usually be detected. Polypi or granulations sometimes spring from the external orifice of these fistulæ, and may require removal before the aperture of the same can be seen. The presence of a fistula in this location is pathognomonic of chronic mastoiditis.

(2) *Functional Examination of the Ear.*—The voice, whisper, and watch tests indicate a loss of the hearing power which varies greatly in different individuals. Even when much destruction of the drum membrane and tissues of the middle ear have taken place, the hearing may be found to be but moderately impaired. When the suppuration is complicated by a labyrinthine involvement the greatest degree of deafness is usually found. Tuning-fork tests will show that the lowest notes are heard but poorly if at all, whereas, unless there is a labyrinthine complication, the higher tones will be heard quite well. Bone conduction is better than air conduction (bc $>$ ac) in uncomplicated cases, and

22

if only one ear is involved in the chronic suppurative process, the tuning-fork will be heard better on the diseased side when placed while vibrating upon the median line of the skull or against the upper central incisor teeth (Weber's test).

In case the labyrinth has become involved, and a mixed deafness is present, both the high and low notes of the tuning-fork will be heard poorly or not at all.   If the labyrinthine deafness predominates over that caused by the damage to the middle ear, the vibrating C_2 fork, when placed upon the center line of the head, will probably be heard better in the better ear, and air conduction will be better than bone conduction—ac > bc, or Rinné, is said to be positive—Rinné+.

The treatment of chronic purulent otitis is both medicinal and surgical, and will be considered in the two succeeding chapters.

CHAPTER XXVII

CHRONIC PURULENT OTITIS MEDIA (Continued)

THE MEDICINAL TREATMENT

In chronic purulent otitis media, as in ailments in other parts of the body, successful treatment must be based upon accurate diagnosis. Hence, before curative measures are attempted a definite conclusion as to the exact character of the disease, its pathology, extent, and situation should first have been determined. An aural discharge may result from an abscess or other affection of the external meatus; from necrosis, inflammation, or new growths in the middle ear, or the pus may have its origin in more than one or even the entire chain of air spaces that communicate with the drum cavity—namely, the mastoid antrum and the mastoid cells. Disease of the Eustachian tube sometimes not only perpetuates a suppurative process within the middle ear, but may itself furnish a part of the muco-purulent material which constitutes the aural discharge.

Considering the widely different sources of the discharge and the varying amount, character, and location of the disease producing the same, it is evident that no single plan of treatment will prove sufficient to effect a cure in all. The several steps of the management, each based upon the well-established principles of aural practise, and the correct diagnosis of the individual case, are therefore given somewhat in the order in which they may be most conveniently studied.

(1) **Constitutional Treatment.**—In a considerable number of cases of chronic aural discharge, it will be found that constitutional conditions exist which are either entirely or partly responsible for the continuance of the local disease. Chief among these are tuberculosis, scrofula, syphilis, and anemia. Impaired nutrition from whatever cause will require the most rational constitutional treatment. If the general symptoms and local pathology point certainly to tuberculosis, all modern knowledge that pertains to the treatment of this disease should, in connection with local medication, be rigidly carried out. Open air, sunshine, suitable food, and exercise in proportion to the physical strength of the patient are essential. Creosote or guaiacol, if well borne by the stomach, must yet be regarded as possessing first medicinal value.

Syphilitic aural complications are rare in chronic suppurative otitis and occur most frequently in the third stage of the luetic disease. Hence, the iodids of potassium or sodium prove most serviceable if given in increasing doses and until their effect on the local ear lesion is noticeably beneficial, after which time gradual reduction of the dosage may be made. The author has no faith in the efficacy of small and infrequent doses of this remedy, but has witnessed satisfactory results after saturation of the patient with the drug has been accomplished.

(2) **Nasal and Nasopharyngeal Management.**—Many aural patients are seldom free from head colds, which materially increase the aural suppuration and hinder or make useless the best-directed efforts of local treatment of the middle ear. These colds are usually caused and maintained by the presence of chronic nasal and naso-pharyngeal inflammation or new growths. In such instances little progress can be made toward the cure of the aural affection until a more healthful condition of the upper air tract is secured. Head colds are also a symptom of vasomotor rhinitis, a nervous state in which the sympathetic control of the circulation in the mucous lining of the nose is lost, resulting in oversecretion and a stuffy feeling about the head— a condition which is exactly similar in its effects on a discharging ear to that just described as resulting from new growths in the nose or nasopharynx.

In all these cases it is imperative to restore free nasal breathing and to subdue the chronic inflammation of the nose and nasopharynx by local applications or surgical measures appropriate to the individual case, the description of which procedures is more fully given in Chapter XIX.

(3) **Local Medication.**—*Syringing.*—Cleanliness of the suppurating aural cavities is the first consideration in the local treatment of any case. The maintenance of absolute sterility of the affected parts is, of itself, often sufficient treatment, and will cure many of the milder affections. This aseptic state may be secured by syringing or by mopping the depths of the auditory canal by means of cotton cylinders of appropriate size held in the jaws of a dressing-forceps (Fig. 203) or by a pledget of sterile cotton on the end of an applicator (Figs. 204 and 205), and of such size as will readily pass to the fundus of the ear. Numerous cleansing and antiseptic solutions have been recommended because of their supposed virtues in the cure of the discharge. Any solution intended for syringing the ear should possess the essential qualities of sterility and non-irritability. The first quality is easily obtained by boiling and the second by avoiding overmedication with

irritating antiseptic substances. The simplest solutions are equal in efficiency to the more complex and expensive ones and the author has secured as good results from the use of normal salt solution or boric acid lotion as from any other he has tried. If the case should seem to

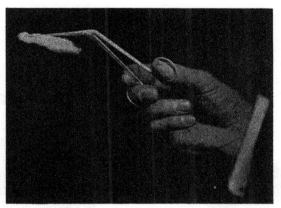

FIG. 203.—DRY METHOD OF CLEANSING THE EAR.

A piece of cotton of convenient size is folded into cylindric shape, grasped near its distal end in the jaws of the aural dressing-forceps, the auricle is retracted in the usual manner and the cotton is inserted gently but firmly to the bottom of the auditory canal. This procedure is repeated until the external meatus and fundus of the ear are thoroughly dry.

require a stronger antiseptic, like bichlorid of mercury, it should not be in greater proportion than 1:5000, and considering the short time that such a weak solution remains in contact with the diseased tissues, it is

FIG. 204.—AURAL APPLICATOR.

clear that the antiseptic qualities of the drug will have little if any more influence over the disease than would the simplest non-medicated, but sterile preparation.

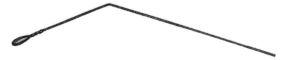

FIG. 205.—DELICATE AURAL APPLICATOR.

The frequency of cleansing the ear is of importance. If the discharge is profuse, foul smelling, and irritant to the tissues over which it flows, it is wise to cleanse it away frequently enough to neutralize its irritant qualities and to abate or lessen the odor. To accomplish this may require three or more daily treatments. In those cases where the discharge amounts to only a drop in the twenty-four hours, the small amount of pus appears but rarely if ever at the meatus, since it dries into a crust over and in the vicinity of the perforation. As previously stated, a crust thus formed is apt to be mistaken for hardened ear wax.

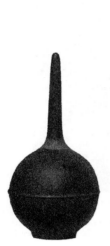 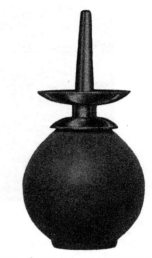

FIG. 206.—COMMON SOFT-RUBBER AURAL SYRINGE, SUITABLE FOR HOME USE BY PATIENT. It is easily sterilized.

FIG. 207.—ALLPORT'S AURAL SYRINGE, WITH SHIELD. No valves or packing to become septic. Easily sterilized; efficient for nearly all purposes of aural cleansing.

Syringing in such cases is only indicated sufficiently often to keep the perforation free from crusting. There is usually present necrosis of the osseous parts, and hence syringing can only yield temporary results.

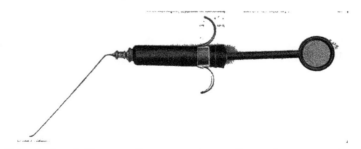

FIG. 208.—BLAKE'S MIDDLE-EAR SYRINGE, WITH ANGULAR TIP FOR CLEANSING THE ATTIC.

When syringing any ear in which there is present a considerable loss of the tympanic membrane, and particularly if the perforation be in the location of the stapes, care should be exercised at the beginning not to inject the fluid too forcibly, since a strong impact of the solution against the inner tympanic wall is likely to cause the patient to be giddy or even to loose consciousness and fall in a faint. This symptom is so constant and pronounced in some individuals that it becomes impossible

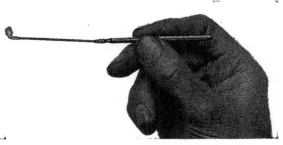

FIG. 209.—COMMON AURAL APPLICATOR BENT AT TIP TO NEARLY A RIGHT ANGLE.
The bent portion should be 4 or 5 mm. in length. When armed with a small tuft of cotton, as shown, this simple instrument is most valuable as a carrier for medicaments into the attic.

to syringe the ear, even though the act be performed with the utmost gentleness. The proper method of cleansing a discharging ear by means of syringing is shown in Fig. 210. The common urethral

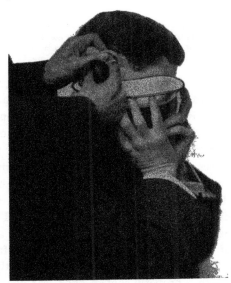

FIG. 210.—METHOD OF EFFECTIVELY SYRINGING THE EAR.
The patient supports the pus basin while the operator retracts the auricle with one hand and uses the syringe with the other. Allport's syringe in use.

syringe which is much in use (Fig. 211), is not an efficient instrument for aural syringing, and should never be recommended for that purpose.

The ear syringes in common use for the injection of fluids into the external auditory canal (Figs. 206 and 207) are not sufficient for cleansing the diseased areas when located in the attic. In this class of cases (see Figs. 196 and 197) a specially devised syringe (Fig. 208) or the attic canula is necessary to clear this portion of the ear from the foul-smelling accumulations of pus or cholesteatoma which are often retained there. By the use of reflected light, with the speculum in position and the auricle retracted, the delicate angular canula can be painlessly passed into the middle ear and upward into the attic behind the remnants of Shrapnell's membrane, in which position the cleansing fluid can be injected through it with sufficient force to dislodge the decomposing masses. After their removal and after the parts have been dried, applications of any desired medicament, as nitrate of silver, can be made to the attic structures by

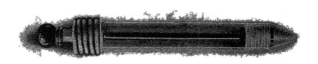

FIG. 211.—COMMON URETHRAL GLASS SYRINGE.

An instrument much used by the laity, some physicians, and even hospitals, as an ear syringe. It is shown only to emphasize the fact that it is useless as an instrument for cleansing the ear, especially if used by the patient himself.

means of a cotton-tipped angular applicator (Fig. 209), which is passed into the attic in the same manner as the irrigating canula.

(4) **Mechanical Removal of Accumulated Septic Matter.—** Syringing, although thoroughly done, is often insufficient to cleanse even the external meatus or the accessible portions of the middle ear. The hardened masses of secretion are sometimes so firmly attached to the walls of the auditory canal or to the irregularities of the tympanic membrane that the injected fluid fails to pass around and behind the accumulations with sufficient force to dislodge them. The parts should therefore be occasionally examined with reflected light as the syringing progresses, and if it be seen that the injections have failed to cleanse them thoroughly, the process can be hastened by gently removing the offending matter with a properly shaped hook, ear hoe, or other instrument especially selected for the case.

The use of peroxid of hydrogen for the purpose of loosening and thus facilitating the removal of hardened masses and of securing the antiseptic action of the drug, is often advisable. It has been charged against this preparation that the gases formed by its contact with pus are apt to carry septic material into the mastoid antrum and cells, where new foci of disease are thus established. Such an occurrence is possible, and therefore certain considerations should govern the use of the remedy. It is most safely employed in cases where the drum membrane is entirely or largely wanting, for in this condition it is not possible for gases to form faster than they escape, and hence the likelihood of infective material being carried to distant parts is scarcely worthy of consideration. On the other hand, if the perforation is small, the reverse is true, and the preparation should not be used.

If, as often happens in the course of a chronic discharging ear, there are present crusts of dried secretion which form a thin casing around the walls of the auditory canal, and which adhere with such tenacity that it is difficult to dislodge them, peroxid of hydrogen is also useful in facilitating their removal and in subsequently sterilizing the skin and hairs of the external meatus. For this purpose the peroxid is most conveniently applied in full strength by means of a proper-sized roll of cotton which has been wet in the solution and is then placed in the canal and allowed to remain long enough—usually only a few minutes—to soften and disintegrate the accumulations, after which they may be easily removed by syringing or by the use of the delicate dressing-forceps or ear-hook.

(5) **Methods of Drying the Parts.**—After the removal of every particle of infective or other material from the external auditory canal and middle ear, all these structures should be thoroughly dried. This is accomplished (a) by the use of the *cotton cylinder* and an ear applicator (see Fig. 203) used as described for mopping the deeper parts of the ear to cleanse them from pus. This of itself is, however, not always sufficient and must usually be supplemented by additional means, one of the best being:

(b) *Heated Air.*—Desiccation by means of the cotton mop can be much facilitated and rendered more thorough and lasting by the additional use of dry and moderately heated air. The benefits derived from the employment of the hot-air current are particularly noticeable in cases where all or a large portion of the drum membrane is wanting. The best method of applying heated air is by means of a specially constructed electric apparatus, the temperature of the current passing through which can be accurately regulated (Fig. 212). The beneficial action of hot air is, no doubt, due to the fact that it produces complete dryness of the affected tissues and thus renders impossible the growth of bacteria so long as the parts remain free from moisture. Although many patients will tolerate a high temperature of the air-blast, the best effects are obtained by moderate degrees of heat, since superheated air is apt to cause an unpleasant inflammatory reaction, and since a milder degree of heat will desiccate the parts equally well if only a little more time is given to its use.

It should be stated that before attempts are made to dry the cavities of the middle ear by any of the preceding methods or by all combined, that the process will often be much facilitated and the effects rendered more lasting if Eustachian catheterization and inflation of the middle ear be first performed. A current of air sufficiently strong to dislodge any pus or other secretion that may fill the Eustachian tube should be blown through the catheter which is inserted in the usual position for inflating the tympanic cavity. The air used for inflating the auditory tract will prove more beneficial if it has also been previously heated. In cases

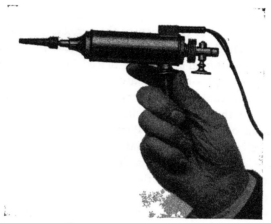

FIG. 212.—ELECTRIC AIR HEATER.
A convenience for thoroughly drying and sterilizing the tympanic cavity.

where the perforation through the drum membrane is large it is sometimes permissible to inject an antiseptic wash through the catheter, into the Eustachian tube and out through the external meatus, thus cleansing the entire tract before applying the drying process as above advised.

(c) *Drying Powders.*—Dusting-powders have, in the past, been quite universally employed, and often without the slightest reason. Hence, frequent disappointment as to results and often danger to life have occurred from their indiscriminate use. The rational employment of powders in aural practise must, like every other remedy, be based upon an exact diagnosis of the condition which is present in the ear as well as upon the therapeutic action of the drug itself. If a large perforation is known to exist in the drum membrane, the moderate application of an antiseptic drying powder to the middle-ear cavity will, in a majority of cases, prove beneficial.   On the other hand, if the rupture is small, it is not possible to blow the powder through it so as to reach the diseased tissues in the middle ear beyond, and in attempting to do so there is danger of filling the perforation with the powder and thus completely blocking the drainage.   The use of powder under the latter circumstances could be of value only in so far as it dries and sterilizes the external meatus.   Since free drainage is a first essential, under no circumstance should any powder be packed into the auditory canal in quantities sufficient to obstruct the outflow of pus.   It seems scarcely necessary to add that the middle ear and external auditory meatus should always be most thoroughly cleansed and dried before the powder is applied.

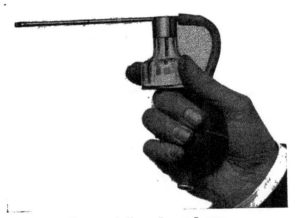

FIG. 213.—DeVilbiss Powder Blower.
The construction of this instrument is such that only the most finely comminuted powder may be blown into the ear.

A long list of powders has been recommended by various authors for aural use, but none is better than finely powdered boric acid if only the desiccating effect of the drug is desired.   By the absorptive properties of the powder the diseased fluids are so taken up that germ life is for the time, at least, inhibited or completely arrested.   Hence, after a discharging ear is cleansed of its septic contents, has been thoroughly dried by mopping with cotton and the application of hot air, the insufflation of a drying powder will continue the purifying and inhibiting process in many cases for a very considerable length of time.

The construction of the powder-blower to be used in aural practise is of much importance.   One with a receptacle which permits the passage of an indirect air current should be employed, since by such an instrument only is it possible to distribute the powder evenly and in finely divided portions over the diseased areas (Fig. 213).

(*d*) *The Gauze Wick.*—When large portions of the tympanic membrane have been lost and there are present neither polypi nor areas of carious bone, the dry and sterile state of the drum cavity which has been secured by the foregoing treatment may be greatly prolonged by the insertion of a sterile or medicated strip of dry gauze to the fundus of the ear in such a manner that the distal end lies in direct contact with as much of the diseased portion of the middle ear as possible. The strips should be ¾ inch wide and 2½ or 3 inches long. They should be specially prepared and in quantity, free from loose ravelings, sterilized, and kept in any suitable jar, from which one is withdrawn by the aural

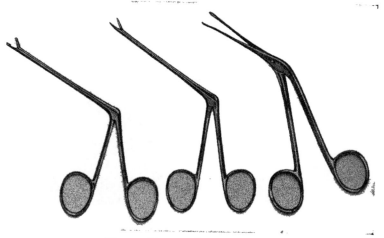

FIG. 214.—HARTMANN DRESSING-FORCEPS.

forceps at the instant it is to be used. The insertion is readily and painlessly accomplished by folding the distal end of the strip into cylindric shape, grasping it ¼ inch from the extremity between the jaws of a delicate dressing-forceps (Fig. 214), when, with the auricle strongly retracted, the gauze is carried at once to the desired position. It is never wise to pack the ear tightly with such a strip, since packing may not only create discomfort to the patient but may also hinder instead of facilitate the drainage. The beneficial effects of the "wick treatment" are, no doubt, brought about by the provision for the absorption of the pus as fast as it is secreted and by the stimulating depletion to which its presence gives rise. The gauze dressing must be changed as often as it becomes saturated with the fluid absorbed from the deeper parts, which may occur several times daily or only once in several days. The above methods of cleansing and drying will, if thoroughly and correctly carried out, often prove sufficient to bring about a speedy cure of the milder and sometimes even of the more severe and troublesome cases.

(6) **Ear Drops.**—Experience has taught, however, that some individual cases of aural discharge are not successfully managed by the dry treatment, owing perhaps to an idiosyncrasy on the part of the patient toward that form of medication. In such cases it can be determined only by trial that the wick method is useless or harmful. There are also those in which the pathologic finding at the time of the first examination will be such that it will be deemed wiser to instil some kind of ear drops from the beginning. If there is uncertainty as to whether the one or the other method should be employed, it is most satisfactory in the majority of cases to choose the dry treatment, at least until its inefficiency or harmful nature is demonstrated.

If the drum membrane has been largely destroyed and exposes a granular mucous lining of the middle ear; if the pus has a foul odor or there are present masses of cholesteatoma, a solution of boric acid in alcohol in the proportion of gr. xx of the former to ʒj of the latter is highly efficacious. After having cleansed and dried the cavity as previously directed, a few drops of this preparation are instilled into the ear and allowed to remain at least five minutes. The solution shrivels the granulations, is antiseptic and astringent, and usually lessens both the odor and the amount of the discharge. When the odor is unusually offensive greater benefit may be derived from the addition of ⅛ gr. of mercury bichlorid to each ounce of the above solution. If used in the strength here advised considerable pain may at first be produced, and the solution should therefore be diluted. As the tissues harden from its continued employment they become less sensitive, and in due time the preparation may be used in its full strength without discomfort to the patient.

During the employment of any liquid medication in aural practise the patient should incline the head far to one side or, preferably, should lie upon a lounge with the affected ear uppermost. All ear drops should be warmed before using. After instillation the auricle should be strongly retracted to the same position in which it is drawn for insertion of the aural speculum and the use of reflected light—namely, upward and backward—until the auditory canal is straightened. Such a movement separates the walls of the external meatus and possibly opens to some extent the perforated tympanic membrane, thus more freely admitting the medicament into the middle-ear cavity. The fluid is then driven deeply into the ear and around the diseased tissues by placing a finger upon the tragus and pressing this structure rapidly and repeatedly into and out of the concha. Siegle's otoscope with the bag attached can also be efficiently used for forcing the ear drops deeply into all the diseased aural recesses. When this instrument is employed for the above purpose, its speculum end is inserted, air tight, into the external meatus, and, beginning with the bag filled with air, compression is gently made so as to drive a column of air inward, and before it the drops intended for the medication. It will be seen that this use of Siegle's otoscope is exactly the reverse of that employed for massaging the drum membrane where adhesions, but no perforation, exist, in which latter method suction only is used.

Solutions of silver nitrate are most beneficial in cases where the mucous lining of the drum cavity is chronically inflamed, thickened, and covered with mucopurulent discharge. The strength of this preparation should not exceed gr. v to ʒj in the beginning, since the reaction from stronger solutions is sometimes severe. The strength should, however, be increased as toleration is established and the necessities of the case demand, until in some instances gr. xc or cxx. to ʒj are most satisfactorily employed.[1]

In order to obtain the full effect of any given strength of nitrate of silver certain precautions in the method of its employment are necessary. This silver salt is exceedingly sensitive to precipitation; therefore its solutions should always be prepared with distilled water. The preceding ear washes should be such as are not incompatible with the silver compound, but if any such have just been used, any remaining portion of the same should be immediately cleansed away by syringing the ear with distilled water. The ear should also be previously dried with the usual thoroughness in order that the silver solution may not be so diluted by secretions or by a quantity of the wash remaining at the bottom of the canal which is sufficient to render the effect of the silver impotent or inert. These suggestions may seem trivial and unnecessary, but are made because frequent failure to cure will result from neglect of their observance.

In the very mild cases, and such as are often seen in children where the perforation is small and posterior to the umbo, and in whom the

[1] D. A. Kuyk, *Transactions Sec. Otol. and Laryngol., A. M. A.,* 1903, advocates the employment in the beginning of a solution of silver nitrate of the strength of 30 gr. to the ounce. This, he states, should be forced into the remotest recesses of the middle ear by means of Siegle's otoscope, the treatment being given every second day. If after a period of two weeks there is no improvement, a solution of 60 gr. to the ounce is substituted, and this is gradually increased until 120 gr. to the ounce are employed.

discharge is stringy, the following lotion has been much and satisfactorily used:[1]

℞. Zinc sulphate,   gr. v;
    Glycerin,   ℥j;
    Saturated sol. boric acid,   q. s. ℥j.—M.

Sig. A few drops of this solution may be instilled two or three times a day after drying and cleansing the ear.

(7) **Caustics.**—Granulations or polypi when present should at once be removed or destroyed. If small, each individual growth may be touched with a bead of chromic acid or of nitrate of silver which has been fused on the end of a delicate aural applicator (see Fig. 209). Chromic acid is much the more potent remedy, and should be used in the middle ear with the greatest care lest severe inflammatory reaction be set up and unnecessary damage be thereby caused to the already crippled hearing organ. If applied to a wet surface any caustic will spread and do mischief to adjoining parts. Therefore the growth to be touched by the destructive agent should be prepared for the caustic application by first cleansing and then thoroughly drying the entire area to be treated according to the methods already outlined. The part which is to be destroyed must also be illuminated and in full view of the operator when the caustic is applied. More than one application is usually necessary, a period of three or four days intervening between treatments.

The destruction of granulations and small polypi may also be accomplished by the use of the electrocautery, a delicate sharp-pointed electrode being used for this purpose. This method, however, is safe only in the hands of the most skilful and under the most favorable circumstances as to location and illumination of the part to be cauterized. The beginner should, therefore, use milder means, even if longer time is required to accomplish the same end.

(8) **Cocain Anesthesia.**—The use of cocain to produce local anesthesia during the action of caustics, as well as of many operative procedures within the middle ear, is highly essential to successful and painless results. The proper method of its employment in the ear is, therefore, important. If the operation is of such nature as to cause hemorrhage in sufficient quantity to obstruct the view of the operative field and thus to hinder the progress of the work, the cocain crystals may be dissolved in the full strength solution of adrenalin chlorid, since this combination will act equally well to benumb the parts and at the same time to exsanguinate them.

[1] Bacon, *Manual of Otology*, 1898.

When large areas of mucous membrane are exposed, as in cases where the drum membrane is largely or wholly wanting, cocain solutions are rapidly absorbed and hence unpleasant or even dangerous symptoms may develop should the drug be carelessly employed. Cocain is sensitive to precipitation by alkaline and other solutions which are often used for cleansing the ear. Hence, if such have just previously been used, any excess of the solution which may have remained in the tympanic cavity should be washed away with some compatible preparation like normal salt or boric acid solution before the application of the cocain is made, since otherwise the anesthetic effect of the latter drug would be greatly lessened or altogether lost. The parts to be anesthetized should also be dried, for if irrigating solutions or secretions remain in the tympanum, the cocain solution will be diluted, and in proportion to the amount of the dilution, its desired action will be lost; 5 drops of a 10 or 15 per cent. solution of cocain, either in adrenalin chlorid or in normal salt solution, according to the effect desired, may be dropped into the ear and allowed to remain from five to ten minutes, after which any excess is mopped away with sterile cotton. If the parts are still sensitive to the manipulation of the probe they may be touched with a cotton-tipped applicator which has been dipped into a stronger solution of cocain.

When the tympanic cavity is highly sensitive the most satisfactory anesthesia is obtained by the direct application of pure cocain crystals to the operative field; 1 gr. of the powdered crystals having been placed upon a glass plate, and a pledget of cotton wound about the end of an applicator, the cotton is first dipped into a solution of cocain and then immediately rolled in the powder until a sufficient amount adheres. A known quantity of the drug can thus be readily carried to the desired spot, the complete insensibility of which is thereby speedily and safely accomplished, since by this method there is no spreading of the cocain and only a small area of mucous membrane can absorb the same; there is, therefore, less danger from toxic effects than when weak solutions are more generously employed. It should of course be remembered that no anesthesia can be obtained from the instillation of cocain solutions into the ear unless there is present in the drum membrane a perforation of sufficient size to admit the drug into the tympanic cavity. If, therefore, the perforation is quite small it will be necessary to inject the cocain solution into the tympanic cavity by means of a small pipet, the canula of which is inserted directly through the perforation.

CHRONIC PURULENT OTITIS MEDIA (Continued)

THE SURGICAL TREATMENT

THE medicinal treatment of chronic otorrhea which was outlined in the preceding chapter will, if systematically and intelligently carried out, cure a large percentage of all cases of this character. Those cases in which there has been destruction of the deeper tissues and in which caries or necrosis of the bony parts has taken place will, however, seldom yield to such mild measures. The accurate diagnosis that should be made prior to the institution of any treatment will at that time indicate the degree of success or failure that is likely to result from mere antiseptic cleansing, local medication, or general therapeutics. Hence, when it is definitely determined that the osseous structures have already been attacked by the aural disease, and that there are present areas of uncovered bone, it is unwise to continue indefinitely with unaided medicinal measures. Therefore, after such means have been faithfully and carefully applied for a few weeks, if the aural discharge is but slightly or not at all lessened, and if the foul odor of the discharge continues despite the treatment; or if it should return immediately after treatment is withheld, there is slight prospect of alleviation or cure of the disease from their further use. In all these cases experience has proved that surgery is the most conservative and logical means of treatment, and that its employment in this class of aural ailments is as rational and is followed by as satisfactory results as when applied to diseases of other regions of the body.

The surgical management of this disease can best be considered in two divisions:

First, the surgery of the middle ear, attic, and parts adjacent, which are accessible to instrumentation through the external auditory meatus, and may be designated intratympanic surgery.

Second, that which embraces all the tissues in and adjoining the ear which are likely to become diseased through extension from the tympanum. This latter includes the intracranial complications. This division is fully included in the radical mastoid operation and will be considered in a subsequent chapter.

INTRATYMPANIC SURGERY

This title should include a discussion of all operative procedures upon the drum membrane and middle ear that are performed for the purpose of securing better drainage, for arresting the discharges, or for improving the impaired hearing by the division of adhesions or other obstructions to the transmission of sound. Sufficient mention has, however, already been made of the milder surgical procedures in the chapters dealing with the treatment of acute and chronic aural inflammations and suppurations, some of which operations have been discarded because found to be of little value. The author believes that the full description of such operations as paracentesis, which as a means of treatment are usually performed in conjunction with the use of important medicinal measures, is best given in the chapters dealing with the treatment of the disease requiring the operation. Intratympanic surgery, however, as related to the management and cure of chronic

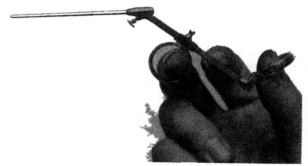

FIG. 215.—BLAKE'S POLYPUS SNARE.

aural suppurations, is so distinctly a method apart from medicinal aid, that it should receive the emphasis and dignity afforded by an entirely separate discussion.

Removal of Polypi by Curet or Snare.—The aural snare (Fig. 215) and curet are the proper instruments to use for the removal of all polypi too large to be destroyed by cauterization. Generally speaking, the curet is best suited for the removal of the smaller tumors, while the snare is preferred for the larger ones. Several sizes of the curet (Fig. 216, a, b, c) are necessary to fit the different sized tumors. Each should have a thin, sharp-edged ring knife. Most aural curets on the market have the serious fault of being so broad at the ring portion that when inserted to the fundus this part of the instrument covers the polypus to such an extent that it is often difficult for the operator to see the growth with sufficient clearness to enable him to perform the ablation as easily and painlessly as could be done with a properly constructed instrument.   In using an instrument with a narrow, thin ring (Fig. 216, C) and a delicate shank the operator is able to observe in most instances the position of the ring at each step of the manipulation.   Little difficulty is, therefore, experienced in passing the ring over the growth to its base, at which

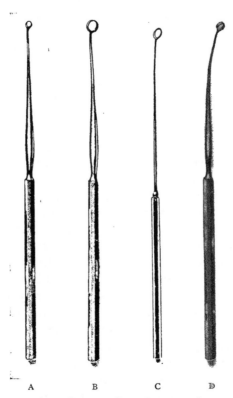

A B C D

FIG. 216.—DIFFERENT SIZES OF AURAL CURETS FOR USE IN REMOVAL OF GRANULATIONS AND SMALL POLYPI FROM THE TYMPANIC CAVITY.
Note thin, fenestrated blades. Curets commonly sold have blades so thick as to render use of instruments difficult or impossible.

time the operator makes firm pressure upon the handle in the direction of the attachment of the polypus and then quickly withdraws the instrument, thus severing and bringing the polypus away with the curet. If more than one polypus is present, the remaining ones may be removed in a similar manner and at the same sitting, provided the hemorrhage is not so profuse as to interfere with further work.

An aural snare (Fig. 215) should be of delicate construction, since little strength is required in any of its parts. The canula should be of the smallest diameter that will admit the small wire used for the écrasement. If the canula is bulky the view of the deeper parts will be so obstructed during its use that precision in encircling the polypus with the wire loop will be interfered with to an extent that may result in an incomplete operation.

Having previously determined the site of its attachment by the use of the examining probe, a large thin-walled speculum is introduced, the auricle is retracted, and the growth well illuminated. A wire loop of appropriate size is inserted and passed along the wall of the meatus opposite to that from which the polypus springs, then over and around the growth, and finally to its base, by the gentle insinuation of the instrument in such a manner and direction as may be indicated by the position and size of the tumor. When the wire loop is believed to have reached the base of the growth it is tightened until a firm grasp is obtained, when it is permissible, provided it does not arise from the tympanic roof, very gently to jerk the instrument and, by so doing, pull the polypus away at its deepest point of attachment. Should the polypi spring from the necrosing tegmen tympani it is entirely possible to expose the dura mater during their complete removal, and thus to open a fresh channel for intracranial infection. Hence, meningitis is a possible early sequence of the removal of aural polypi from the attic, and a certain amount of care should, therefore, be exercised in the performance of this operation. If diseased bone can be detected in the midst of polypi which spring from the tegmen tympani, it is safer to perform the radical mastoid operation than to rely upon intratympanic measures directed toward the removal of the disease.

After any remaining growths have likewise been removed, the blood is dried from the meatus and a strip of sterile gauze is inserted to its bottom. But little pain either accompanies or follows these operations, and the wounded areas usually heal rapidly. If any remnant of the polypus is left behind by the snare or curet, the same should be touched with chromic acid once each week until it is completely destroyed. Following the removal of polypi the probe should be used to detect, if possible, the nature of the tissue from which they grew. If found to have sprung from the hypertrophied mucous membrane the polypi are not likely to return; whereas, if uncovered bone is found at the seat of their origin, a speedy recurrence may be expected. In any case, the patient should be informed that the polypi are only a symptom of the aural affection, and that, therefore, their removal is only one step, and often the least important one, in the cure of the suppurative disease.

Ossiculectomy and Curetage of the Middle Ear and Attic in the Treatment of Chronic Suppurative Aural Diseases.—When the violence of the acute disease, together with the resulting chronic suppuration, has caused the death of a portion or all of one or more ossicles (see Fig. 202) the necrosed part becomes in effect a foreign body in the tympanic cavity, and its presence sets up an additional irritation. Good surgery indicates the early removal of such an ossicle, together with the polypi, granulations, or thickened mucous membrane in which it is usually imbedded.

Ossiculectomy is not indicated if there is present, in addition to the diseased ossicle, an extensive implication of the osseous walls of the more inaccessible parts of the attic, or if a suppurative process is already well established in the mastoid antrum as well as in the middle ear; because in such cases it is obvious that removal of the accessible portions of the disease could only improve but not cure the aural ailment. Ossiculectomy is also contra-indicated in cases where the lumen of the external auditory meatus has become greatly narrowed as a result of chronic eczematous or other inflammatory thickening of its walls or from the projection into it of an osteomatous or other growth. Under such circumstances it is impossible to see the parts to be operated upon with sufficient clearness or to manipulate the instruments within the limited space with that degree of precision which should characterize intra-tympanic surgery. The radical mastoid operation is better suited to such cases, since by it the disease can be more intelligently and thoroughly removed and the results are certain to be more satisfactory.

If, however, the previous examination of the ear has made it fairly certain that the disease is limited to the structures of the middle ear, ossiculectomy with thorough curetage of the hypertrophied mucous membrane will effect a cure in a large proportion of cases.

The operation of ossiculectomy may be performed either with or without a general anesthetic. Determination of this point must be based upon whether or not the patient possesses that amount of self-control necessary to endure the moderate pain attendant, and upon the extent of the diseased tissues to be removed. The author has, in selected cases, frequently removed the malleus and incus, chipped away a considerable portion of the external attic wall, and accomplished an entirely satisfactory curetment of the thickened mucous membrane under the local cocain anesthesia. When the perforation in the drum membrane is large, local anesthesia may be secured as described on p. 351. If the tympanic opening is small, the solution may be dropped through it into the cavum tympani by means of a delicate ear pipet.

The occurrence of even slight bleeding at any stage of the operation will so hinder the progress as to make the operative work both uncertain and unsafe. The use of adrenalin chlorid in 1:1000 solution is, therefore, of the greatest assistance since it produces a nearly bloodless field. For the reason that chloroform causes less venous stagnation and therefore less bleeding than ether, the former anesthetic should be the choice when general narcosis is desirable.

Aside from the position of the patient, which should be prone under general anesthesia and upright when cocain is used, the steps of the operation are the same in both. The preparation of the ear, hands, and instruments should be in accordance with the strictest interpretation of the modern methods of asepsis. The sitting posture of the patient is somewhat advantageous from the fact that when the patient is erect the operator sees the field of operation in that position with which he is most familiar; whereas, with the patient lying down, it becomes necessary to bear the changed position constantly in mind. In addition to the instruments required, a half-gross of sterile cotton mops especially prepared should be at hand. These are made by twisting appropriate sized pledgets of cotton about one end of long, smooth toothpicks. Each mop is rapidly used when needed to absorb secretions or blood and is then thrown away. A darkened room and a good source of light are essential. The electric head light shown in Fig. 89 is satisfactory, but an ordinary head mirror can be used equally as well. The largest ear speculum that can be inserted into the meatus ought always to be selected, since as much space as possible should be provided through which to see the field and in which to manipulate the instruments necessary for the performance of the operation.

The *first step* consists in liberating any remaining portion of the drum membrane from its attachment to the malleus. In many cases this remnant of membrane, as well as the mucosa of the middle ear, is greatly thickened and highly vascular, in which condition sufficient bleeding will be caused, if the greatest care be not taken in making the necessary incisions, greatly to hinder the progress of the work. The knife shown in Fig. 141 is inserted through the membrane 1 mm. from the annulus tympanicus, at a point on a level with and posterior to the umbo. The incision is carried rapidly upward to the posterior fold, then along the lower margin of this fold to the short process, after which it follows the manubrium into the perforation. On account of the troublesome hemorrhage it would cause, much caution should be exercised not to insert the knife too deeply and thereby wound the mucous membrane covering the inner wall of the drum cavity. The anterior attachments of the drum membrane to the malleus handle are likewise incised, after which the portions so detached can be turned down or entirely removed. Any tendency to bleed as a result of the foregoing procedure is now checked by the use of the cotton mops or cylinders of cotton, applied accurately and under moderate pressure to the bottom of the canal, where they are allowed to remain for a moment. The fundus of the ear is thus dried so that definite inspection of the work is again possible.

Disarticulation of the incudostapedial joint and severance of the tendon of the stapedius muscle constitutes the *second step*. The head of the patient must now be placed in the position most favorable for the inspection of this joint (see Fig. 198). The angular knife shown in Fig. 217 is passed just inward to the long process of the incus and in

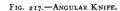

FIG. 217.—ANGULAR KNIFE.

front of the joint to be severed, when, by rotation of the knife-handle, the blade of the instrument slides along the inner surface of the long process of the incus till the joint is reached and disarticulated.

The instrument is then inserted posterior to the head of the stapes in order to detach the stapedius muscle from the stirrup. Since any violence to the stapes may not only produce a more profound deafness but may also cause distressing dizziness or even permit septic material to enter the vestibule, it is highly important that no unskilful or rude manipulation be made when operating on this or adjacent structures.

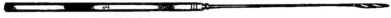

FIG. 218.—BLUNT-POINTED KNIFE.

It is largely for the protection of the stapes that it is advisable completely to separate the incus from the stapes before any attempt is made to extract either the malleus or incus.

Any hemorrhage that may have been set up is again checked in the former manner, after which the *third step*, the detachment of the ligamentous supports of the malleus, is accomplished. The blunt-pointed knife (Fig. 218) is selected for this purpose and passed under the posterior fold into the tympanic cavity at a point immediately behind the short process of the malleus. With the cutting edge turned upward the instrument is carried firmly into the tissues above, while, at the same time, the handle of the knife is depressed. This procedure is repeated by making an upward incision through the anterior fold just in front of the short process. The anterior and posterior ligaments are thus severed and the malleus is detached everywhere except from the suspensary and annular ligaments, each of which readily yields when traction is applied in removing the malleus. At this juncture it is once more necessary to deal with some bleeding, after which the malleus is seized at the uppermost part of the manubrium by a delicate but strong forceps (Fig. 219), and traction is made, first downward until the bone is dislodged from the attic, and then outward through the meatus.

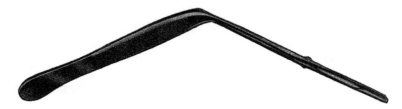

FIG. 219.—McKAY'S FORCEPS, WITH TEETH GROUND SHORT.

The incus, if present, is next extracted. The preceding manipulations may have displaced this ossicle forward, backward, or downward into a position which will require searching to discover it. For this purpose the incus hook (Fig. 220) is inserted into the postero-inferior quadrant, immediately behind the tympanic ring, and with its concavity looking forward. In this position, and keeping the hook close to the annulus throughout the course, it is carried around the tympanum either until the ossicle is encountered and withdrawn or until a complete circuit has demonstrated that it does not lie in the path pursued by

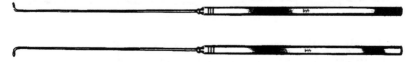

FIG. 220.—INCUS HOOKS, RIGHT AND LEFT.

the hook. If not found, the reverse incus hook is tried and the drum cavity is explored in the reverse order to that just described. This last movement, in which the concavity of the hook is directed toward the mastoid antrum, makes it entirely possible for the operator to drive the ossicle into the mouth of the aditus ad antrum, and thus to lose it in a most unfavorable situation. The surgeon should, therefore, always have such an accident in mind, and by the exercise of care and gentle manipulation avoid its occurrence.

It sometimes happens that, even when known to be present, the incus is difficult to find. If not removed, its presence must continue to excite trouble, and the condition of the patient will, therefore, continue unimproved because of the incomplete operation. Time spent in gently searching for the little bone is, therefore, essential to the cure, and thoroughness in every respect is due the patient who has entrusted his case to the surgical procedure.

Owing to the free blood supply to the stapes this ossicle is seldom necrosed. Its situation in the pelvis' of the oval window, however. seems a favorable one for the formation of connective tissue, which, during the long inflammatory process, is often deposited in this locality in sufficient amount to imprison the tiny bone and to render it immovable to such a degree as greatly to impede the passage of sound-waves into the labyrinth. After the larger ossicles are removed and the field of operation thoroughly dried, the condition of mobility of the stapes should be determined by means of the probe used under direct inspection and illumination. If the foot-plate is unduly covered by adventitious tissue and adhesive bands are found stretching from the pelvic walls to the crura and head of the ossicle in such a way as to render it immovable, the hearing power of the patient may in some cases be considerably and in others surprisingly improved by severing the bands that fix the stapes immovably in the oval window. This is accomplished by circumcising the new tissues of the foot-plate with a straight knife (Fig. 141), the blade of which will at the same time sever any adhesive bands attached to the head or crura. After such incisions the ossicle may be moved in different directions by means of a cotton-tipped probe, in order completely to break up any partly severed adhesions and to secure the greatest freedom of motion; or, in some cases, if it is thought quite probable that the adhesions will speedily recur, the ossicle may be completely removed by lifting it from the window by means of a hook inserted between the crura or by seizing the head with forceps and making traction, while at the same time a rocking motion is given to the hand.

Much experience in intratympanic surgery is requisite to remove the stapes without serious injury to the labyrinth. If the incisions about the foot-plate should be made too deeply or if the stapes is torn from the window by violence, the fluid of the labyrinth will escape and a distressing dizziness and difficult locomotion will result. Furthermore, since the tympanic cavity in these cases is the seat of a chronic suppuration, the subsequent probability of a labyrinthine infection of traumatic origin should be borne in mind.

After the removal of the diseased portions of the ossicular chain has been satisfactorily accomplished, the tympanic walls are examined by means of the probe, in every accessible part, to determine if there are carious areas; and, if such are present, to ascertain their location and extent. The thickened, granular, or polypoid areas of mucous membrane should be thoroughly cureted away. To efficiently reach every portion of the diseased mucosa a number of different sized curets, with varying curves of shank, will be needed. The author prefers the small sharp ring curets with malleable shafts that may be bent to the exact angle required to reach the diseased areas (Figs. 216, *c*, *d*). With

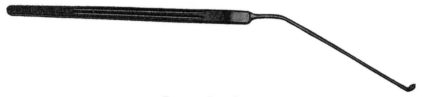

FIG. 221.—ATTIC CURET.

these sharp and accurately fitting instruments the thickened membrane is quickly removed from every part. Any carious portions of bone that have previously been detected are also honed smooth with the stout sharp curets. Curettage of the attic is frequently best accomplished by the employment of the curet shown in Fig. 221 which is operated from within in an outward direction; or by those shown in Fig. 222, *a*, *b*, which are operated anteroposteriorly or vice versa.

It is frequently found necessary, in order to carry out in a thorough manner the removal of all the diseased structures, to chip away the

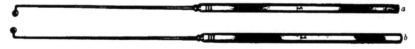

FIG. 222.—ATTIC CURETS.

upper portions of the outer wall of the attic. This is indicated because this portion lies in immediate contact with the neck of the necrosing malleus, over which the products of attic suppuration have passed for an indefinite time. This is best accomplished by means of Hartmann's cutting forceps (Fig. 223), with which the outer attic wall can be bitten away to such an extent as greatly to enlarge the communication between the tympanic cavity and the external auditory meatus. This step will greatly facilitate the after-treatment and drainage of the attic space.

While the after-treatment is in most instances simple, nevertheless success or failure of the operation depends, in no small measure, upon

the efficiency and persistency with which the case is subsequently managed. Immediately following the completion of the operative work
the fundus of the ear is thoroughly dried and a strip of borated gauze
·is inserted to the bottom of the canal in such a way that the most distal
part lies in direct contact with the entire inner wall of the middle ear.
Coils of the strip are then loosely packed over this till the concha is
reached and filled. Since it is usually not desirable to disturb the first
dressing under twenty-four or thirty-six hours it is safest in most cases
to cover the entire auricle with several pads of gauze, over which, as a
completion of the dressing, a roller bandage is applied as shown in
Fig. 255. Such a dressing not only insures against further infection of
the ear through meddlesome interference on part of the patient or
attendant, but also secures the best possible drainage and the greatest
degree of comfort to the patient.

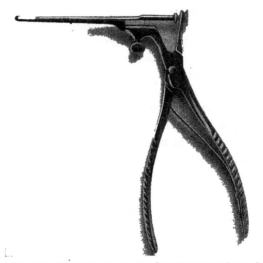

FIG. 223.—HARTMANN'S BONE GOUGE FOR THE REMOVAL OF THE OUTER ATTIC WALL.

In case the hypertrophied tympanic mucous membrane has been
removed from a considerable area by the curet, a very profuse serosanguineous discharge occurs for the first few days. During this time
the method of making the first dressing should be repeated at the first
and possibly the second subsequent dressing, since no better provision
can be made for catching the discharge and providing against the
entrance of sepsis from without than the plan here advised. At the
time the first dressing is removed if the strip taken from the meatus is
free from odor and if, upon inspection, the middle-ear cavity is found

free from blood-clots or retained secretion, no syringing or other medication is indicated, since better results will be obtained if only a fresh sterile·
gauze strip be inserted. Even after several days, if the discharge has
greatly subsided, the daily insertion of a fresh strip of gauze may constitute the only necessary treatment.

If, however, the purulent discharge continues and the foul odor
persists, antiseptic cleansing is indicated. The continuance of such a·
discharge for any considerable length of time after the operation and
during subsequent treatment would indicate that the disease had not
all been reached by the operation, and that the continued suppuration
comes from the mastoid antrum or cells. The disease in such cases
can be satisfactorily removed only by the radical mastoid operation
which is fully described in Chapter XXX.

After the performance of ossiculectomy and curetment, granulations
and small polypi are sometimes formed during the healing process.
These must be destroyed at once by caustics, as already described on
p. 351. As the discharge lessens in the cases that progress satisfactorily,
there springs out a growth of epithelium from the dermal side of the
tympanic ring, which under the most favorable circumstances will
ultimately cover the drum cavity, thus "dermatizing" the mucous
membrane and rendering a further discharge impossible. From the
standpoint of curing the discharge, such dermatization is highly desirable, but from that of the hearing function it is unfavorable, since
usually there is some loss of hearing, resulting from the completion of
the process of dermatization of the mucous lining of the tympanic
cavity.

If the curetage of the Eustachian tube has proved unsuccessful
in shutting off the communication of the tympanic cavity from the
nasopharynx, some discharge arising from the tube itself may continue
indefinitely or may be intermittent and occur only in cases of an acute
nasopharyngitis with an accompanying tubal catarrh.

After the cessation of a chronic aural discharge, either spontaneously
or as a result of medicinal or surgical treatment, there remains permanently, in the large majority of cases, an opening through the drum
membrane. In such cases a recurrence of the discharge may be brought
on by the entrance of water into the ear either intentionally from syringing or accidentally from bathing. Individuals with large perforations
through the drum membrane should, therefore, be warned as to the
possibility of a recurrence of the former disease under these circumstances,
in order that care may be exercised to prevent the entrance of water
into the ear.

CHAPTER XXIX

CHRONIC MASTOIDITIS

CAUSATION, PATHOLOGY, SYMPTOMS, AND DIAGNOSIS

CHRONIC inflammatory affections of the mastoid are of more frequent occurrence than has heretofore been recognized. While the disease is commonly referred to as a mastoiditis and thus leads to the assumption that the inflammatory and suppurative processes are limited to the mastoid portion of the temporal bone, in reality the extent of the affection is often much more widely reaching, as will be pointed out in the section on the pathology of the disease, and may involve not only the osseous structures of the middle ear and mastoid process but also those of the petrous portion of the temporal bone, including, of course, the labyrinth.

Few divisions of medicine have received more careful study from the standpoint of their anatomy, pathology, and technic of operative treatment than has been bestowed in the recent past upon the chronic suppurative diseases of the temporal bone. Much of the knowledge thus obtained is already settled and accepted as a standard of guidance in practise, whereas much is still in the developmental state and remains to be further worked out, or is yet to have the correctness of its principles more satisfactorily demonstrated.

Causation.—Excluding traumatism, the cause of chronic mastoiditis is always a preceding suppurative process within the middle ear. The mastoid antrum, when considered either anatomically or pathologically, must be regarded as a part of the cavity of the middle ear, because the large channel of communication between the two, which is provided by the aditus ad antrum, renders it certain that any disease which may originate in one will be rapidly carried to the other, either by the direct extension of the causative inflammation or from the transportation by gravity of the pathologic products from the one to the other space. Both post-mortem findings and clinical evidence teach the truth of this statement. The mucous membrane which lines the Eustachian tube and middle ear is continued in a modified form directly into the mastoid antrum and cells. This membrane forms the normal barrier against erosion by the invading pus and hence, so long as it is intact and free from ulceration, the damage resulting from entrance of purulent material into the mastoid antrum is not likely to be great. When, however, any portion of this protective membrane becomes necrotic from the contact of violently septic pus or from the retention of pus or other fluid under pressure, the underlying bone is then open to invasion and its death by necrosis will in due time take place.

Normally, the cells of the mastoid process from antrum to tip are in communication with each other, and, therefore, pus that has once

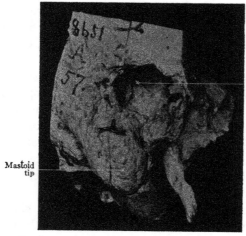

Bone destroyed
by cholesteatoma

Mastoid
tip

FIG. 224.—CHOLESTEATOMA OF MASTOID. CARIES OF JUGULAR FOSSA.
(Warren Museum, Harvard Medical School. J. Orne Green Collection.)

entered the antrum may find its way by gravity into all these air spaces, where, because of its dependent situation, it is most likely to be retained to establish that pathologic condition which is characteristic of chronic mastoiditis.

Pathology.—*Caries and Necrosis of the Temporal Bone.*—Of all the cranial bones the temporal bone is the most commonly attacked by osteitis. Circumscribed areas may be destroyed or sometimes destruction of the whole temporal bone occurs.[1] Caries is common in

[1] "Necrosis means, in contradistinction from caries, complete death of the bone, which is brought about through a disturbance in the nutrient vessels with final abolishment of the circulation. A reactive inflammation takes place in the region immediately around the area of diseased bone. The bone, robbed of its nourishment, dies within the walls of reactive granulation tissue and for lack of vessels no resorption takes place, so that the dead bone lies in a cavity.

A third process stands between caries and necrosis, called caries necrotica, which process is common in the temporal bone, found principally in the region of its pneumatic cells, where through caries the continuity of the thin bony plates are dissolved and the bone becomes filled with granulations."—*Suppuration of the Labyrinth,* E. P. Friedrich.

the recessus epitympanicus, the antrum, and in the malleus and incus. The stapes is rarely attacked. First, the mucous membrane becomes infiltrated with pus and just as soon as the disease has reached a certain intensity the mucoperiosteum is in no condition to nourish the bone

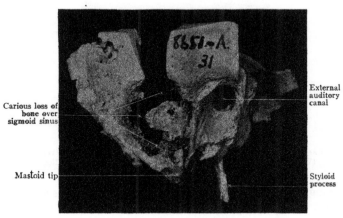

FIG. 225.—CARIES OF WHOLE MASTOID.
(Warren Museum, Harvard Medical School. J. Orne Green Collection.)

sufficiently. As a result the superficial part of the bone dies, appearing whitish, porous, crusty, and chips off easily. Then the caries extends deeper and deeper into the bone until it breaks through the cortex, forming one or more fistulæ (see Figs. 223 and 224). By carious soften-

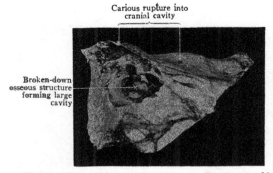

FIG. 226.—CARIES OF TYMPANIC ROOF. MASTOID OPERATION AND TREPHINING; MENINGITIS; FATAL.

ing the normal middle-ear spaces may be greatly enlarged or be united to other cavities by destruction of dividing septa; thus, caries of the antrum may break through into the middle cerebral fossa (Fig. 226); the posterior cerebellar fossa (Figs. 227 and 229); the tympanic cavity

(Fig. 228); the external lateral semicircular canal to the vestibule; the mastoid cells, and external auditory canal. Pressure necrosis may take

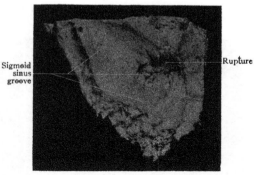

FIG. 227.—CARIES OF SIGMOID AND PETROSAL GROOVES, ALSO OF EXTERNAL CORTEX. MENINGITIS.
(Warren Museum, Harvard Medical School. J. Orne Green collection.)

place through insufficient drainage of the products of secretion (Fig. 230). Bone is especially attacked in tuberculosis, scarlet fever, and measles, less often in typhoid fever, influenza, and diphtheria.

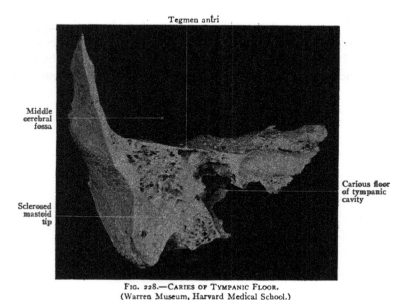

FIG. 228.—CARIES OF TYMPANIC FLOOR.
(Warren Museum, Harvard Medical School.)

Through pressure by cholesteatomata (see Fig. 231) necrosis of the bone takes place and great cavities are sometimes formed, even extending far into the cranial cavity. Of the general diseases syphilis causes caries especially in the gummatous stage, next most common is tuberculosis causing cheesy destruction of the tuberculous inflamed tissue. In syphilis and in tuberculosis there may be periostitis of the squama without disease of the middle ear.

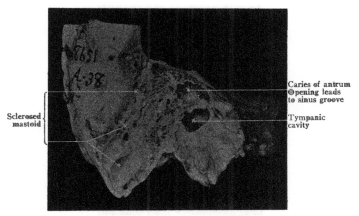

FIG. 229.—CARIES OF SIGMOID GROOVE. PHLEBITIS OF LATERAL SINUS.
(Warren Museum, Harvard Medical School. J. Orne Green Collection.)

Symptoms.—Many individuals who suffer from chronic mastoiditis make no complaint whatever concerning the ailment, except it be of the aural discharge. Of this latter some speak trivially, while others because of the insignificant amount deny the presence of the discharge. Except

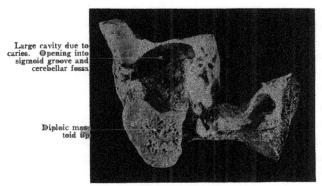

FIG. 230.—LARGE CAVITY IN MASTOID PROCESS DUE TO PRESSURE NECROSIS.

at the time of an acute exacerbation of the chronic trouble, at which time inflammatory swelling and retention of the pus results in pain either deeply in the ear or over the mastoid—should a rupture have taken place through the cortex and a periostitis and postaural swelling

24

be set up—the patient is comfortable and follows his usual voca-
tion. There is, therefore, seldom any definite forewarning of the
fact that a slowly advancing necrotic process is taking place in the
deep-seated parts of the ear, and in the very midst of structures

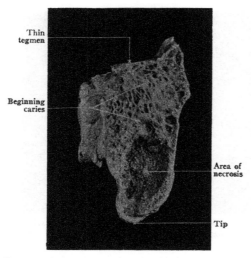

Thin
tegmen

Beginning
caries

Area of
necrosis

Tip

FIG. 231.—CASE OF PRESSURE NECROSIS FROM CHOLESTEATOMATA.
(Warren Museum, Harvard Medical School.   J. Orne Green Collection.)

the invasion of which may, at any time, lead to serious or even fatal
consequences.

The character of the aural discharge, the presence and appearance
of granulations, polypi or fistula, or, indeed, of all the objective symptoms
that are found in the middle ear and auditory canal of those who are
subjects of chronic suppurative otitis media, are observed in cases of
chronic mastoiditis; for, as previously stated, the one disease is a sequel
to the other, and the symptoms of each are, therefore, in a large measure
identical and often entirely inseparable.

Although, as has already been intimated, mastoiditis may have
been present many years in a given case, its existence may not be suspected by any one unless something occurs to interfere with the previously
free drainage from the middle ear or unless there is an extension of the
disease to the meninges or lateral sinus; unless the facial nerve, periosteum, or cervical lymphatics are involved; or, finally, unless there is
absorption of septic material into the general circulation with resulting
systemic disturbances.

In addition, therefore, to the symptoms already narrated in connection with chronic suppurative otitis media (see p. 325), the occur-

rence of the following symptoms will be diagnostic, not of the fact that mastoiditis is present, for that should have already been known, but of the fact that something of additional gravity in the progress of the disease has taken place which indicates a new invasion of territory and the possible approach of danger to the life of the individual.

1. *Pain.*—So long as free drainage from every infected cavity connected with the middle ear is maintained, pain is seldom present. Its appearance, therefore, is indicative of swelling in some portion of the drainage tract, of other obstruction due to the growth of polypi, cholesteatoma or dried pus, and, finally, to an extension of the mastoid disease to the meninges, to the cerebral or cerebellar structure, or to the periosteum covering the external surface of the mastoid process. The pain may be sharp and intermittent or dull and continuous. It is always limited to the affected side of the head unless general meningitis is present. The patient locates the pain in the depths of the auditory meatus or in the deeper portions of the mastoid. If of cerebral origin it may be limited to a small but definite area at some point far distant from the ear, as at the outer end of the supraorbital ridge or over the parietal region above the auricular attachment. When it is present superficially over the mastoid region it is usually due to an infection of the periosteal covering of the part, and hence sensitive areas may be detected early if deep pressure be made over the usual seats of mastoid tenderness (Fig. 151).

2. *Localized swelling,* which takes place over the postauricular region (Fig. 181) or within the auditory canal. This is due to a periostitis and a collection of pus which is the result either of the superficial inflammation or of a rupture of the mastoid abscess through the bony cortex. The tumefaction which sometimes occurs within the meatus is seen on the posterosuperior wall at its junction with the tympanic ring, and if sufficiently large may obscure a view of the posterosuperior quadrant of the membrana tympani. The cause, appearance, and significance of such a swelling differs in no way from that which occurs in acute mastoiditis, and this has already been described (see p. 278). Glandular infection of the neck is occasionally a cause of swelling in the cervical region and, as a symptom, is seen most frequently in cases where the aural discharge has been irritating and has eroded the skin of the external meatus, through which the absorption of septic material takes place. Cervical adenitis of adjacent lymphatic vessels and glands is also common in tuberculous individuals, particularly children.

3. *Dizziness and Profound Deafness.*—In a case that has previously been symptomless, the sudden onset of marked or total deafness, together with tinnitus aurium and dizziness, is indicative of an invasion of the labyrinth. The dizziness will possibly amount only to an unsteadiness of gait that requires constant attention on the part of the individual when on his feet, or it may be accompanied by vomiting and be of such severe nature that the patient must keep the recumbent posture (see Chapter XLIII.).

4. The *pulse* and *temperature* are sometimes affected in the more severe complications of mastoiditis. While dangerous infection of the pneumatic spaces of the temporal bone may have long been present, yet usually if the drainage is good neither the pulse nor temperature are greatly affected. Should, however, a local or general meningitis set in or should a sinus infection occur, both pulse and temperature will be elevated, and show disturbances somewhat characteristic of the respective diseases (see Chapters XXIV. to XXXVII.). Likewise, in cases of brain abscess resulting from the infected mastoid, the temperature and pulse are both at first raised, but later both may become very decidedly subnormal and may remain so for a considerable time.

5. *Nystagmus* or *strabismus* occurring in any case of chronic aural discharge, either of itself or accompanied by one or more of the above symptoms, should be regarded as a suspicious symptom of an intracranial extension. The occurrence of choked disc is also an indication of cerebral or of cerebellar complication.

6. *Cessation of the Aural Discharge.*—Sudden cessation of the discharge from an ear that has long been suppurating profusely is usually due to the fact that a rupture has taken place which has allowed the pus to enter the cranial cavity; or in case the rupture takes place outward, the pus collects under the periosteum over the mastoid; or, possibly, as in Bezold's abscess, it dissects its way downward through the deep tissues of the neck (see Figs. 179, 224, 226 and 267). In this connection it must not be forgotten that in any discharging ear the cessation of the flow may occur gradually as a consequence of the natural healing of the parts or from the assistance due to local treatment, and under such circumstances this occurrence should not be construed as of evil omen. But in a case where the discharge has been persistent and of long duration; where it has been foul smelling, and perhaps accompanied by the presence of carious bone or polypi of the middle ear, the sudden cessation, particularly if coincident with or quickly followed by the above symptoms of pain, fever, vertigo, etc., would be highly

diagnostic of the fact that the pus had found a new outlet, and that the resulting condition of the patient is more than likely one of great danger.

Diagnosis.—To determine merely that chronic mastoiditis is present in any given case should not be a difficult matter; but to ascertain the exact nature and extent of the mastoid infection, and the presence or absence of dangerous possibilities that have already developed or are likely to occur at any time, is a far more difficult task although one of vastly greater importance. Briefly stated, the one consideration most essential to the practical side of the diagnosis is the definite determination of the question as to whether or not there is present in any given case a sufficient amount of disease to positively justify the performance of a difficult operation for its cure, an operation which will disqualify the individual for business or pleasure for at least a month, and one upon which some probability of failure and some possibility of danger are attendant. With this one consideration foremost in mind, the following points in the examination should all be carefully weighed before the diagnosis is made and before an operation is finally determined upon.

1. The history of the case; the original cause of the aural affection; whether or not the patient has previously received efficient treatment for the discharging ear, and whether or not the discharge has been constant, intermittent, odorless, or foul smelling.

2. The absence or presence of aural polypi, bloody or sanious discharges, necrosed ossicles or tympanic walls, aural or postaural fistula.

3. The presence or absence of pain, and of normal, subnormal, or elevated temperature.

4. Whether or not there are acute exacerbations of the ear disease in which pain, swelling, tenderness, and fever are present; also as to the presence or absence of vertigo, tinnitus aurium, and sudden deafness.

5. The information obtained by the most thorough examination of the fundus of the ear, the tympanic attic, and as much of the aditus ad antrum as can be reached. In this examination every accessible diseased area should be inspected by sight if possible, and this should always be supplemented by the exploring probe which is passed into the attic and over every portion of the tympanic walls in the effort to make certain concerning the presence or absence of denuded areas, detached sequestra, or collections of cholesteatoma.

Valuable and necessary as is the preceding history of the case as

an item which enters into the diagnosis, much more ﹀
exact information which the surgeon obtains durin
inspection of that considerable portion of the seat
which is subject to examination by sight and the t
instruments.

CHRONIC MASTOIDITIS (Continued)

TREATMENT. THE RADICAL MASTOID OPERATION

Preliminary Remarks.—As has been stated in a previous chapter (see p. 353) many cases of chronic aural discharge are incurable by either medicinal means or by operative procedure performed through the external auditory meatus. A study of the anatomy of the temporal bone by the method of making many sections through it in such direction as will best show the great extent of its cellular interior—or, one might

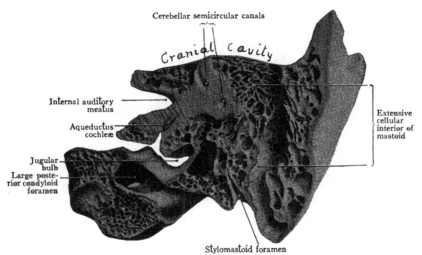

Cerebellar semicircular canals

Cranial Cavity

Internal auditory meatus

Aqueductus cochleæ

Jugular bulb

Large posterior condyloid foramen

Extensive cellular interior of mastoid

Stylomastoid foramen

FIG. 232.—SECTION NEARLY PARALLEL TO SUPERIOR PETROSAL SINUS GROOVE.
Shows the wide extent of pneumatic spaces connected with the middle ear.

more accurately say, the cavernous arrangement of the labyrinth of air spaces of the bone, and at the same time show their relation to each other and to the vital structures in close proximity to them—is necessary to a correct appreciation of the fact above stated—namely, that many suppurative aural affections are entirely incurable except by the most radical operative measures (Figs. 232 to 237). It is evident that, should infection and subsequent suppuration once extend from the

375

tympanic cavity into a labyrinth of connected air spaces, such as that shown in Fig. 232, that the natural drainage through the antrum and middle ear, which lie at the top of the system of cavities, would not furnish a sufficiently good outlet to bring about a cure, and that

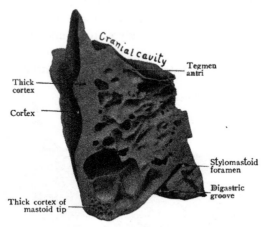

FIG. 233.—VERY THIN TEGMEN TYMPANI   NOTE LARGE, THICK-WALLED CELLS IN THE TIP OF THE MASTOID PROCESS.

surgical assistance in such instances is entirely necessary to rid the structures of the disease.

The radical mastoid operation may, therefore, be defined as a surgical procedure which is intended for the cure of that class of chronic suppura-

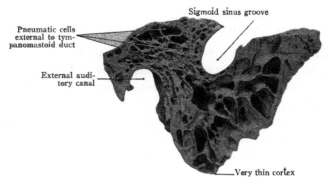

FIG. 234.—SECTION OF TEMPORAL BONE ON A PLANE EXTERNAL TO THE MASTOID ANTRUM AND TYMPANIC CAVITY.
The section is made at an angle that includes the knee of the sigmoid sinus groove, and hence shows the very close relation of the cells to the sigmoid sinus.

ting ears in which the seat of the suppurative process cannot be effectively reached by measures directed through the external auditory meatus.   The radical mastoid operation is essentially one that is intended to remove the suppurative products, which are the result of necrosis of both soft and osseous tissues from every accessible portion of the

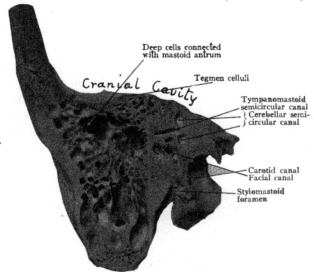

FIG. 235.—VERTICAL SECTION OF TEMPORAL BONE IN A PLANE POSTERIOR TO THE TYMPANIC CAVITY AND MASTOID ANTRUM.
Deep cells are seen extending backward as far as the sigmoid sinus, from which they are separated by a very thin osseous lamella.

temporal bone. The operation, therefore, includes the diseased struc-tures of the middle ear as well as those of the mastoid antrum and

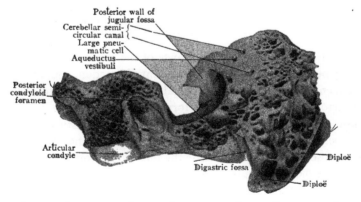

FIG. 236.—SECTION OF TEMPORAL AND OCCIPITAL BONES THROUGH JUGULAR FOSSA SHOWING LARGE PNEU-MATIC CELLS SURROUNDING THIS FOSSA.
Note the great depth of these cells and their connection with superficial mastoid cells.

cells, and from all these cavities sequestra, carious bone, polypi, choles-teatoma or, indeed, every pathologic accumulation of whatever kind that has either invaded or resulted from the invasion of the original disease must be removed.

It will be seen from the wide scope of the radical operation that it differs greatly from the simpler one which is performed for the cure of acute mastoid suppuration. The simple operation should, of course, always be radically performed, in the sense that it ought, in every in-stance, to be carried out in a thorough manner; but in cases where the simple operation is indicated the disease has been of short duration, has only involved but not hopelessly destroyed the parts of the middle ear that are intended for the conduction of sound-waves, and, as stated in the chapter descriptive of this operation, these essential parts of the organ

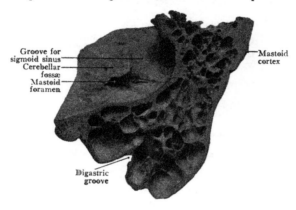

FIG. 237.—PERPENDICULAR SECTION OF THE TEMPORAL BONE POSTERIOR TO THE STYLOMASTOID FORAMEN. The specimen shows the great extent of cellular development with which the operator may meet. Note that the cells surround the sigmoid sinus for a long distance.

of hearing can, by the timely performance of the simple mastoid opera-tion, usually be saved from serious impairment of function, and, therefore, the subsequent hearing of the individual will be preserved to a useful and satisfactory degree. In the performance of the simple procedure the middle ear is not entered nor are its contents disturbed. The operation performed for the relief of acute mastoiditis has, therefore, a twofold purpose—namely, to evacuate the pus and necrotic accumulation within the mastoid and to preserve and restore the patient's hearing.

The radical operation is largely concerned in ridding the patient of pyogenic tissues, and the consequent prevention of sequelæ dangerous to life, which are likely to arise from their continued presence in the temporal bone. In other words, it is intended as a life-saving measure rather than one in which improvement of hearing is concerned; for usually by the time the radical mastoid operation is indicated the damage already done within the middle ear—and not infrequently to the labyrinth also—has been sufficient to destroy or at least very seriously to·impair the function, and hence the operation itself will most probably affect the remaining hearing power neither for better nor worse. It has been considered necessary to state the above differences between the simple and radical mastoid operation for the reason that some confusion exists in the minds of many physicians concerning the nature and purpose of each procedure.

Indications for the Performance of the Radical Mastoid Operation.— 1. Failure to cure a chronic aural discharge after following out in a painstaking and thorough manner for a period of six weeks to three months the measures set forth in the chapter devoted to the treatment of chronic suppurative aural disease (see p. 399).

2. The occurrence of pain over the mastoid, within the ear or radiating over the side of the head, particularly if this becomes persistent and severe and can be connected with the chronic otorrhea.

3. Continuous or frequently repeated attacks of dizziness when associated with chronic aural discharge, the presence of aural polypi, or with necrosed bone in the middle ear or attic.

4. The presence of a postauricular fistula or of a fistula of the posterosuperior wall of the external auditory meatus, which, upon examination with a probe, is found to extend deeply into the mastoid interior.

5. The occurrence of postauricular mastoid tenderness and swelling in connection with chronic aural suppuration.

6. In any case of chronic suppurative otitis media in which there is present a more or less complete occlusion of the external auditory meatus, due to diffuse external otitis, osteoma, or other tumor.

7. When symptoms of meningitis, sinus thrombosis, or abscess of the brain appear.

8. The presence of cholesteatoma in the attic or mastoid antrum.

9. The sudden cessation of a profuse aural discharge coincident with the development of one or more of the above symptoms.

The radical operation will prove unsuccessful as a curative measure unless all the diseased tissue is by it removed; and, as has already been seen (Figs. 232 and 234), the suppuration may include very extensive and deepseated portions of the temporal bone, in which case an operation to be as thorough and extensive as the condition demands is not without danger to life. It becomes a debatable question, therefore, in cases where no severe pain is present, and when no visible danger is threatening the life of the individual, whether it is wiser to advise immediate operation or to permit the disease to continue until some more urgent necessity for surgical interference arises. In these comparatively symptomless cases the surgeon should obtain every possible amount of information concerning the exact condition of the disease in the middle ear and mastoid process, such information being secured, of course, by an actual examination by every known means, before he may consider that he is justified in undertaking to perform the radical mastoid operation. While, as stated in indication number 1 above, it is usually thought advisable to treat a chronic discharging ear for a few weeks before resorting to radical measures, yet, in practise, this preliminary treatment which is administered in the hope of curing the suppuration and thus averting the necessity for surgical interference, is often given without the slightest expectation by the surgeon of any permanent relief, because it is clear from the beginning that he is helpless to cure the disease which his first examination had positively proved to lie entirely beyond the reach of any trivial method of treatment. When, therefore, the presence of necrotic osseous areas is definitely determined in any case, and there is every probability that the pus which is discharging from the ear has its origin in the deeper mastoid cells and antrum, it is no doubt the wisest plan not to advise operative postponement because delay is unsurgical, and prompt determination in attacking the seat of the disease in a rational way will not only cure the suppuration but may also prove the means of saving the life of the patient.

The fact that cases are frequently observed who have passed from childhood into old age with a suppurating middle ear or mastoid without developing any serious symptoms, and with apparently no danger to life, is not altogether good argument against the necessity for the radical mastoid operation in other cases that are, apparently, similarly diseased, because numerous cases have been reported in which an individual so affected was able to work at hard manual labor up to the very hour that violent and fatal symptoms first manifested themselves. Furthermore, during the performance of the radical mastoid operation on persons who previously had manifested absolutely no dangerous symptoms, it is frequently found that the dura mater over the tegmen antri or tympani, or over the lateral sinus in the sigmoid groove, has been laid bare by the necrotic process, and that the sinus itself or the exposed portion of the dura mater is covered with granulations and bathed in pus. Certainly these cases are in constant danger of general infection and should, therefore, be dealt with according to the well-established principles of surgery.

In those who are past sixty years of age and in cases where pulmonary tuberculosis or other cachectic disease accompanies a chronic aural discharge, the radical mastoid operation is not indicated except when severe pain or other symptoms arise that urgently demand relief.

Technic of the Radical Mastoid Operation.—The preparation of the field of operation is exactly the same as that advised preliminary to the operation for acute mastoiditis. In addition to this if it is probable than an intracranial complication exists which would require opening the skull at some point, the whole scalp or at least the whole of the affected side of the head should be shaved, scrubbed, and dressed with a bichlorid pack on the evening previous to the day of the operation. Since it is usually the intention to close the postauricular incisions immediately in the radical operation, and since in some cases grafting of the uncovered portions of the osseous wound can be immediately and successfully performed after the removal of all the disease, it is highly essential to have an absolutely sterile operative field, both inside the old suppurative cavity and on the skin covering the mastoid region. To secure this end it is necessary in the cases where no emergency exists not only to thoroughly syringe the external auditory canal with antiseptic solutions but also to use the attic syringe (see Fig. 208) for the purpose of dislodging any masses of cholesteatoma or dried secretion that may be concealed in this location. This should be followed by filling the external auditory meatus three times a day for several days preceding the mastoid operation with the alcohol and boric acid preparation (see formula, p. 227).

Immediately before the commencement of the operation additional antiseptic precaution may be advantageously taken by applying a solution of bichlorid of mercury, 1:1000 in alcohol, to the walls and hairy parts of the external meatus. This solution should be vigorously rubbed into the skin by means of cotton twisted upon a stout applicator. A wick of narrow gauze which has been previously saturated with the same solution is then inserted into the canal to its bottom or even into the cavity of the middle ear if the drum membrane is wanting. This strip is removed as soon as the primary incisions are completed.

Whereas it is permissible to perform the simple mastoid operation in the home of the patient when the surroundings are clean and the operator can secure good light, it is seldom advisable either in the interest of the patient or surgeon to undertake the radical procedure outside of a well-equipped hospital, for the reason that in doing a complete operation it frequently becomes necessary to expose or open the cranial cavity or lateral sinus; or either may be uncovered accidentally. In either instance the necessary after-treatment can be carried out antiseptically in the modern hospital, but is usually questionable and therefore often dangerous when attempted even in the best appointed household.

The primary incision is begun at the tip of the mastoid process exactly as in the simple operation, and is likewise carried upward parallel to the furrow in the skin which indicates the attachment of the pinna and ¼ inch posterior to it.   This curvilinear cut is carried upward over the superior attachment of the auricle further than in the simple case, for, as will be presently stated, it is necessary, as the operation proceeds, to detach the soft tissues of the superior as well as those

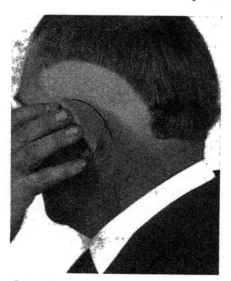

FIG. 238.—THE LINE OF PRIMARY INCISION FOR THE RADICAL MASTOID OPERATION.
This line may be extended forward or downward, if found necessary, at any time during the progress of the operation.   An additional backward incision may also be made from the center of the first if thought advisable. See also Fig. 276, line A B.

of the posterior wall of the external meatus; and to do this easily requires that the skin, superficial fascia, and sometimes the fibers of the temporal muscle and underlying periosteum be incised to the point above the ear shown in Fig. 238. Advantage is gained in most cases by making, in addition to this, the horizontal backward incision shown in Fig. 240.   This can be done either at the time of making the primary curvilinear cut or at any subsequent period when it may be decided that a more exposed area of the mastoid is for some reason necessary.

The anterior and posterior flaps are then detached from the bone and turned respectively backward and forward by means of the sharp periosteal elevator (see Fig. 161); the anterior being reflected to a point sufficient to expose clearly to view the posterior margin of the mouth of the auditory meatus. The blunt periosteal elevator (Fig. 239) is then substituted for the sharp one. This latter instrument is so constructed

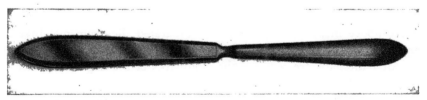

Fig. 239.—Periosteal Elevator for the Separation of the Soft Tissues of the External Auditory Meatus from the Underlying Bone.
The shape of the tip is adapted to that of the osseous auditory meatus.

that its shape and size adapts itself to that of the meatal walls of the osseous portion of the auditory canal, and hence with it the skin and periosteal lining of the posterior and superior walls of the canal can be quickly separated from the bone down to the tympanic ring (Fig. 240).

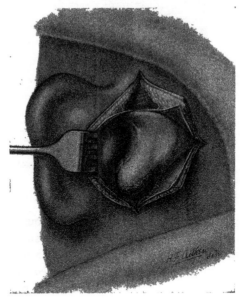

Fig. 240.—The Osseous Mastoid Field Denuded Preparatory to the Performance of the Radical Mastoid Operation.
The boundaries of the suprameatal triangle show clearly beneath the linea temporalis. Note that the soft tissues are completely separated from the posterior and upper walls of the bony meatus. Compare Fig. 163 in which the soft tissues are reflected for the operation suitable for acute mastoiditis.

If the drum membrane was previously found to be wanting the dissection is continued to the bottom of the auditory meatus and until the inner end of the separated portion of the tube lies loosely at the seat of its former attachment to the annulus tympanicus. In case the tympanic membrane is partly present it is advisable to incise the canal walls at a right angle to its axis just exterior to the tympanic ring, since if one or more of the ossicles are present and attached to the remnant of the drum membrane, it would be possible to wrench the stapes from its position if the above incision had not already separated the drum membrane and its ossicular attachment from the integumentary lining of the canal.

After the flaps are reflected the landmarks of the exposed mastoid are discernible, provided all the bleeding points have been clamped and the accumulated blood has been absorbed by the gauze. The chiseling of the bone is begun at the same point and the mastoid antrum

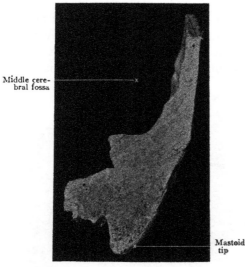

Fig. 241.—Eburnated Mastoid Process, not a Single Cell Appearing in the Whole Section.

is opened in exactly the same manner as previously described and illustrated (Fig. 168). If desired, however, the superoposterior wall of the external meatus may be cut away together with the adjoining bone at the same time that the wound is deepened in the direction of the antrum. In operating on the acutely inflamed mastoid it is quite a common occurrence to uncover superficial cells immediately after the cortex is chiseled off; but such cells, lying so near the surface, are much more rarely met with in the chronic case when performing the radical mastoid operation. In this latter class of cases where there has been a long-continued inflammation in the bone, granulation tissue sometimes fills the mastoid cells; this later becomes fibrous, and after a long time ossification takes place and many of the cellular spaces become

finally obliterated (see Fig. 241). When the last stage of the inflammatory process is reached, osteosclerosis, or eburnation of the mastoid, is
said to have taken place (Fig. 241). The mastoid antrum itself and the
posterior meatal wall may be involved in the osteosclerotic process, and
when this is the case the cavity of the antrum may be greatly lessened
in size and the deeper portion of the external auditory meatus may, as
a result, become very much narrowed.

Should osteosclerosis have taken place the operator must expect
to chisel from cortex to antrum through the ivory-like bone without
encountering any cellular structure. He must also bear in mind the

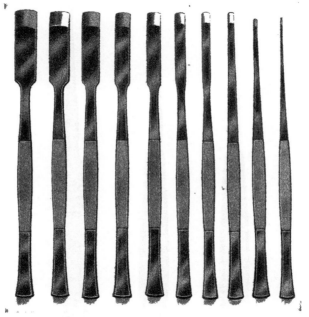

FIG. 242.—JANSEN'S SET OF MASTOID CHISELS. (See also gouges shown in Figs. 167 to 172).

fact that the mastoid antrum will very likely be much smaller than
normal; moreover, because of the encroachment upon this cavity by
the sclerosed surrounding bone, the antrum may be displaced slightly
upward or inward and forward toward the middle ear, and therefore
may be very difficult to reach. It may be profitably stated here that
chisels made of the finest steel, the edges of which are in perfect order,
are necessary to penetrate the dense bone, and that, therefore, in performing the radical operation it is wise to have an additional number of
different sized chisels and gouges (Figs. 242 and 167 to 172), so that no
delay may result from compulsory chiseling with dull instruments.

25

The precaution previously given as to the proper method in the employment of the gouges should be observed in this operation, and it is highly essential to the safety of the patient that the osseous cavity shall, as the work progresses, be kept entirely free from collections of bony chips or blood, so that the operator may at all times be able to recognize the earliest approach to any cell, mastoid or otherwise, and to use at once the exploring instrument in order to determine the nature and extent of the space that is uncovered. Should these rules be followed

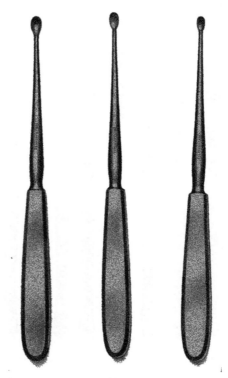

FIGS. 243, 244, AND 245.—HAMMOND'S MASTOID CURETS.
Each is provided with a sharp, curved beak.

in all radical mastoid operations the danger areas which are normally situated close to portions of bone which must be chiseled away may usually be successfully avoided, whereas otherwise they would be almost certainly encountered and injured.

As the wound deepens the sharp curet (Figs. 243 to 247 *a* and 247 *b*) should be employed when possible in the further removal of bone. Should the bone be soft enough the opening can, by the use of this instrument driven in the direction of the antrum, be very rapidly deepened,

and the mastoid antrum be thus uncovered.   The operator may know
that he has entered the antrum when the exploring probe (see Fig. 173)
can be passed for a distance of several millimeters in the direction of
the middle ear, and perhaps for a considerable distance under overhanging ledges of bone in every direction.   When it becomes certain
that the cavity which has been partially uncovered is the antrum, the
opening is at once sufficiently enlarged to permit the thorough explora-

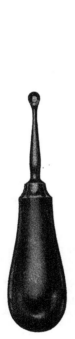

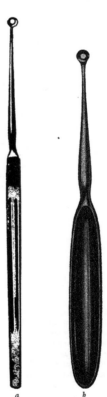

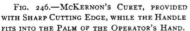

FIG. 246.—McKernon's Curet, provided
with Sharp Cutting Edge, while the Handle
fits into the Palm of the Operator's Hand.

FIG. 247.—*a*, Small Sharp Mastoid Curet; *b*,
Convenient Curet for Clearing Small Angles of
Mastoid Wound.

tion of its walls on every side.   The contents of the cavity may be found
to consist of thickened, polypoid, or necrotic membrane, of inspissated
pus, or of cholesteatomatous material.   Its walls may be found denuded
in places, so that rough and carious bone is visible or can be felt with
the explorer.   In the worst cases it is sometimes discovered that the
bony partition separating the antrum from the cranial cavity above is
wanting and that the dura mater lies exposed to direct infection; or that

the lateral sinus may have been encroached upon posteriorly and is bathed in pus; or, possibly, the osseous covering is eroded and the dura is covered with necrotic granulation tissue. In short, any of the conditions which have been detailed in the section on the pathology of this disease may be exposed and determined at the time of uncovering the antrum.

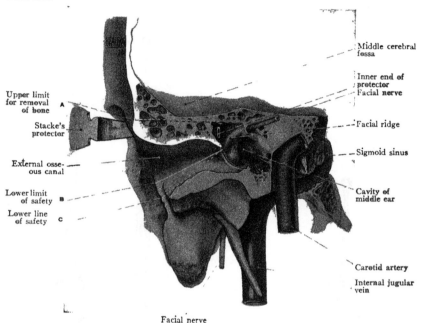

FIG. 248.—PERPENDICULAR SECTION OF THE RIGHT TEMPORAL BONE IN THE PLANE OF THE EXTERNAL AUDITORY MEATUS AND MIDDLE EAR, SHOWING THE SURGICAL RELATION OF THE POSTEROSUPERIOR WALL OF THE OSSEOUS AUDITORY CANAL TO THE ADITUS AD ANTRUM AND FACIAL NERVE.

A complete tympano-mastoid exenteration has been performed on the specimen, and a Stacke protector has been inserted through the osseous opening from without inward; the inner end of the protector is seen lying in the aditus ad antrum external to the facial ridge. The illustration is intended to show the extent to which the inner end of the posterosuperior wall of the osseous meatus may be removed without risk of injury to the facial nerve. The portion of the osseous meatus which is commonly removed during the radical mastoid operation lies between lines A and B, but in any case in which it is found necessary to do so, all the bone between lines A and C may be safely removed. It should be observed, however, that the *inner termination* of lines B and C are *at the same point*, and it should always be borne in mind that the width of bone at the inner termination of lines A and B represents the greatest width of bone that should ever be removed at the inner extremity of the external auditory meatus. The illustration accurately shows that any greater width of osseous removal would injure the facial nerve as it passes under the inner extremity of points BC.

If the posterosuperior margin of the posterior meatal wall has been cut away at the same time the bone has been removed in penetrating to the antrum, there will now be left a bridge of bone between the antrum and the middle ear which forms the outer wall of the aditus ad antrum (Fig. 248), and in order to connect these two cavities and convert them into one it is necessary to remove this intervening bridge.

To accomplish this is one of the most difficult and dangerous steps of the whole operation—not dangerous to life, perhaps, but what is almost equally serious, namely, danger to the function of the facial nerve, with subsequent facial paralysis. Every precaution in the use of one's anatomic knowledge and skill in the manipulation of instruments is therefore necessary at this part of the procedure, in order that no violence be done to either the facial nerve or the external semicircular canal. The Fallopian canal, through which the facial nerve passes, runs directly under the bridge of bone to which reference has just been

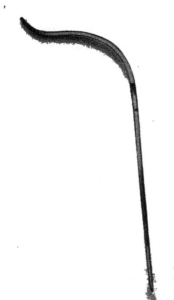

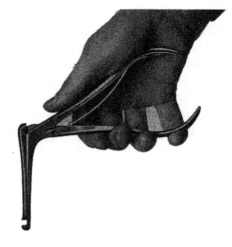

FIG. 250.—KERRISON'S BONE-FORCEPS, FOR THE REMOVAL OF THAT PORTION OF THE INNER END OF THE EXTERNAL OSSEOUS MEATUS WHICH OVERLIES THE ADITUS AD ANTRUM.

As will be seen by reference to Fig. 248, the facial canal lies immediately under the bone at this place and the nerve is therefore exposed to great risk of injury during this step of the radical mastoid operation. The lower jaw of the instrument here shown is inserted through the aditus, is lifted until it hugs the ledge of bone, is then closed, and the bone is bitten away without danger to the underlying nerve.

FIG. 249.—STACKE'S PROTECTOR.

made, but the lumen of the aditus ad antrum lies between the nerve and the bridge. Therefore, in chiseling this bridge away a protector should be placed under the bridge, in order to cover the nerve and insure against the penetration of the deeper parts by the chisel (Fig. 249).

Instead of using the chisel and protector in removing the bridge of bone overlying the facial ridge as above described, the Kerrison cutting forceps (Fig. 250), which are made in three sizes to suit the various sizes of the aditus ad antrum that may be met with, either on account of diseased conditions that are present or of the age of the individual, may be employed. The beak of this instrument, which serves as a protector, is inserted through the opening of the aditus, when, by compressing the handles, the cutting surfaces of the upper jaw are driven through the bone which is thereby ʻbitten away without the possibility of danger to the facial nerve. Injury to this nerve, however, may arise from the rude or forcible introduction of either the Stacke protector or the Kerrison forceps, and therefore the operator must be gentle in his efforts to insert either through the opening under the bridge. The assistant who holds the Stacke protector in place after its introduction and while the operator is removing the bone can also injure the underlying nerve should he make too much pressure upon the handle, which, acting upon the facial ridge as a fulcrum, may crush or otherwise injure the nerve.

It will be observed that when the removal of the posterior wall of the meatus is not accomplished coincident with the deepening of the bony channel that is made in entering the mastoid antrum, that the thin plate of bone left standing between this opening and the meatus will be shaped like the side of a truncated pyramid, the base of which is represented by the posterior margin of the external meatus. This can be best understood by a reference to a specimen of the temporal bone upon which the operation has been thus completed (see Fig. 248). Special attention is called to the shape of this wedge for the reason that its inner extremity forms the outer wall of the aditus ad antrum and constitutes the bridge of bone, of which mention has already been made, that overlies the facial nerve and semicircular canal. In the removal of the postmeatal wall, therefore, this triangular piece of bone here described may be cut away as broadly as the whole width of the external meatus at its external end, but as the inner or antral end is approached the facial nerve will be injured if a greater width is removed than is represented by the actual width of the outer wall of the aditus ad antrum.

Immediately after the removal of the outer wall of the aditus, as just described, the overhanging ledge of the squamous portion of the temporal bone (see Figs. 248 and 263), which forms the outer wall of the attic chamber of the middle ear, should be ablated. The exploring instrument is first passed into the attic, and by this means the depth and height of this portion of the tympanic cavity are determined. Since the transverse portion of the facial nerve traverses the inner wall of the attic, this nerve may be easily injured during the removal of the outer osseous wall of this cavity. Therefore the greatest caution must be observed, both in the choice of instrument used and the method of employing the same, in conducting this essential part of the operation. When the small chisel or gouge is used the Stacke protector should be inserted behind the overhanging attic wall and the chiseling should be done directly down upon it. The Kerrison forceps are also safe for this purpose, but it is sometimes impossible to use them, owing to the thickness of the cutting parts and the consequent difficulty of inserting the same into proper position. Whatever method is selected it is necessary to continue the removal of bone until no overhanging ledge exists, and the bent explorer when introduced into the attic may be withdrawn in any direction without meeting any obstruction.

Following this exposure of the attic all oozing of blood should be checked by packing the interior of the wound tightly for a few seconds. When thus dried the entire middle ear is visible, and therefore if any of the drum membrane, or the ossicles, or their fragments still remain, they can now be easily removed, and this should always be attended to at this stage of the procedure. In doing this it is usually not desirable to disturb the stapes, and hence, in order to prevent its injury, this ossicle should be disarticulated from the incus before the others are removed.

Time will be gained and the subsequent curetment of the middle ear be made both easier and safer should the operator now pack the cavity of the middle ear tightly with gauze and return to the antral portion of the wound, which has by this time ceased actively to ooze, and can, therefore, be better inspected than at any previous period of the operation.

The amount of bone that should be removed from the mastoid process varies in almost every case, and is determined largely by the extent of the necrotic process which has taken place and by the surgical principle which requires that all the diseased cavities shall be left free from pockets or irregularities of surface that would interfere with the successful application of the skin flaps, of the skin grafts, or with the subsequent process of healing by granulation. In the sclerotic mastoid (see Fig. 241), which has already been described, it is frequently not required to remove more bone than that which must necessarily be cut away to freely expose the antrum, aditus, and attic of the middle ear; whereas, should fistulous channels have previously extended from the interior of the mastoid to its surface, or should the pneumatic spaces, instead of undergoing the osteosclerotic process, have broken down (see Figs. 224 and 230), the greater part or even the whole of the mastoid process may require removal. Sometimes, as stated in the section on its pathology, the presence of a cholesteotoma in the antrum will cause an extensive absorption of the surrounding bone; in these cases it will usually be necessary to remove the osseous structures beyond the line of the cavity or until healthy bone is encountered in every direction. A wide experience in the surgical management of these cases and an extended observation of the behavior of carious bone under different degrees of its surgical treatment is frequently necessary in determining just how far the disease has extended, and consequently just how much of the osseous structure needs to be cut away. In general, however, it may be said that when bone has been reached that seems hard and firm under the curet, and when there is capillary oozing from every portion of its freshly cut surface, it is safe to presume that the operation has been carried far enough, and that nature will repair the parts rapidly if the after-care be conducted according to good surgical principles.

When satisfied that the diseased portions of the mastoid process which lie below the antrum have been dealt with thoroughly, the operator again returns to the tympanum and mastoid antrum. The withdrawal of the gauze packing which was placed there some minutes before leaves these parts dry and easy of inspection. Every portion of the walls and bony edges of these cavities should at this time be inspected with the explorer, and any overhanging ledge or any suspicious looking area of bone should be removed wherever found. A proper sized curet is selected and all polypi, granulations, or thickened mucous membrane that may be found in either antrum or middle ear should be scraped away. Most writers agree that the tympanic end of the Eustachian tube should be thoroughly cureted and its mucous membrane removed, to the end that the subsequent healthy granulation within the tube will close it and thus shut off the cavities of the middle ear from further infection through an extension from the nasopharynx. However thoroughly the mastoid operation may be performed in every other particular, if the Eustachian tube is not closed by some such procedure as above stated, the patient will be subsequently liable to attacks of aural discharge whenever he suffers from an acute nasopharyngitis; the influence of the tube in thus keeping the mastoid wound infected may cause an indefinite continuance of the aural discharge and to some extent, at least, defeat the purpose of the radical operation. A burr has been devised for the purpose of removing the tympanic portion of the tubal membrane and of stimulating the adjacent bone to the production of granulation tissue; and this instrument may be employed instead of the curet if so desired. During the use of the curet for the purpose above stated, deplorable injuries may be caused unless the operator is gentle in its use, and keeps the situation of all important anatomic structures constantly in mind. By rude and careless manipulation of the curet in the tympanum the horizontal portion of the facial nerve may be readily injured, the stapes may be scratched from the pelvis of the oval window, or the dura mater may be exposed over the tegmen tympani. Puncture of the jugular bulb while cureting the floor of the middle ear or of the carotid artery while cureting the Eustachian tube are also possibilities that should not be forgotten. The chief reason for a successful result in one radical mastoid operation and failure in another often lies in the fact that one operator is not satisfied to close his wound until every little nook and corner of the entire wound has not only been freed from disease but is also made smooth and regular in contour, whereas another,

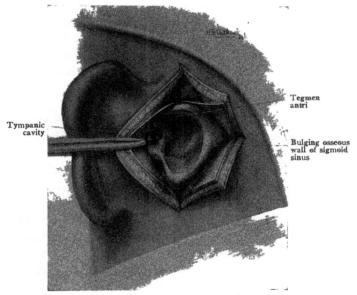

Tympanic cavity

Tegmen antri

Bulging osseous wall of sigmoid sinus

FIG. 251.—TYMPANOMASTOID EXENTERATION COMPLETED.
Note that the cavity is smooth and free from overhanging ledges of bone.

either from carelessness or lack of training in the principles of bone surgery, ignores such minute detail and closes the wound over a cavity so badly prepared to receive the skin flaps or grafts that failure is inevitable from the first. Hence, it cannot be said that the bony wound is properly prepared until every pocket of infection, every overhanging ledge of bone or sharply angular ridge, has received such careful attention that the resulting cavity is clean and smooth in every direction (Fig. 251).

The next step of the radical mastoid operation is directed to the repair by plastic methods of as much of the denuded bone as possible to the ends that deformity may not result and that the wound will heal in the shortest length of time and with the least suffering and inconvenience to the patient.

For this purpose the posterior half of the fibrocartilaginous canal is utilized, and from it skin flaps are so cut that when properly placed in the wound they will line as much of the osseous cavity as possible with actual integument. These skin flaps will, in addition, furnish areas from which new epithelium will spring that will ultimately cover the remaining denuded area and provide a permanent non-secreting lining for the entire wound.

Two principal methods of cutting the skin flaps are in general use, and whether the operator shall employ the one or the other depends much upon whether the bony cavity which has resulted from the operation is large or small, and also upon whether or not the postauricular wound is to be immediately sutured or is to be left open for subsequent inspection and treatment. In general, it may be said that the Körner flap (Fig. 252) is preferable when the mastoid cavity is small and when the postauricular wound is to be immediately closed.

Method of Making the Körner Flap.—An incision is made through the entire thickness of the posterosuperior wall of the fibrocartilaginous meatus, beginning at its deepest or tympanic end and continuing outward along the posterosuperior portion as far as the concha. A second incision, exactly similar and parallel to the first, is made along the posteroinferior portion and from 6 to 8 mm. distant. A tongue-shaped flap is thus cut from the canal which has an attachment only at the concha (see Fig. 252). Usually a free hemorrhage results from these incisions and sometimes one or more spurting arterioles will need clamping, torsion, or possibly ligation. In order to insure accurate and permanent apposition of this flap to the posterior wall of the mastoid wound, where it should be ultimately placed, it is necessary to dissect the skin of the cartilaginous meatus entirely away from the cartilage and other soft parts, all of which latter are cut off close to the base of the remaining skin flap at the concha, after which the integumentary portion which remains is pliable and can be pushed backward to the desired position in the osseous wound of the mastoid. In order to prevent kinking of this flap during subsequent dressings and to assure its permanency of position, a suture should be passed through the periosteum of the adjoining auricular flap, then through the posterior portion of the Körner flap, and the latter is thus anchored in a position which will be most favorable to its immediate adhesion to the bone. If it be determined that a skin graft shall be applied at the primary operation, this should be done as the next step, after which the postauricular flaps are completely closed by

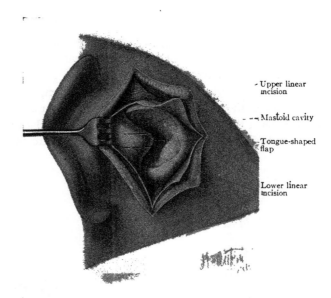

FIG. 252.—THE KORNER FLAP.

The incision through the soft tissues is extended below the mastoid tip further than is usually necessary.

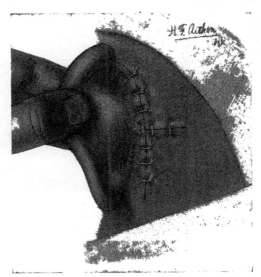

FIG. 253.—THE RADICAL MASTOID OPERATION COMPLETED.

Drainage is secured through the external auditory meatus, which is somewhat enlarged by the reflection of the flaps.   In case the dura has been exposed over sinus or tegmen it is not wise to suture the entire wound, as here shown.

catgut sutures (Fig. 253) and a strip of gauze is inserted into the newly made cavity through the greatly enlarged meatus.   The soft-tissue flaps are most conveniently sutured by means of half-curved needles which are held in the jaws of a medium-sized needle-holder (Fig. 254). The method of applying the strip of gauze is of considerable importance. By means of reflected light it must first be seen that the Körner flap is in proper position. The narrow strip of gauze is then seized at one end by the dressing-forceps and, under continued illumination, it is carried to the deepest portion of the wound. Over this, one fold after another is packed up to and against the Körner flap in such a way as to slightly stretch and spread it out to its full extent and to gently press it into snug apposition

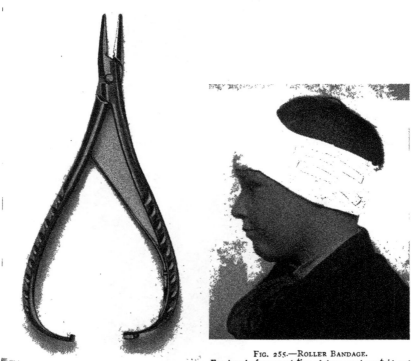

FIG. 255.—ROLLER BANDAGE.
Employed after completion of the several mastoid and
other operations upon the ear.

FIG. 254.—NEEDLE-HOLDER.

to the raw surface of the bone. Tightly packing the cavity must be avoided since it is unnecessary, causes pain, and may result in the death or sloughing of the flap. The first dressing is completed by the plentiful application of gauze over and about the auricle and by a roller bandage over all (Fig. 255).

The Panse Flaps.—These flaps are best suited to cases in which it has been found necessary during the operation to remove a large amount of the osseous structure of the temporal bone, in consequence of which a large cavity remains to be healed. They should also be chosen when either by accident or intention the sigmoid sinus or dura mater has been exposed or opened. The Panse flaps are formed from the posterior wall of the fibrocartilaginous canal by making one incision through the entire thickness of the soft parts, exactly in the center line of this wall, and from its deepest portion well out into the concha. At the conchal end of the incision a second cut is made at right angles to the first and in an upward direction for about 6 mm.; this is followed by a third cut, beginning at the end of the first, and extending downward through the concha for 6 mm., the three incisions forming a ⊤, which bounds

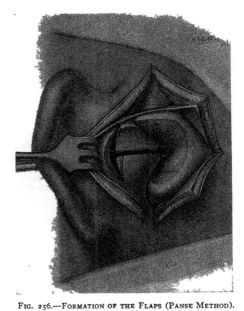

FIG. 256.—FORMATION OF THE FLAPS (PANSE METHOD).
Note the situation of the T-incision. Note that the cartilage has been removed from the upper flap. The lower flap should be treated likewise before it is stitched in place.

the two quadrangular flaps that are thus constructed from the post-meatal soft structures (Fig. 256). The distance to which these incisions should extend into the concha depends upon the size of the osseous cavity that is to be lined. When this is very large the first incision, or stem of the ⊤, should be carried to within a short distance of the antihelix, and the other two should follow the curvature of this fold respectively upward and downward to a slightly greater distance than has been previously designated. After the Panse flaps have been properly shaped by the above described incisions, and after the cartilaginous portion of each flap has been removed by careful dissection, the

remaining or integumentary portion of each should have its denuded
surface placed into direct contact with the osseous portion of the adjoining mastoid wound, and in this position should be anchored by one
or more catgut sutures to the adjacent periosteum (Fig. 257). Success
in the employment of the Panse method is, like that of the method of
Körner, somewhat dependent upon the complete removal of the cartilaginous portion of each flap on either side. To dissect out the cartilaginous portion of each flap requires a few minutes, but the advantages
derived from it are so great that this should not be neglected in any
case. Even when the Panse method of making the flaps has been

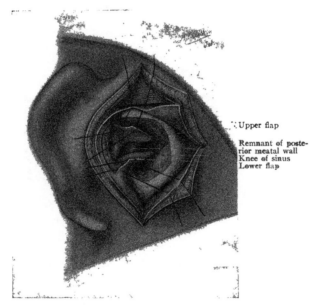

Upper flap

Remnant of poste-
rior meatal wall
Knee of sinus
Lower flap

FIG. 257.—METHOD OF SUTURING THE PANSE FLAPS.

employed the author has, in the great majority of his cases, been able
successfully to close the postauricular wound at once (see Fig. 253)
and to secure a union of all the flaps by first intention. When a considerable part of the concha has been utilized in the formation of these
flaps the external auditory meatus is, of course, subsequently much
larger than normal, but this slight deformity, if such it might be called,
is preferable to the long-continued treatment by the postauricular open
method, which will also be likely to result in a scar that is more noticeable than the enlarged meatus. The provision of a large meatus serves
the excellent advantage of enabling the surgeon to at all times see every
part of the mastoid wound through this channel and to thus be able to

carry on the after-treatment in an intelligent and most satisfactory manner. In all cases of large mastoid wound where the Panse flaps have been employed, and enough of the concha has been included to leave a large meatus, the results have been so good in the author's cases that he has never regretted the immediate closure of the post-auricular wound. When skin-grafts are to be used primarily the same should be applied immediately after the flaps have been properly placed and the external wound has been sutured. The insertion of the gauze packing and the final external dressing differs in no essential respect from that described as proper after the Körner flaps have been employed.

Skin Grafting.—The length of time necessary for the complete healing of the cavity of the mastoid wound after the radical mastoid operation may be greatly shortened by the application of skin grafts to all those portions of the osseous wound which it has been impossible to cover by means of the skin flaps heretofore described. These grafts may be applied either at the time of the mastoid operation or a week or ten days subsequently, and after the surface of the cavity has begun to granulate. If at the primary operation it is possible to eradicate all the foci of suppuration, to sterilize the resulting cavity, and to leave a smooth osseous surface in all parts of the wound, the probability of success resulting from the application of the graft at this time is sufficient to warrant its trial, for should it fail to take, no harm has been done by the attempt; and should it succeed it will save much time in the healing and will obviate the unpleasant necessity for a second general anesthetic, which must be given should the grafts be applied on some subsequent occasion.

Should it have been impossible at the time of operation to remove all infectious areas from the mastoid, and therefore a cavity be left which cannot be completely sterilized, it would be wiser under such circumstances to wait a week or ten days before applying the grafts, and in the interval to make the necessary efforts to secure a cleaner field for their reception. Some operators, however, prefer to do the grafting as a secondary measure under all circumstances.

Technic of the Skin Grafting.—On the evening preceding the day of the mastoid operation, and at the same time that the head is surgically prepared, the area from which the skin graft is to be taken, the front or inside surface of the patient's thigh, should likewise be sterilized. An area 6 inches square on one or the other of these regions should therefore be shaved, scrubbed, and finally prepared by the application of a bichlorid dressing (1 : 1000), which latter is bound over the sterilized field and allowed to remain until the mastoid wound is ready to receive the grafts. At the time this dressing is removed from the thigh the skin is rubbed with alcohol, which is in turn bathed off with warm normal salt solution. The knife which is to be used for cutting the graft is first dipped in warm saline solution, and while the skin of the prepared area on the patient's thigh is rendered tense by the operator's left hand, its edge is made to penetrate the layers of epidermis, after which the blade is turned flat against the skin, when by means of a rapid sawing motion an epidermal graft 2 inches square may be quickly removed. This was formerly transferred to a spatula made for the purpose and of convenient size to enter the mastoid wound; and when in proper position in the deep portion of the latter the graft with the freshly cut surface presenting toward the bone was slid from the spatula by means of a sharp needle, and was then spread over the cavities of the middle ear and antrum and, indeed, all remaining uncovered surfaces. This manipulation of the graft should, of course, be done under the guidance of reflected light, and should any blood or air collect under the same it should be sucked away by means of a small pipet upon the outer end of which is a suction bulb. Upon the graft are gently packed pledgets of sterilized cotton or small gauze sponges until the meatus is completely but loosely filled.

A more recent and easier method of application, also an equally successful one, is to use instead of the spatula a 2 × 2 inch piece of sterilized crape lisse, upon which the graft is evenly spread with its cut surface outward. The crape is then gathered from all its edges into a somewhat cylindric shape, and with the graft still upon its outer surface, it is inserted into the depths of the wound *via* the auditory canal, after which, by means of a probe, it is spread over all the denuded surfaces. It seems not to be absolutely necessary to the successful taking of the graft that every portion of it shall come into direct contact with the denuded bone, for wherever any area of the graft touches the bone, adhesion takes place and in this way many islands of epidermal covering are formed, which soon run together and cover the whole surface of the wound. Those portions of the graft which are not brought into immediate contact with the wound will quickly die and are brought away on the crape when it is withdrawn at the first dressing.

Following either method the graft is left undisturbed for about five days unless symptoms should arise which indicate an earlier change of the dressing. When undisturbed for the full time an odor, usually very foul, will be present. This is due to the decay of those portions of the graft which were not in contact with the wound and which consequently could not adhere and grow. The odor is not, therefore, necessarily indicative of failure of the taking of the graft.

At the first dressing the ear may be gently syringed with an antiseptic fluid, after which the cavity is dried and a gauze wick packing is loosely inserted into every part. This treatment must be subsequently repeated each day in order to keep the cavity sufficiently dry to favor that complete epidermization which is so necessary to the permanent cure of the mastoid disease. At the first dressing subsequent to the mastoid operation, provided all has progressed normally and the dressing has been undisturbed for five or six days, it is usually found that the primary mastoid incisions through the soft tissues have united by first intention. If any suture has become infected the same should be removed and the pustulating track of the stitch be at once disinfected, dried, and powdered with boric acid. It is advisable to continue the use of the roller bandage for at least a week subsequent to the first dressing, even though the wound at that time seems well united, because by its longer application provision is made not only against infection from without but also against injury to the tender mastoid and auricle, which might result from unconscious movement of the patient during sleep.

At each subsequent treatment the wound is syringed, if thought advisable, with antiseptic fluids. Some cases seem to do better if the cavity is only mopped dry and is afterward lightly powdered with some antiseptic. Whatever the mode of treatment, the interior of the wound must each day be inspected by means of reflected light in order that the surgeon may at all times know that the progress of the healing is as it should be. If the skin grafts have failed or have only taken over insular areas, exuberant granulations may spring up, septic material be retained, and additional death of bone occur. Any such tendency should, of course, be detected at once during the after-management. Painstaking care of the wound during the healing process is always sufficiently well rewarded by good results to amply justify its bestowal upon every case.

Accidents and Dangers that may Occur during the Performance of or Subsequent to the Radical Mastoid Operation.—A study of the anatomic relations of the mastoid process, mastoid antrum, and middle ear to the cerebrum, cerebellum, sigmoid sinus, facial nerve, and semicircular canals must always lead the observer to the conclusion that accident and danger may lie in the path of the radical mastoid operation during nearly every step of its performance. This conclusion becomes the more confirmed by a large experience in operating, and from an examination of a great number of temporal bones, in both of

26

which ways it is learned that frequent anomalies of all the structures involved occur, and that the operator can therefore never determine beforehand, with a helpful degree of certainty in any case, whether the dangerous structures are normally placed beneath the cortex or whether they traverse the very paths that are usually followed through the bone by the operator in reaching the diseased tissues which he desires to remove. As examples of what is meant, it may be cited that it is not uncommon to find the sigmoid sinus running directly through the field covered by the suprameatal triangle—the normal safety route for opening into the mastoid antrum (see Fig. 183). Or the middle cerebral fossa may lie so low that it overhangs the mastoid antrum and thus occupies a plane below the linea temporalis, the landmark that is given as a safe line below which the operator may chisel without endangering the brain at this point. Fortunately, the course of the facial nerve seldom, perhaps never, varies from the normal, but its close proximity to the most frequent seats of the carious processes renders it necessary in almost every radical mastoid operation to remove diseased bone in the immediate vicinity of the Fallopian canal, perhaps often within $\frac{1}{2}$ mm. of it, and thus the function of the nerve is constantly endangered even in cases of average severity. Furthermore, the necrosis of the temporal bone may extend to the petrous portion and include the semicircular canals or cochlea, the removal of which from these locations would require the most exact anatomic knowledge and operative experience, as well as the most delicate touch in the handling of instruments; otherwise the operator may wound these deep-seated structures.

The first and most essential requirement in the avoidance of these accidents is that before an operator undertakes a surgical procedure involving so many accidental and dangerous possibilities, he should have acquired the most perfect knowledge of the anatomy of the temporal bone by having personally made many sections and dissections of its structure. In addition, he should have performed the radical operation on the cadaver many times and should also have witnessed its performance a number of times on actual patients by an operator of great experience.

The next essential in the avoidance of danger is that the primary incisions through the soft tissues should always be sufficiently extensive to permit an amount of exposure of the skull over the mastoid region that at the beginning, as well as throughout the entire procedure, will render it easy for the operator to be certain of his landmarks, and to enable him to recognize them with certainty at any period of the operation (see Fig. 240).

The third essential is that bleeding from all the larger vessels must be controlled by clamping, ligature, or torsion, and the capillary oozing by pressure when necessary, in order that the wound may be sufficiently clear to enable the operator to recognize the landmarks and the nature of the structure upon which he is operating. The bony chips and necrotic débris must be kept out of the wound as rapidly as dislodged by the chisel, for skill in operating and anatomic knowledge of the structures will be of little service in dealing with parts that are filled with blood or obstructed by the products of the operation. And, finally, a good light during all stages of the operation, either natural or artificial must at all times be available.

Always begin the chiseling far forward in the suprameatal margin. This will usually avoid direct entrance into an abnormally placed sigmoid sinus. By removing the osseous chips immediately after their detachment, by directing the edge of the gouge toward the meatus, and by observing constantly the surface from which each chip is removed it will be possible, in all cases, to approach either the sinus or dura and even lay them bare without risk of injury to the dural structure. In this connection it should again be pointed out that the frequent use of the exploring probe will often avoid error.

In addition to the above precautions, injury to the facial nerve may usually be avoided by exercising the greatest care possible in the removal of the posterior portion of the osseous meatal wall. It is at the deepest portion of this wall that the danger to the nerve is greatest, and hence in cutting away the inner third of its length the operator should be goverened by the rules previously given for this step of the operation. The point here to be emphasized is that unless it can be actually demonstrated that the ridge of the Fallopian canal lies more deeply, the greatest width to which the postmeatal wall can be removed at its inner extremity is represented by the diameter of the aditus ad antrum (see Fig. 248).

The dangers arising to the facial nerve, oval window, and large vessels which lie in close proximity to the middle ear from a too vigorous curetment have already been pointed out, and it is now only necessary to again call attention to the possibilities of grave error from this cause and to suggest a caution in the performance of this necessary, though delicate part, of the operative procedure.

Facial paralysis (Figs. 258 and 259) may follow the radical mastoid operation as a result of the penetration of the Fallopian canal by the chisel or curet and of the consequent injury or severance of the facial nerve; or it may be the result of a serous effusion into the Fallopian canal in sufficient amount to compress the nerve and in this way to abate its function. In case the latter is the cause, the paralysis of the muscles supplied by the nerve will usually be gradual in its development,

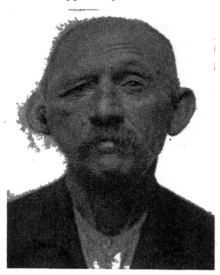

FIG. 258.—FACIAL PARALYSIS RESULTING FROM EPI-
THELIOMA.
(See Fig. 69.) Shows appearance of face when patient attempts to wrinkle the forehead.

and the loss of facial movement may not be noticed for from one to several days following the mastoid exenteration. Should the nerve trunk be severely contused or entirely severed during the operation the facial paralysis will be complete at once, although it will probably not be detected until the patient begins to arouse from the anesthetic.

The prognosis as to the restoration of function in postoperative facial paralysis depends upon the nature and severity of the cause. If the injury to the nerve is trivial or if there is only a traumatic neuritis with effusion into the sheath of the nerve, a partial or complete restoration of function may be expected in from six months to a year. If, however, the nerve has been greatly contused or completely severed

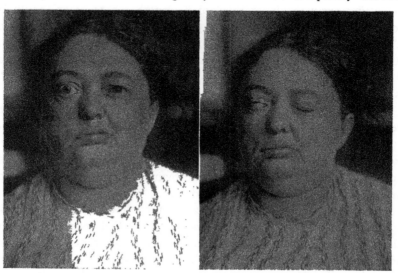

FIG. 259.—VARYING FACIAL EXPRESSION AFTER DISEASE OR INJURY TO THE FACIAL NERVE.

or if a portion of its trunk has been entirely destroyed, the prognosis is not favorable since the function will not likely be restored, and the muscles supplied by the facial nerve will in time undergo more or less atrophy. The peripheral portion of the nerve itself will finally atrophy until its trunk will be difficult or impossible to find when dissections are made for that purpose. Many operators whose observation is worthy of quotation have reported cases of recovery of function after severe injury or even after the division or destruction of a portion of the facial nerve. Bezold (*Z. f. O.*, Vol. XVI.) reports the complete restoration of the nerve, and consequent return of function to the facial muscles, after destruction of the greater portion of the Fallopian canal including the facial nerve. Pierce (*Trans. Am. Laryngol. Otol. and Rhinol. Soc.,* 1906) states that in a case in which $\frac{1}{4}$ inch of the facial nerve was destroyed restoration of function occurred after a period of nine years.

The treatment of the resulting facial palsy is medicinal, mechanical, and surgical. In cases where it is definitely known or strongly believed that the nerve has been but slightly injured or that there is no injury at all, but only an effusion into the nerve sheath, surgical treatment is not indicated and the internal administration of drugs, together with well directed massage of the facial muscles, should be advocated. The bowels should be kept freely open by the administration of salines to favor the absorption of exudates from the sheath of the nerve, and later strychnin in $\frac{1}{40}$-gr. doses, three times a day, may be given to stimulate the nervous system. Massage of the affected muscles is essential to prevent their atrophy and this should be given once or twice a day for a period of at least five minutes, the manipulations including the deep-seated as well as the more superficial muscles. The application of the interrupted electric current twice or three times a week will also be of service in preserving and restoring the deficient muscle-tone.

When the facial paralysis occurs immediately after the mastoid operation and the operator knows that the nerve was extensively injured during the procedure, surgical measures may be instituted at once with a view to the restoration of the lost muscular function.

The Surgery of the Facial Nerve.—It has been demonstrated by experiment that regeneration will occur in the peripheral portion of a nerve that has partly degenerated as the result of an injury to its trunk, and that its former function can again be exercised if this segment of the nerve be grafted upon the central segment of a healthy nerve. Practical use has been made of this fact, and the injured seventh nerve has been many times united with the spinal accessory or with the hypoglossal nerve, and with a fair degree of success provided the operation is performed sufficiently early, and before wasting of both the nerve-fibers and the muscles supplied by them is too far advanced. Experience seems to show that it is better to unite the facial with the hypoglossal than with the spinal accessory, for when the latter has been united with the facial there has followed an associated movement between the groups of muscles that produce shoulder movement and those which produce face movement, which was very annoying to the patient and noticeable to the observer. In other words, after the operation of splicing the facial and spinal accessory nerves has been performed, whenever the patient either voluntarily or involuntarily moves the face, the shoulder of the corresponding side is also moved, and vice versa. After uniting the facial and hypoglossal nerves, persistence of the former function of the hypoglossal nerve also gives rise to associated movements of the tongue, but since this movement takes place within the mouth, and is therefore hidden from the public, it is not nearly so annoying to the patient.

The hypoglossal nerve is exposed in the neck by making an incision along the anterior margin of the sternocleidomastoid muscle, extending downward from a point opposite the anterior border of the mastoid process to a point opposite the cricoid cartilage. The parotid gland is exposed and held forward while the sternocleidomastoid muscle is pulled backward. The deep fascia is opened throughout the whole extent of the wound, exposing the trunks of both the hypoglossal and facial nerves. Each should be freed from its connections to adjacent structures for a sufficient distance to provide a combined length of the nerves which will enable the operator to bring the two ends together after their trunks have been completely severed. The facial nerve should be cut off squarely near the point of its exit from the skull and the hypoglossal should be divided at a point just beyond where it crosses the external carotid artery. The peripheral portion of the facial is turned downward and the proximal end of the hypoglossal is turned upward, so that the two meet over the posterior belly of the digastric muscle (Fig. 260). The respective ends of the nerve trunk are then united by means of a small curved needle and catgut. The sutures, four in number, should include only the sheaths of the nerves. It is needless to say that the stumps of each nerve should have been previously cut squarely off so that the two ends can be most accurately coaptated and retained in contact with each other until union has occurred, because the success of the operation depends entirely upon the accuracy with which this step is performed. Should infection of the wound occur and suppuration in or about the grafted nerve take place during the process of union, failure to restore the function would most certainly result. Every precaution must, therefore, be taken, both in the preparation for and the performance of the operation itself, to the end that the most perfect asepsis is secured. The external wound

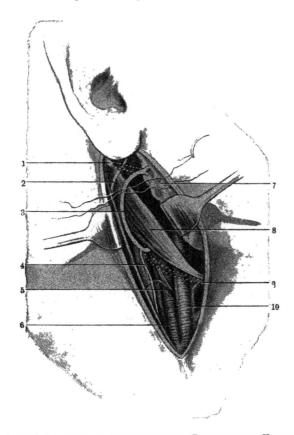

FIG. 260.—FRAZIER'S OPERATION FOR ANASTOMOSIS OF THE FACIAL WITH THE HYPOGLOSSAL NERVE.
1, String of the central segment of the facial nerve; 2, spinal accessory nerve; 3, reflected portion of the hypoglossal nerve; 4, descendens noni; 5, occipital artery; 6, internal carotid; 7, parotid gland drawn forward with a retractor; 8, digastric muscle; 9, course of hypoglossal nerve before it was reflected; 10, external carotid artery (Frazier).

should be closed at once because a primary union of every tissue is desirable.

Results.—Complete restoration of the function of the facial nerve as exhibited by the movements it is capable of imparting to the muscles of the face which it supplies has not as yet been attained by this operation. When successfully performed, however, two grades of improvement may be expected, as follows: In the first the muscle-tone of the

affected side of the face is so improved that the muscles are no longer
flaccid and the facial expression during a state of repose is no longer
asymmetrical. A still further improvement may take place in time,
whereby the patient will be able to control certain groups of facial
muscles, as, for example, those that close the eye, those that wrinkle
the forehead, or those that pucker the lips, as in whistling. This latter
improvement is most gratifying to the patient, and can be secured provided the antiseptic and surgical technic of the operation is not faulty,
and the grafting has not been delayed until the peripheral fibers of the
facial nerve have degenerated and the muscles supplied by them are
atrophied.

CHAPTER XXXI

THE INTRACRANIAL COMPLICATIONS OF SUPPURATIVE PROCESSES WITHIN THE TEMPORAL BONE

General Considerations.—Mention has already been made in the several sections of this work which deal with the suppurative aural diseases of the fact that when an infection of the pneumatic spaces of the temporal bone has once taken place, an extension of the same to the meninges, brain, or lateral sinus may occur at any subsequent time.[1] When we examine this bone in section and note the very intimate relation its cellular interior bears to the sigmoid sinuses and brain coverings, and then recall the frequency and persistency with which the mastoid cells suppurate, we are led to marvel not that intracranial complications frequently occur, but that they do not take place much more often than is at present recognized. (Examine Figs. 261 to 264, and note especially the very thin osseous partitions which separate the cells from the intracranial contents.)

As a result of the examination in section of 100 temporal bones the author found that the tegmen antri, tegmen tympani, and tegmen celluli, which form the compact but exceedingly thin roof of the pneumatic temporal structure and a small portion of the floor of the brain, are on the average not more than one-third as thick as is the bony cortex which separates the mastoid cells from the exterior surface of this portion of the skull. There are some exceptions to this statement, occurring chiefly in those cases in which there were one or more large pneumatic cells at the tip of the mastoid process (Fig. 232), in which instances the shell of bone separating the air space from the digastric fossa was about the same thickness as the tegmen. It follows, therefore, that in the average case of suppuration occurring within the temporal labyrinth of cells, that the pus when confined under pressure, would meet with much less resistance when pursuing a brainward direction than it would in traveling in an outward direction, provided,

---

[1] Concerning this point C. R. Holmes states: That after excluding cerebrospinal and tuberculous meningitis and trauma and a small proportion of cases that may have had their origin from the head and neck outside of the nasopharynx and sinuses, practically all cases of inflammation of the brain and its membranes are caused by extension of purulent inflammation from the ear and from the nose and its accessory sinuses.

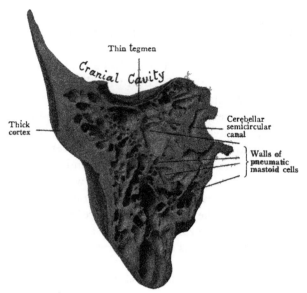

FIG. 261.—PERPENDICULAR SECTION OF TEMPORAL BONE IN A PLANE POSTERIOR TO THE TYMPANIC CAVITY
AND MASTOID ANTRUM.
Note the very thin tegmen and the comparatively thick cortex.

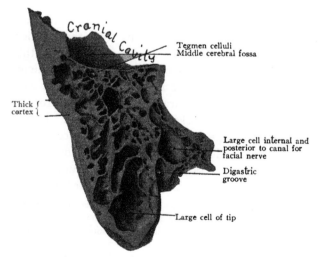

FIG. 262.—VERTICAL SECTION OF TEMPORAL BONE ON A PLANE BETWEEN THE MASTOID ANTRUM AND SIG-
MOID GROOVE.
The specimen shows a thick cortex and a thin tegmen. The pneumatic spaces extend back almost to the occipi-
tal bone and one very large cell is internal to the digastric groove and facial nerve.

of course, that the meninges on the cranial side of the tegmen and
the soft tissues covering the outer cortex of bone are not considered
factors in the resistance. Experienced mastoid operators are aware that

perforation of the bone outward often takes place, whereas, perforation through the tegmen into the cranial cavity or into the groove of the sinus

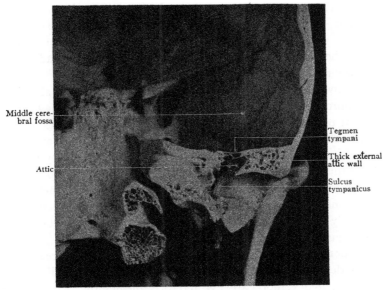

FIG. 263.—SECTION OF SKULL IN PLANE OF EXTERNAL AUDITORY MEATUS AND TYMPANIC CAVITY. Note thinness of tegmen tympani and thickness of bone external to tegmen over external auditory canal.

is perhaps more rarely observed. This being contrary to what should be expected concerning the direction of the perforation in view of the

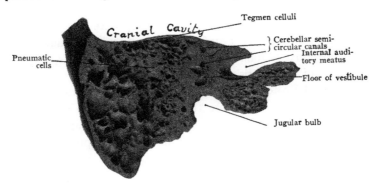

FIG. 264.—SHOWS FIRST, A PAPER-THIN TEGMEN CELLULI AND SECOND, THE SOLID AND THICK BONE IN WHICH THE VESTIBULE AND SEMICIRCULAR CANALS LIE. Compare thickness of the tegmen with that of cortex.

anatomic facts stated above, it must be that either the erosion through the tegmen or sigmoid groove is sometimes overlooked by the operator or else the resistance of the dura mater to the invasion of pus is greater than that of the periosteum. It is highly probable that a greater number of perforations take place into the cranial cavity than are ever recognized, because these patients very often die without a correct diagnosis having been made, without operation or post mortem, and the cause of death in such cases is usually reported as meningitis. Too often the physician in charge has had no suspicion that the cause of the death had its origin in a suppurating ear.

The advancement of medicine is perhaps nowhere better shown than in the improvement that has taken place in the methods of diagnosis and treatment of suppurative aural diseases and their complications, for in his earnest efforts to cure these affections the otologist has of late followed the necrosing processes into whatever depth or direction they may have led, and thus he has discovered the origin of and has developed a treatment for a class of diseases that has created an entirely new field in otology, one which lies beyond the ear, but which is nevertheless so inseparably connected with aural affections that it should be included in the domain of otology.

Frequency.—Hassler states that of 81,684 ear cases treated there were 116 deaths due to intracranial extension. Of these 48 died of sinus thrombosis, 28 of cerebral abscess, and 40 of meningitis. Körner reports that in 115 necropsies after death from ear extension, 41 died from sinus thrombosis, 43 from brain abscess, and 31 from meningitis.

In an exhaustive article on the statistics of this subject, Pitt reports that of 9000 autopsies made in the hospitals of London, the record representing the consecutive ones, and therefore was for deaths from all diseases, just as they naturally occurred, 57 were due to suppurations in the temporal bone, or 1 such death in every 158 running hospital cases, distributed as follows: 48 died of sinus thrombosis, 28 of cerebral abscess, 40 of meningitis.

Körner, of Rostock, who has compiled most extensive statistics on this subject, shows that more than 6 of every 1000 deaths from ear diseases are the result of brain abscess. Jansen found abscess of the brain once in 2650 cases of acute middle-ear suppuration, whereas, the same author found 6 cases of brain abscess in 2500 cases of chronic aural suppuration.

The records of the Manhattan Eye and Ear Infirmary show that of 12,744 cases of suppurative aural discharge treated from 1895 to 1905, 60 were complicated by intracranial extension. Of these 60 cases, 23 were affected by a sinus thrombosis, 30 by meningitis, and 7 by brain abscess.

The cause of the several intracranial diseases which result from aural suppuration is the same for each of the diseases—namely, the entrance into the cerebral or cerebellar fossæ of infectious products from the suppurating foci within the temporal bone. The extension may take place either directly, as in instances where the necrosis spreads from the mastoid interior, uncovers the dura at some neighboring point (as in Fig. 226), and thus admits the pathogenic fluid directly into the cranial cavity; or the septic material may be indirectly carried to the meninges or to the sigmoid sinus contents through the medium of the intercommunicating veins, in which instance there is no visible path between the infected area of the temporal bone and that resulting within the cranial cavity. Oppenheimer, (*Medical Record*, Aug., 1902), in a study of the venous system of the temporal bone, with a view of establishing the part these vessels play in the transmission of pathogenic material from the diseased cellular structure of the bone to the cranial contents, states that it is his belief that such transmission is in the majority of cases directly through an opening provided by previous necrosis of the intervening parts; nevertheless, meningitis, sinus thrombosis, and brain abscess are often the result of the carriage of septic matter by means of these venous channels. Infection of any portion of the cerebral contents through the medium of the vascular channels most frequently follows an acute suppurative process within the temporal air spaces, whereas the direct extension of the sepsis through necrotic or carious channels is more frequently met with in chronic cases. When the dura mater has been exposed by the destruction of the thin osseous lamella against which it lies, the pus is thereby admitted to direct contact with this brain structure. The localized meningitis which follows results in the production of granulation tissue which no doubt frequently forms an effectual barrier against the further invasion of the pus, and thus the further spread of the infection is limited. The dura becomes thickened over the exposed area and adhesions take place over its inner surface to the arachnoid and over its outer surface to the edges of the fistulous opening in the adjacent part of the temporal bone. By this means leptomeningitis is prevented on the one hand and pachymeningitis on the other. Because of the efficient protection offered by these adhesions and by the thickened dura a perforation may exist through the tegmen or into the sigmoid groove for a long time without the occurrence of symptoms indicative of its presence further than the usual aural discharge. In infants and young children infection of the temporosphenoidal lobe of the brain may occur as a result of the passage of the pathogenic fluids from the middle ear or mastoid antrum directly through the squamopetrosal suture (Fig. 10), early life is filled only with soft tissues through which pass th ous veins connecting the cavity of the middle ear with th structures.

The symptoms, diagnosis, and treatment are best given in the discussion of each individual intracranial disease.

CHAPTER XXXII

INTRACRANIAL COMPLICATIONS (Continued)

SINUS PHLEBITIS AND SINUS THROMBOSIS

THIS is the most frequent of the intracranial complications and, like the others, occurs oftener than has heretofore been recognized. The occurrence of a sinus thrombosis in any given case of suppuration of the mastoid cells must depend largely upon the location of such cells in relation to the sigmoid sinus groove. Hence, if the cells are large and are separated from the groove of the sinus by only the

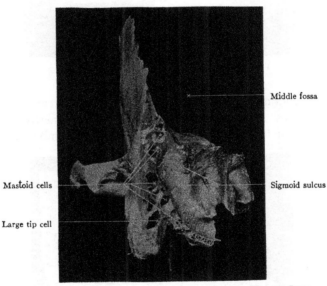

FIG. 265.—SHOWS THIN WALL BETWEEN SIGMOID SINUS AND MASTOID CELLS.
(Warren Museum, Harvard Medical School. J. Orne Green Collection.)

thinnest osseous partitions, as shown in Figs. 265 and 266, a sinus infection would be very probable in case of mastoid suppuration, whereas if the mastoid process is eburnated, as in the illustration shown in Fig. 241, it is scarcely probable that sinus infection would ever occur as a result of mastoiditis.

Pathology.—Sinus thrombosis is usually secondary to diseased bone overlying the sinus (see chapter on Bacteriology). The most common site for the infection is the sigmoid portion of the lateral sinus (Fig. 267; see also Figs. 224 to 227). The diseased bone or extension of thrombi through small vessels leading from the diseased focus to the sinus causes a sinus phlebitis (Körner), and the phlebitis may set up a mural throm-

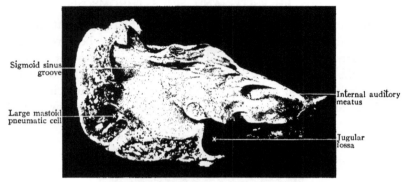

FIG. 266.—LARGE CELL INTERNAL TO DIGASTRIC GROOVE.
Note very thin bony partition between cell and sinus.

bus which continues to grow either with the blood stream or against it. This thrombus is always infectious, although the newly formed advancing end of the clot may be sterile. The thrombus may cause

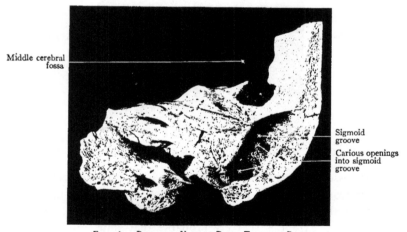

FIG. 267.—POSTERIOR VIEW OF RIGHT TEMPORAL BONE.
Caries extending from the mastoid into the sigmoid sinus. (Warren Museum, Harvard Medical School. J. Orne Green Collection.)

sudden obliteration or may gradually block the sinus. The thrombus may extend backward to the torcular Herophili and even into the lateral sinus on the other side. The thrombus may extend into the superior or inferior petrosal sinuses (Figs. 268 and 269), to the cavernous sinus, and thence to the ophthalmic vein. Extension to the jugular bulb and the internal jugular vein, with involvement of the lymphatic glands along the vein, may take place. Thrombosis may extend from the internal jugular into the facial vein. Extension through the mastoid emissary vein or through the anterior condyloid vein may also occur (see Fig. 269).

Optic neuritis occurs in 35 to 50 per cent. of cases according to Jansen. Paralysis of the hypoglossal nerve, through pressure on the

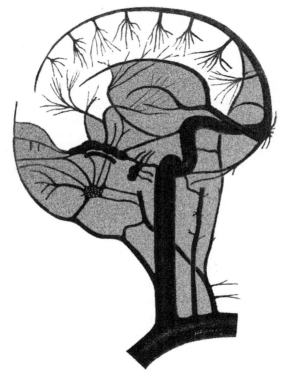

Fig. 268.—The System of Venous Intracranial Sinuses and Connections with the Veins of the Neck.
Compare with Fig. 269.

condyloid vein as the nerve comes through the anterior condyloid foramen, may occur. Thrombosis of the jugular bulb may cause pressure upon adjoining structures, and thus paralysis of the vagus, spinal accessory, or the glossopharyngeal may result. Thrombosis of the cavernous sinus, with extension to the ophthalmic vein, always gives positive ophthalmoscopic pictures. There may be paralysis of the abducens, trochlearis, oculomotorius, or trigeminus nerves, either a

27

single nerve or more than one of the above being affected in the same case.

Diagnosis and Symptoms.—The formation of a clot in the sigmoid sinus is attended by symptoms that vary so widely in different cases that diagnosis in the early stages is always difficult and often impossible. That a diagnosis should be made in each case at the earliest possible moment is a matter of great importance to the welfare of the patient. The attendant upon any case of suppurative aural disease should be ever alert to the possibility of a sinus infection, and should, therefore, take note of all unusual symptoms in order that he may immediately call to his aid every diagnostic means, to the end that recognition of the sinus affection may be made before the infection has been disseminated by the blood-current to distant parts of the body and before a general sepsis has been established.

Since sinus thrombosis nearly always results from an existing aural infection, all the symptoms that usually accompany a suppurating ear may be present. Except in those acute cases where infection of the jugular bulb takes place through the floor of the middle ear, there is a preceding mastoiditis, the symptoms of which may obscure or even be entirely mistaken for those of the lateral sinus thrombosis. Pain, swelling, and tenderness in the mastoid region, while present in some cases of lateral sinus thrombosis, are not of themselves a diagnostic indication that the sinus is involved.

The symptoms of sinus thrombosis are typic and atypic. Of the typic manifestations the behavior of the temperature is of greatest diagnostic importance. In any case of suppurative middle-ear disease the temperature may be normal or only slightly elevated, but should infection of the sinus occur it will at once rise to 102°, 104°, 106° F., and not infrequently higher, and after a short time will drop to normal or near the normal. One or more such fluctuations may occur during the twenty-four hours, depending entirely upon the rapidity with which the septic matter from the diseased vessel is thrown into the general system. The rise in temperature is usually preceded by a chill, and the fall, especially if the disease is well advanced, is followed by exhaustive sweating. More than one chill may occur in the twenty-four hours, the character of which may amount to a pronounced rigor or may be so mild that it will be recognized as only a coldness of the extremities; the fact that a chill has occurred may pass unobserved by the attendants and may only be learned by inquiry directed to the patient. In all suppurative aural cases that run a fluctuating temperature the development of chilly sensations should always be looked for by the nurse,

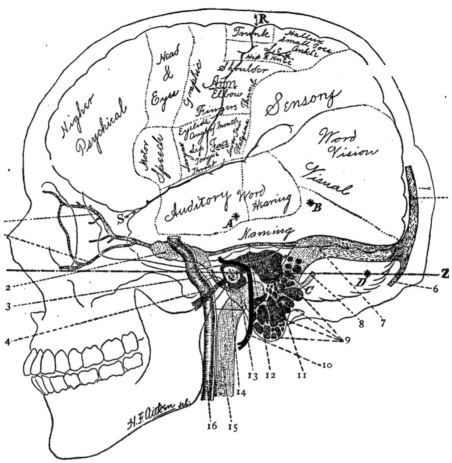

FIG. 269.—KEY TO TRANSPARENT HEAD. Y, Z, REID'S BASE-LINE.

hthalmic veins; 2, cavernous sinus; 3, inferior petrosal sinus; 4, Eustachian tube; 5, superior longitudinal sinus; 6, occi
7, lateral sinus; 8, mastoid vein; 9, mastoid cells; 10, course of facial nerve; 11, mastoid antrum; 12, superior petros
enter of external auditory meatus; 14, membrana tympani; 15, internal jugular vein; 16, internal carotid artery.

Points of election for trephining the skull in exploration of the cerebral structures adjoining the tegmen antri, tegm
d the neighboring surface of the petrous portion of the temporal bone. (See Fig. 277.) Point A lies 1 inch abo
-line at the center of the auditory meatus. Point B lies 1¼ inches above Reid's base-line and 1¼ inches posterior to tl
e external auditory meatus. C is a point on Reid's base-line ⅞ inch posterior to the center of the external audito
lies over the sigmoid sinus when the latter follows the normal course. This would be the point of election for removir
cortex in case it is desirable to enter the sinus without first having performed a mastoid exenteration. The very variab
e sigmoid sinus may in any given case place it either anterior or posterior to point C. Point D represents the posteri
loratory operation on the skull over the cerebellar fossa. A point on Reid's base-line, midway between points C and
at 1½ inches posterior to the center of the auditory meatus and ¼ inch below the base-line, is the one of election f
; cerebellar fossa. S, Fissure of Sylvius. R, Fissure of Rolando. Note the position of the several sensory and mot
; brain located along the course of these fissures.

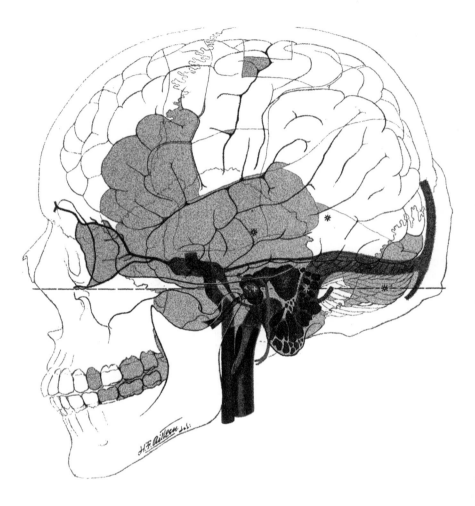

FIG. 269.—TRANSPARENT HEAD, SHOWING SYSTEM OF VENOUS SINUSES, THE SURGICAL RELATION OF THE STRUCTURES OF THE TEMPORAL BONE, AND THE MOTOR AND SENSORY AREAS OF THE BRAIN.

and frequent inspection of the hands, feet, and knee-caps should be made with a view of ascertaining this important information, because the mere chilly sensations are as important in a diagnostic way as are the pronounced chills.

Severe sweating is not always present, but in the typic case is frequent and often most pronounced. During the earlier stages of the vein involvement it may attract but little or no attention, but as the general infection becomes more marked, the amount and persistence of the perspiration becomes one of the most prominent features of the disease, since it is often sufficient in quantity to wet the bedclothing and thoroughly drench the patient. At first the sweating occurs only during the subsidence of the temperature, but in the worst cases it may continue, though lessened, throughout both the highest and lowest temperatures. The patient, thus exhausted by excessive body heat and rapid loss of fluid, becomes quickly emaciated and presents a most typic septic appearance.

Pain on the affected side of the head is usually present and may be localized in the mastoid or occipital regions. The pain may also be referred to the neck in case there is an accompanying cellulitis of the cervical tissues; or in the event that the cervical glands have become infected and are consequently enlarged and inflamed. This infection of the lymphatic glands and cellular tissue of the neck may give rise to a general tumefaction of the affected side, all the structures being finally massed together by the inflammatory process. Should resolution not promptly take place, a deep abscess may be the ultimate result. This general infection and infiltration of the cervical tissues gives rise to a condition that was once described as a sausage-like lump in the neck, to which condition great diagnostic significance was attached. Such a symptom is observed only in the later stages of sinus thrombosis, and if the case has been under observation from the first a diagnosis of the true condition should have been made long before the appearance of the neck infiltration.

The pulse-rate varies with the temperature. When the fever is only moderate the rate may not greatly exceed 100, but when the temperature rises to 104° or 106° F. the pulse-rate may rise to 150 or 180 per minute. It should not be forgotten in this connection that sinus thrombosis and brain abscess may both be present in the same individual, and that when such is the case the influence of the abscess upon the circulation will lower the pulse-rate to normal or even less.

The mentality of the patient is unaffected in the beginning and often remains so during the course of the disease. In many cases, however, drowsiness comes on as exhaustion increases and the patient finally dies in a coma.

Vomiting is a symptom to be expected in any intracranial complication. It is present at some stage of sigmoid sinus thrombosis in the large majority of cases. The vomiting is of a cerebral character and usually takes place without reference to the time of taking food.

Constipation is the rule in the early stages, but as systemic infection becomes marked, and when nature is making every effort to eliminate the poison, a diarrhea often accompanies the profuse sweating that has already been mentioned.

Vertigo is seldom present in uncomplicated cases. Epileptiform convulsions have been several times reported. In from one-fourth to one-third of all cases of sinus thrombosis there are intracranial changes which are discoverable by ophthalmoscopic examination, and when other evidences of the suspected sinus disease are not sufficient for diagnosis the eye findings will prove most helpful.

During the later stages of the sinus thrombosis the septic clot within the vein may disintegrate and particles of the same may be cast off into the general blood stream. Emboli thus formed are carried first to the right side of the heart and thence to the lungs, where they lodge in the smaller pulmonary vessels and set up new foci of infection with quickly resulting pneumonia. This occurrence at first gives rise to a dry and irritating cough that is most trying to the already wasted energies of the patient, who frequently dies at this period from the multiplicity and severity of his ailments. Occasionally, however, the infection is carried through the lungs into the arterial circulation, where it is finally deposited in one of the extremities, as a result of which multiple abscesses quickly form and death finally takes place from the general pyemia which occurs.

Atypic Cases.—A number of cases have recently been reported in which few, sometimes only one, and in several cases not a single one of the above symptoms was present, although exposure of the vein at the operation or post-mortem examination has proved without doubt the existence of a thrombosed sinus. Although the behavior of the temperature is regarded as one of the most reliable symptoms of sinus thrombosis, instances are recorded in which the temperature has remained normal for a considerable length of time after the thrombosis had taken place. While large statistics as to the frequency with which a chill occurs are not available, the records at hand indicate that a decided rigor is not a symptom in over 50 per cent. of the cases. Chilly sensations are, however, present at some time during the progress of the disease, so that it may be stated as probable that either a decided chill or chilly sensation is a symptom in 80 or 90 per cent. of all instances of sinus thrombosis. It should be remembered that the patient may not complain of the chilly sensations and that, therefore, it may not be known that they have occurred unless the attendant has frequently sought information on this point.

In the atypic case the temperature may suddenly rise from normal or near the normal to 104°, 105°, or 106° F., and remain steadily at that point or remit but slightly. Sweating will likely not occur and no other symptom be present except the high continuous fever and the mastoiditis. If, as is sometimes the case, this latter gives rise to external symptoms, the diagnosis cannot be readily made and the patient must be watched and frequently examined for additional information.

Since it is highly essential to efficient treatment that the diagnosis should be made in the early stage of the thrombosis, advantage must be taken of every available aid to this end. The blood-count should be early made and afterward repeated in all suspected but doubtful cases. A high leukocytosis is considered by many to be of value and, certainly when demonstrated in the presence of other suspicious symptoms, is helpful. A high percentage of polymorphonuclear cells also aids in the diagnosis because the presence of this blood condition would indicate the existence of a collection of pus in some part of the body, and with all other symptoms pointing to sinus involvement, this information would be of first value.

In infants and young children the thrombosis of the jugular bulb may take place as a result of the direct transmission of septic matter from the middle ear through the lamella of bone which separates the tympanic cavity from the jugular fossa. This osseous partition is always very thin in the infant, sometimes no thicker than parchment. Rarely a dehiscence exists in the bone, and in such cases the mucous membrane of the middle ear and the wall of the jugular bulb lie in immediate contact. In every instance, therefore, of suppurative otitis media in the infant it would seem an easy matter for pathogenic material to find its way into the jugular bulb without following the usual route through the mastoid antrum and cells and finally into the sigmoid sinus.

Children so affected present atypic symptoms and unless the attending physician is aware of the possibility of the occurrence of jugular bulb thrombosis in any case of middle-ear suppuration in early life, the developing sinus thrombosis may be entirely overlooked. The most important symptom denoting jugular thrombosis in the infant is a sudden rise in the temperature from normal or near the normal to 104°, 105°, or 106° F., after which the decline is as precipitous as the rise. The fluctuations in temperature occur with some regularity. The child is fretful and shows evidence of severe illness during the height of the fever, but during the remissions, especially of the first few days, it looks well, plays with its toys, asks for food, and in every way deceives all concerned as to the gravity of the illness. The pulse-rate varies with the temperature, and is high when the fever is up, but approaches the normal when the fever recedes. A distinct chill is seldom present, but if examination of the hands and feet of the child be made just when the temperature begins to rise it will usually be found that they are cold. After several days the patient becomes more prostrate, the tongue becomes white and dry, and the child takes on a septic appearance that may be accompanied by a pneumonia which quickly terminates in death.

Excepting the advanced and typic cases of sinus thrombosis, the diagnosis is always attended with difficulty. The disease may be mistaken for malaria, typhoid fever, pneumonia, and in children, for digestive disturbances. The chill, high fever, remission of the temperature and interval of profuse perspiration which accompanies it may be identical with that of a typic attack of malaria. An examination of the blood and a determination of the presence of the plasmoidum malariæ would be necessary and helpful under such circumstances. A central pneumonia sometimes complicates a discharging ear, in which case the chill and sudden rise of temperature produced by the lung involvement may be very misleading, for it is admitted that this form of pneumonia cannot always be diagnosticated by means of auscultation and percussion, and that therefore the expectoration of rusty sputum must be awaited to determine the exact nature of the ailment. The course of typhoid fever during the first week presents many symptoms that are almost identical with those of sinus thrombosis and, when occurring in any case which has a suppurating ear, might prove very misleading; and here again blood tests may give information which, when carefully compared with all other obtainable facts concerning the case may, together, be sufficient to enable the diagnostician to say that it is clearly the one or the other disease. If dietary and digestive causes are suspected in the child a purge of castor oil, a limitation of the food to proper substances, and the administration of enzymes to aid the feeble digestive powers, should prove sufficient in most instances to reduce the temperature to normal, where it will permanently remain provided the cause of the disturbance lies in the digestive tract.

In many instances of suspected sinus thrombosis the otologist will do wisely to seek the help of practitioners in other departments of medicine before he is willing to decide with certainty that a patient is suffering from a thrombosed vein, because the deciding information must frequently be obtained from those who are skilled in general diagnosis—from the neurologist, oculist, and laboratory expert.

Since sinus thrombosis is nearly always secondary to mastoiditis, it is good surgery in strongly suspected cases to open the mastoid antrum and cells in most instances, both as a measure that is necessary to secure proper drainage, and in addition, if conditions within the bone should justify it, of exploratory enlargement of the wound to the extent of uncovering the sinus for purposes of immediate inspection. If after this is accomplished and it is believed that the sinus is not involved, the wound may be treated as hereafter described and the symptoms of the patient be subsequently watched most carefully, with a view of opening the sinus and dealing with it in a radical manner at any time that the evidence of its involvement seems sufficient to justify the measure. Exploratory operations upon the mastoid and sinus must, therefore, be regarded among the important diagnostic measures, particularly in the early stages of the formation of the clot.

INTRACRANIAL COMPLICATIONS (Continued)

TREATMENT OF SINUS INFECTION AND SINUS THROMBOSIS

THE treatment of sinus thrombosis is almost wholly of a surgical nature. During the early stages of the disease when there is yet doubt as to the exact nature of the trouble, the treatment may be conducted upon any expectant plan which seems best suited for the relief of the symptoms which are present; but after it has been definitely determined that an infected blood-clot has formed in the sigmoid sinus or jugular bulb, from which it has perhaps extended downward into the jugular vein itself, surgical interference is at once indicated for the reason that the continued discharge of septic material from the seat of the thrombus into the general circulation will rapidly add to the already infected state of the patient and will quickly lessen his chances of recovery. The objects of operative treatment, therefore, should be to rid the individual at the earliest moment of the obstruction within the vein and to prevent as far as possible the further entrance of infected emboli into the general circulation.

The patient is prepared in an exactly similar manner as for a mastoid operation, with the additional precautions of shaving the hair for a greater distance around the ear and of sterilizing the neck of the affected side from the mastoid tip to the clavicle.

The steps of the operation that are necessary to accomplish the desired ends are: First, the ablation of the mastoid and the exposure of the sigmoid sinus from its knee downward. Second, the exploration of the sinus with a view of discovering the nature and extent of its thrombosed contents. Third, the ligation and perhaps the removal of a portion of the jugular vein in the neck, provided the information obtained during the performance of the second step is such as to indicate with certainty that the safety of the patient depends upon the isolation of the infected region from the general circulation. Fourth, the removal of the clot from the sinus and bulb, and, lastly, the dressing of the mastoid wound, including the sigmoid sinus.

In all cases of sinus thrombosis which occur as a complication of a coexistent mastoiditis, the first step of the operation for the relief of the thrombosis consists in opening the mastoid antrum in the usual way, since this not only rids the patient of the original foci of infection but also provides an avenue through which the sinus may be more readily and widely exposed. In cases in which the mastoid operation has been previously performed and in which the sinus thrombosis has subsequently developed, the mastoid wound must again be opened and the cavity thoroughly disinfected. In either case the intervening bone between the mastoid cavity and the wall of the sigmoid sinus should be removed to the extent that 1 inch or more of the vessel is exposed. It may be found necessary to uncover the sinus as far downward as the jugular bulb or as far backward as the torcular, but until such extensive removal of the bone in these directions is seen to be actually required by the great extent of the thrombus, the smaller opening over the vessel, as above stated, should be considered sufficient. It is, however, never wise to depend upon a trivial exposure of the sinus, either for diagnostic or operative purposes, for it is obvious that if but a small portion of the course of the vessel is uncovered for inspection and palpation, that the results of both of these important aids to diagnosis would be incomplete and therefore unreliable. Moreover it is not possible to carry out any operative measures on the sinus unless a sufficiently wide exposure of the vessel is provided, for the reason that the very free hemorrhage which is incident to opening the sinus cannot be controlled and any contained clot could not be safely or efficiently removed through the narrow opening thus provided. When a small area of the sinus wall has been uncovered by the mallet and gouge, it is safest to continue the removal of the bone by means of a rongeur or, preferably, the Jansen forceps (Fig. 269). In order to lessen the liability of puncturing the sinus with the beak of the instrument, the wall of this vessel should be separated from the bone for a considerable distance over the course from which the bony covering is to be removed. This may be accomplished by inserting a blunt spatula between the sinus wall and the overlying bone and thus carefully separating the one from the other. When this has been accomplished the jaw of the bone forceps when introduced will pass between the two structures without the necessity of applying undue force directly to the sinus wall. A perisinuous abscess may be associated with the thrombosis, and when this is the case pus will pour from the direction of the sinus as soon as the chisel penetrates the sigmoid groove. A fistulous tract may be found leading from the suppurating mastoid cells directly into the groove for the sigmoid sinus (Fig. 167), or the abscess which occupies this site may have resulted from an infection which was carried from the mastoid through the intercommunicating veins, in which instance no communicating sinus will be found. In either case the vessel wall at the seat of the abscess is usually thickened and seminecrotic granulations may have already covered the most exposed portion of the dura. Whatever may be the condition in which the sinus wall is found, any collection of pus or other fluid which may be present should be dried away with small gauze sponges, after which all possible information concerning the sinus contents should be gained by means of a study of the appearance of the vessel and by the palpation of its contents.

If the sinus is normal and is therefore carrying its usual amount of venous blood, it will probably present a dark bluish appearance. In

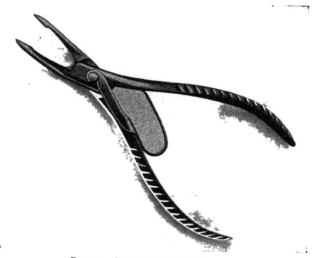

FIG. 270.—JANSEN'S GOOSE-NECK FORCEPS.

case it is completely thrombosed, and there should be in addition an inflammation of the sinus walls, the vessel will appear darker and its walls will seem unduly thickened. Should the contained clot be in a state of decomposition the walls of the vessel may look necrotic and grayish. On palpation the vein, if normal, will feel soft and usually some pulsation can be detected. If the finger be placed transversely across the sinus at the lower end of its exposed portion and sufficient pressure be exerted on it to occlude its lumen, dilatation will take place above the finger, provided the vein had been previously patent.[1]

[1] It was formerly thought advisable to insert a hollow exploring needle into the exposed sinus and to make the attempt to aspirate blood from the vessel. In case fluid blood could be thus aspirated this fact was regarded as sufficient evidence that the sinus was not thrombosed. Absence of such evidence is worthy of consideration in cases where the vessel is completely filled with the clot, but since the diagnosis should be made before this

While the information thus obtained is of some value it should not be forgotten that it is impossible by such means alone to determine with a reliable degree of certainty whether or not an infected clot lies within the vessel. The importance of the above phenomena as a means of determining the existence of a thrombus was emphasized at a former time when other and more reliable diagnostic aids and a larger experience were not available to enable the operator to make a diagnosis until a late period of the disease, and not until after the vein had become so completely filled with the clot that it could be both easily seen and felt by the examiner. At the present time, however, the diagnosis should, if possible, be made long before such visual and palpable evidence of thrombosis is present in the vein; and therefore at this early stage, when the surgeon is given opportunity to look and feel for evidence of disease within the sinus, the thrombus is yet small, and in fact may amount to little more than the agglutination of a trivial amount of septic material upon the site of the invasion of the vessel wall or to a larger but soft clot which only partially fills the lumen. In either case the blood continues to flow through the vessel in a more or less normal volume and the clot cannot be felt through its walls. Furthermore, the thrombus may not be located in the sigmoid sinus at all, but in one of the petrosal veins; or, that which is more commonly the case, and especially in children, it may have occurred primarily in the jugular bulb; in which latter situation because of its inaccessible position it could not be palpated. Therefore unless the clot is large enough to completely block the vessel the latter may appear normal in every respect, may feel soft, and pulsation may be made out. Furthermore pulsation may be imparted to a completely occluded sinus and the same be detected by the examining finger, in case there is an active inflammation of the adjoining cerebellar structure.

If the previous history of the case, when taken in connection with the evidence acquired by the examination of the exposed vein as just described, is not sufficient to convince the surgeon that thrombosis is present, the author believes that the wisest course to pursue would be that of packing the mastoid wound at this juncture and awaiting further development in the case. This advice would seem particularly the proper one to follow in cases where the patient's vital powers are yet good, and in whom, therefore, a delay of further operating for a period of from twenty-four to forty-eight hours would make but little difference as to the outcome, but might add much to the certainty of a diagnosis.

time, if possible, this method has fallen into disuse. Aspiration is not free from danger since several operators have reported infection of the sinus contents as a result of the insertion of the aspirating needle.

However, if the previous history and symptoms of the patient have led to the very conclusive opinion that the sinus is thrombosed and this is in sufficient measure confirmed by the inspection of the uncovered vein, the latter should at once be opened and its contents inspected. Before this is undertaken the entire wound and all instruments should be again most thoroughly sterilized. The sinus is best opened by means of a curved and pointed bistoury, the entire thickness of the wall being slit for a distance of 1 inch or more. If the vessel is not completely obstructed by the thrombus in both directions a free hemorrhage will follow. Since this hemorrhage may be so profuse as to at once obscure the entire operative field and thus greatly hinder the progress of the operation, some provision should be made before the sinus is incised to control the troublesome bleeding which would be otherwise certain unless the sinus is completely occluded by a blood-clot. Two small but firm rolls of sterile gauze should, therefore, be prepared and placed across the sinus, one above and the other below the proposed incision in the vessel; the management of these should be intrusted to an assistant whose duty it shall be to make pressure upon each at the proper moment. The assistant, therefore, places the forefinger of each hand upon the respective upper and lower cylinders of gauze, but does not exert firm pressure upon either until the surgeon has freely incised the sinus wall, when, should a free hemorrhage occur, first one and then the other roll of gauze is compressed in order to check the flow of blood and to determine from which direction it comes. If the lower portion of the sinus is completely thrombosed while the upper end is still patent, the bleeding will be profuse from the upper end only. If the thrombus is situated below the entrance of the inferior petrosal vein, the hemorrhage will be free from both directions; that from the direction of the bulb coming through the inferior petrosal vein. If the mastoid emissary vein (Fig. 269) is large, a copious flow of blood may take place from this source even though the jugular bulb and lower portion of the sigmoid sinus be completely thrombosed. Free hemorrhage from the torcular end is evidence that the vein in this direction is not thrombosed, and hence curetment in this direction should not be made. When any clots which may be present in any part of the sinus have been thoroughly removed by the curet and the blood is observed to flow normally from both dircetions, the two flaps that result from the slit in the sinus wall are then folded inward into the lumen of the sinus and pressed against the adjacent tissues by means of a little roll of iodoform gauze, which latter is left in place until the first dressing. This procedure is sufficient to check all hemorrhage, after which the mastoid wound is filled with iodoform gauze strips in the usual way and the operation may be considered finished.

If when the slit is made into the sinus it is found that the vessel is filled with a thrombus extending in both directions, no bleeding will, as a matter of course, take place, and it will be necessary to empty the vein both in the direction of the torcular and toward the bulb. But before undertaking this an important and often difficult question must be decided, namely, whether or not the jugular vein should be tied in the neck before attempting to remove the extensive thrombus from the sinus. This question must be settled somewhat according to the previous symptoms of the case, but largely upon the condition of the thrombosed vein as may be determined at the moment the thrombus is exposed by the incision through the walls of the vessel. If the symptoms of the case have been severe, if the cervical glands are enlarged, and the tissues of the neck thickened, these general indications would suggest the necessity of ligation. If in addition to the above information the thrombosis is found upon opening the vein to be extensive, if the same should show signs of disintegration, or should give evidence that it has already broken down and is suppurating, there should remain no question concerning the surgeon's duty to ligate the jugular and perhaps to dissect out and remove as much of the same as is found to be diseased before he attempts to curet the thrombus from the sinus above. By the previous ligation of the jugular only can the septic thrombus be completely removed, for the obvious reason that curetment of the sinus cannot be effectively performed through the incision in the vessel to a point as far distant as the jugular bulb without first having extensively removed the bone in this direction; and, moreover, even if it were possible to satisfactorily cleanse the vessel by means of this procedure, there is great danger of dislodging particles of the clot into the general circulation, unless this has been provided against by the previous ligation of the jugular. It is, therefore, advisable in most cases of complete thrombosis to tie off the jugular as a preliminary step to the removal of the thrombus. When this decision is reached the mastoid wound should be temporarily packed with iodoform gauze, while the operator proceeds at once with the ligation of the jugular.

Technic of the Ligation of the Internal Jugular Vein.—The antiseptic dressings that were applied to the neck on the previous evening or at the time the patient was prepared for the general operation, are now removed, while the hands of the surgeon and assistants, as well as all instruments to be further used in the completion of the operation, are thoroughly sterilized. A sand-bag is placed under the patient's head to render the sternocleidomastoid muscle tense and to place the deeper structures in the most favorable position for the operation. The vein in the upper part of the neck runs parallel to the course of the anterior margin of the above-mentioned muscle (Fig. 271), and hence the latter is used as a landmark. The vessel is most usually ligated below the entrance of the facial vein, and hence the incision into the neck is begun at a point on the anterior margin of the muscle horizontally posterior to

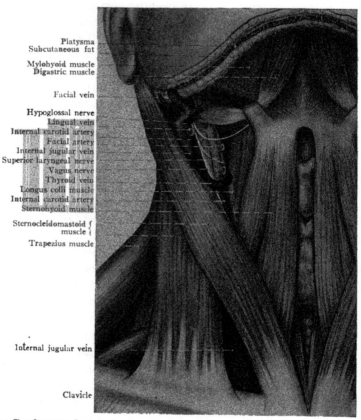

Platysma
Subcutaneous fat

Mylohyoid muscle
Digastric muscle

Facial vein

Hypoglossal nerve
Lingual vein
Internal carotid artery
Facial artery
Internal jugular vein
Superior laryngeal nerve
Vagus nerve
Thyroid vein
Longus colli muscle
Internal carotid artery
Sternohyoid muscle

Sternocleidomastoid {
muscle {

Trapezius muscle

Internal jugular vein

Clavicle

FIG. 271.—THE INTERNAL JUGULAR VEIN AND ITS SURGICAL RELATIONS IN THE TRIANGLES OF THE NECK.

the angle of the jaw and is extended downward parallel to the sterno-mastoid for 1½ or 2 inches. In the worst cases it will be necessary to carry the incision to the clavicle. The skin and superficial fascia and the platysma myoides muscle are divided by the scalpel, but as the deeper structures are reached the dull dissector or handle of the scalpel should be substituted; finally, the common sheath of the jugular, carotid, and pneumogastric nerve is opened upon the grooved director (Fig. 272).

The divided superficial vessels are all immediately clamped and perhaps ligated. The deeper ones are pushed aside or torn across by the blunt dissector, but should they bleed, must have the torsion applied at once or be ligated, because it is entirely essential to safe operating that the entire wound be dry, so that the operator may at all times clearly see the structures with which he deals. The wound is meanwhile held widely open by means of two retractors, the posterior one of which is hooked deeply under the sternocleidomastoid muscle, by which means the latter is pulled backward and well away from the common sheath of the above-mentioned vessels and nerve. The internal jugular vein lies external to the carotid artery and pneumogastric nerve and will, therefore, come into view first when the common sheath of the vessels

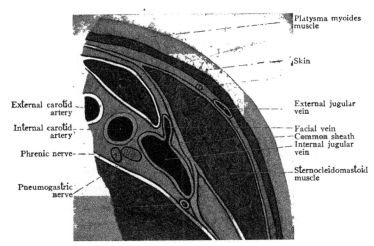

FIG. 272.—SEGMENT OF CROSS-SECTION OF THE NECK IN THE UPPER CERVICAL TRIANGLE, SHOWING THE DEPTH AND RELATION OF THE INTERNAL JUGULAR VEIN.

is opened. The vein may be recognized by its dark blue color unless there has been present a cellulitis with resulting inflammatory exudate, which has obliterated, to a great extent, the normal appearance. Lying as it does upon the carotid artery, the throbbing impulse of the latter is imparted to the vein, even when the latter is thrombosed; and for this reason pulsation in the vessel is not an indication that it is unobstructed by a thrombus, but if patent to the blood-current the respiratory effect upon the vessel will always be evident to the observer. The vein is elevated from the nerve and artery by separating the cellular tissues in which all are imbedded by means of a slightly curved dull dissector, the greatest care being always taken that no injury be done to the other structures which lie within the common sheath.   In cases where the vein has been completely occluded by the thrombus, either in the sigmoid sinus or jugular bulb, that portion in the neck will probably be collapsed and, therefore, much more difficult to find than if it were either normal or filled with a coagulum.   A double catgut ligature is passed around the vessel below the entrance of the facial vein, or still lower if the clot extends further down the vessel, by means of an aneurysm needle, and the jugular is tied in two places 1 inch apart.   The surgeon must never fail to lift the vein up and inspect its whole circumference carefully in order to be sure that nothing but the vein itself is included in either ligature.   Negligence concerning this precaution might result in tying the pneumogastric nerve together with the vein.   Following the double ligation the intervening portion of the vessel is completely severed by a straight scissors.

Subsequent to the ligation and severance of the vein in the neck, equally experienced operators differ as to the disposition that should be made of that portion which lies between the upper ligature and the jugular bulb, one class believing that it is best to tie off all the intervening contributory veins and then to dissect out the trunk of the vessel as high toward the jugular bulb as possible, again ligate at the upper limit of the dissection, and then to sever and remove this portion of the internal jugular entirely from the neck.   The other class maintains that equally good results are usually obtained if only the circulation of the infected part is cut off from the general system by means of the simple ligation and division of the vein.   If the thrombosed contents of the vein are infected and breaking down of the clot with suppuration is likely to result in any case, undoubtedly good surgery requires that much of the vein, together with its contents, be gotten rid of as soon as possible, and hence the plan of dissecting the vessel out of the neck should be followed.   On the contrary, if the condition of the vessel at the time of operation indicates that the lower end of the thrombus is not infected and will therefore not likely disintegrate or give rise to local or general infection—and this is more probable in the cases whch are operated on early—then the vessel may be safely left *in situ* after once it is ligated and divided.   When the deep cervical glands have become infected and consequently enlarged, they will be easily distinguished during this operation, and should be removed in order to avoid subsequent infection from this source.

Ballance, of London, advises that the upper end of the vein be brought out through the wound and used as a drainage-tube.   This disposition of it would seem decidedly proper in cases where suppuration had already taken place or was imminent.   When the plan of resection of the jugular is chosen it will be found necessary to ligate all the large tributary veins before these are severed from the main trunk. In case the thrombus extends down the jugular for a considerable distance it may be found that several of the entering veins are themselves thrombosed. When this is the case the ligatures should be applied to these vessels, and the same should be divided and removed beyond the occluded portion when possible.

Whether a portion of the vein is or is not removed from the neck after ligation, the cervical wound should be freely flushed with normal saline solution and a gauze wick or cigarette drain inserted from the upper to the lower end. Deep sutures are then introduced and the whole incision is closed over the drain with the exception of a small opening at each end for the entrance and exit of the drain. In case the cellular structures of the neck are infected and perhaps suppurating no sutures should be introduced, and the whole cervical wound should be packed with iodoform gauze until healing by granulation has been completed. The chief avenue through which septic material can enter the system having now been closed by the ligation or removal of the internal jugular, the final step of the operation—namely, the removal of the thrombus from the sigmoid sinus—should be undertaken. The operator, therefore, removes the gauze from the mastoid wound, exposes the sinus, and proceeds to curet the clots away. It is better to empty the vessel in the direction of the bulb first for the reason that if the inferior petrosal sinus is implicated no hemorrhage will occur from below, and the work of the removal can, therefore, be more easily performed; and should the petrosal be patent and free bleeding occur, no advantage is lost by beginning on the lower portion first. A curet of proper size and curvature is, therefore, inserted into the sinus in the direction of the bulb and the infected contents of the vessel are thereby removed. It may be necessary to reinsert the instrument several times before all of the clot can be withdrawn. If the sinus walls have been infected for several days it is possible that softening of their structure has taken place, and, therefore, the curetment must be gently performed, since otherwise the instrument would penetrate into the cerebellar fossa and result in rapid spread of the infection with almost certainly fatal consequences. If after the thrombosed vein has been emptied by the curetment no bleeding occurs from the direction of the jugular bulb, it may be safely inferred that the inferior petrosal vein is implicated; and, therefore, if the condition of the patient will permit of further operating, the bone should be removed from the sinus in this direction as far as the jugular fossa if necessary. This will

28

enable the operator to empty the bulb of any remaining clots, and possibly to expose the mouth of the petrosal vein to an extent that a flow of blood from this direction may be secured. Should portions of the infected thrombus be left in the sinus subsequent danger of general infection may arise, although this is greatly lessened by the previous ligation of the jugular.

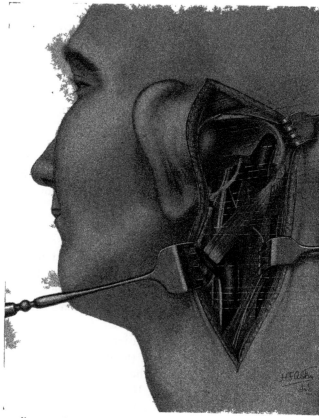

Temporal muscle

Periosteum

Linea temporalis
Fibrocartilaginous canal
Tympanomastoid duct

Sigmoid sinus

Jugular bulb
Facial nerve
Glossopharyngeal nerve
Sternocleidomastoid muscle
Spinal accessory nerve
External jugular vein
Hypoglossal nerve
Vagus nerve
Digastric muscle
Internal carotid artery
External jugular vein
Areolar tissue
Ascending cervical artery

Scalenus anticus muscle
Facial vein

Hypoglossal nerve
Internal jugular vein
External carotid artery
Desc. branch of hypoglossus
Vagus nerve
Sternocleidomastoid muscle

FIG. 273.—DISSECTION OF THE MASTOID AND CERVICAL REGION SHOWING ALL THE STRUCTURES WITH WHICH THE OPERATOR MUST DEAL IN PERFORMING THE SEVERAL OPERATIONS CONNECTED WITH THE SURGERY OF THE EAR.
In duplicating this dissection on the cadaver the student will better comprehend the many difficulties with which the operator may meet in executing the necessary steps of these operations.

The upper or torcular end of the sigmoid sinus should next receive attention, and is emptied of its clots by inserting the curet backward and then gently withdrawing the instrument along first one wall of the sinus and then another until the whole has been cleansed from any obstruction. When the sinus is reopened this fact may be known by the free flow of blood which immediately occurs from the torcular end. If it is found impossible to remove all the obstruction and to establish the blood-current by working through the osseous opening that was earlier provided, the bone should be removed for any necessary distance over the backward course of the sinus, and the cureting be then continued until the blood flows in an unobstructed stream. When this has been accomplished the edges of the sinus walls are folded together as above described, and the sinus itself is pressed against the adjacent structures by means of a properly shaped compress of iodoform gauze. The mastoid wound is dressed by means of a separate gauze packing, the same methods being followed as have heretofore been described. The surgical relation of all the structures with which the surgeon must deal in performing the several operations for the relief of sinus thrombosis is very excellently shown in the dissection represented in Fig. 272.

The first dressing is allowed to remain forty-eight hours and often longer, depending altogether upon the subsequent symptoms of the patient. When the jugular has been ligated in the neck the dressing of this portion of the wound will usually require attention at the same time. In case the vein has been dissected out of the neck and a cigarette or gauze drain has been inserted the whole length of the cervical wound, 1 inch or more of this gauze should be pulled from the lower angle and the extracted portion cut off at this and each subsequent dressing until the drain is wholly removed. At the first dressing the sigmoid sinus may be found collapsed and its inner walls adherent; it may be suppurating or granulations may be found already springing up which will in time obliterate its lumen. If suppuration occurs a free outlet must be provided for the pus and its rapid absorption secured by means of frequent dressings and the liberal use of iodoform gauze. Unless the vein has been brought out of the upper end of the wound after it has been ligated, according to the method of Ballance, and is used as a drainage-tube, it would be unsafe to employ irrigation as a means of cleansing, for the reason that by so doing there is danger of washing septic matter into the general circulation through anastomosing vessels (see Fig. 268).

CHAPTER XXXIV

INTRACRANIAL COMPLICATIONS (Continued)

OTITIC BRAIN ABSCESS.—PATHOLOGY, SYMPTOMS, DIAGNOSIS, AND PROGNOSIS

Pathology.—Of all brain abscesses those of otitic origin are the most common. In the first years of life cerebral and especially cerebellar abscesses are much rarer than in adults. Abscess is most common in the second and third decennial, according to Bezold. However, every brain abscess in the presence of disease of the temporal bone is not necessarily thus originated. The abscess may be situated far from the focus of suppuration in the temporal bone and even on the opposite half of the brain. Infection may be carried by pyemic metastases from the lungs or from putrid processes in other organs, as, for example, empyema of the pleura, endocarditis, osteomyelitis, or tubercular disease. Extension of suppuration may occur either from the labyrinth or sigmoid sinus, and rarely from the hiatus subarcuatus, according to Hinsburg. Körner states that otitic brain abscess is situated in the immediate neighborhood of the primary seat of the disease in the temporal bone. Accepting this rule, the collection of pus must be in the temporal lobe of the cerebrum or in the cerebellum. This class of abscess is usually single, whereas abscesses not of otitic origin are often multiple. The primary suppuration in the temporal bone is more often chronic than acute and, as a rule, is preceded by extensive disease of the bone, as caries, necrosis, and erosions by cholesteatomata. Hammerschlag states that about 25 per cent. of brain abscesses occur after acute middle-ear suppuration. Otitic abscesses in the temporal lobe are twice as frequent as those in the cerebellum, according to Körner. Suppuration can progress directly or indirectly from the original focus to the brain. Eulenstein says that direct progression is rare, in which case the purulent inflammatory process attacks the bone and passes by continuity to the dura; the dura agglutinates with the pia and surface of the brain and suppurative softening of the latter takes place. As a rule a thin layer of brain substance lies between the abscess and the brain membranes (see Fig. 273). In the indirect progression of the disease from the infected foci in the temporal to cranial cavity,

436

bacteria gain entrance from the primary focus by way of the lymphatics, the sheaths of arteries, the perforating veins, or along the nerve-sheaths of the facial or auditory nerves. The infection may follow the blood paths, as Körner suggests, by extension of thrombosis and phlebitis in the pial vessels. In this indirect way the tissue between the brain abscess and the dura does not show any macroscopic changes. After the bacteria have gained an entrance either red or white softening may take place, according to whether there is much hemorrhagic extravasation or little; the brain tissue disintegrates with the formation of pus, and then, if the surrounding brain substance

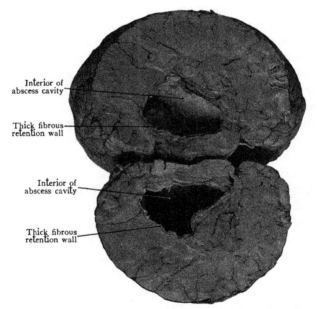

Interior of
abscess cavity

Thick fibrous
retention wall

Interior of
abscess cavity

Thick fibrous
retention wall

FIG. 274.—CASE OF LARGE CHRONIC TEMPOROSPHENOIDAL BRAIN ABSCESS WITH THICK FIBRINOUS RETEN-
TION WALLS.

possesses sufficient vitality, fibrin and leukocytes are thrown out which form a capsule around the collection of pus. The thickness of the abscess capsule varies from 1 to 5 mm. or more (Fig. 274). The capsule may become calcified, vessels may penetrate it from the brain tissue, and the abscess may be absorbed; or the capsule may be replaced by granulation tissue with increased formation of pus, the pressure from which may thin the capsule and cause rupture of the abscess into the ventricles of the brain or into the subdural space.

Symptoms.—The symptoms of acute and chronic brain abscess differ greatly in violence. In the acute variety all the symptoms are usually more pronounced in the beginning and grow more rapidly worse than is the case in the chronic form of the affection. When brain abscess is chronic the pus may become encysted and the symptoms of the disease remain vague and indefinite throughout a period of many months or even years. The most prominent symptoms of both acute and chronic abscess of the brain are pain, vomiting, slow pulse, normal or subnormal temperature, rigors, intra-ocular changes, cessation of the aural discharge, slow cerebration, and perhaps paralysis of certain groups of muscles. All of these symptoms are seldom present at one time or in any one case, but if careful note be made of the entire progress of the abscess, many and perhaps the majority of those above noted may be observed in a large percentage of cases.

The pain in the beginning may occur only in the depths of the ear of the affected side, from which point it later radiates over the temporal and mastoid regions, and finally concentrates upon some small area which may be located at quite a distance from the affected ear. The pain during the early stage of the abscess formation is partly the result of faulty drainage, and should the pus by its own pressure break into some new and larger channel, temporary relief may at once occur. In cases of chronic brain abscess the pain may intermit for several hours or even days, only to return with its former severity. During such intervals of freedom from suffering the patient believes great improvement has taken place, and he may resume his occupation until such time as he is again compelled, on account of his suffering, to abandon his task and remain indoors or even in bed. The author has observed two cases through long periods in which this pain recurred at irregular intervals of from one to several hours. Both would industriously read any convenient book with seeming interest and pleasure or would engage in games enthusiastically and successfully; would laugh and talk as vigorously as though they enjoyed life to its fullest extent, until suddenly, when seized with the pain over the temporal region, they would abruptly cease what they were doing, hold the head between the hands, and would cry out in great agony. At a later period in the disease the pain became constant though less severe, and frequent attacks of screaming occurred in one case for a few days preceding the fatal termination.

Vomiting is a symptom which occurs in nearly all intracranial diseases in which inflammation is present or where there is pressure from fluids or tumors upon the cerebral or cerebellar structures. While, therefore, vomiting occurs in many cases as a symptom of brain abscess at some period during the progress of the disease, this symptom is helpful in a diagnostic way only when taken in connection with other and more important ones.

The course of the temperature has a much greater significance. In the beginning of the brain abscess, when there is likely to be present a complicating localized meningitis, the temperature is elevated, but not high, and seldom exceeds 101° F. It is likewise elevated toward the close of the disease should the latter end fatally, since usually a leptomeningitis or cerebritis is added at this stage. In the intermediate period, however, when the abscess has developed to a sufficient size to produce pressure upon the adjacent brain structure, the temperature is often normal or subnormal, and in some instances falls as low as 97° F., at which point it may persist for several days. This behavior of the temperature is strikingly different from that of either sigmoid sinus, thrombosis, or meningitis, and when accompanied by other symptoms of brain complication is most significant of brain abscess.

The pulse rate is of equal diagnostic importance to the low temperature, and in uncomplicated cases it bears a close relationship to the latter. Thus, in the early stages, when a localized meningitis of sufficient extent exists over the abscess cavity to produce a rise in temperature, the pulse is also somewhat quicker than normal; but as the size of the abscess increases to the extent of producing considerable pressure in the portion of the brain which it occupies, the pulse-rate is reduced and may be as low as 40 per minute, although the average rate is between 60 and 70. Both the slow pulse and lowered temperature are attributable to the pressure exerted upon the brain structures by the accumulated fluid, and, therefore, small abscesses may produce but little change in this respect, while the same is true of a large chronic abscess that has become encapsulated, and consequently is separated from healthy brain tissue by a thick protecting wall of fibrous or connective tissue, and will, therefore, be incapable of creating a pressure upon its environment to a degree that will affect either the pulse or temperature.

When the pulse is slow because of an intracranial pressure it is usually also full and strong, but should the disease approach a fatal termination the heart's action becomes both rapid and weaker. General meningitis sometimes complicates a brain abscess, and when this is the case a rather curious phenomena may arise, in so much as the pulse remains abnormally slow, whereas the temperature is high. Should the abscess rupture into the ventricles or break upon the surface of the brain, the pulse will almost immediately become weaker and faster and the temperature will rapidly rise.

Chills are not of as frequent occurrence in this disease as in sinus thrombosis, and when they do take place are usually not so severe, and are not followed by profuse and exhaustive sweats. A brain abscess may run its whole course to a fatal termination without a single chill or even chilly sensation having been complained of. On the other hand, a rigor will almost certainly occur when the abscess makes each advance. Thus, should a rupture of an abscess take place in any direction, the occurrence will in all probability be marked by a chill of some degree of severity. The establishment of a secondary abscess or of a general meningitis of either variety will likewise be announced by a rigor.

The general appearance of the patient while not in any sense characteristic, is often indicative of the presence of a severe illness. The face may be sallow and worn, the body emaciated, and every feature be one such as to impress the observer that the individual has undergone much suffering. Macewen has called attention to the presence, when the abscess is fully established, of a putrid odor to the breath, and states that the odor persists even after the suppurating ear and the foul tongue and mouth of the patient have been thoroughly cleansed. The author has seen one case of brain abscess in which this odor was markedly present. The hair of the scalp sometimes seems lifeless over the affected side of the head, and the scalp itself is wrinkled and has a tendency to become scurfy over the diseased area.

Ocular symptoms in the form of photophobia, inequality of pupils, diplopia, or optic neuritis are present at some stage of the abscess in a large proportion of all cases. Photophobia is most often seen in the first few days of the abscess, whereas the other eye symptoms above enumerated develop as the abscess enlarges and sets up inflammation or pressure on adjoining structures. Optic neuritis may be present in both eyes, but not with the same intensity in each. Vision is not seriously affected by the occurrence of this affection, and does not occur at all if the abscess is only of short duration or if it is small. This particular eye complication may be the result of other intracranial diseases—namely, tumor of the brain, meningitis, and cerebritis—and its presence cannot, therefore, be considered as highly diagnostic of brain abscess except when with it are associated such other important symptoms as a discharging ear, localized pain, vomiting, a slow pulse, and a normal or subnormal temperature. The pupils are not usually affected when the abscess is small, but when large and located in the temporosphenoidal lobe the pupil of the eye on the same side may be greatly dilated and fixed. When only moderately dilated it may be found that the pupil of the affected side will react to light with such sluggishness when compared with the behavior of its fellow in this respect as to furnish a valuable symptom.

Another symptom which is sometimes observed is the cessation of the aural discharge at a time coincident with the development of symptoms of the intracranial disease. When cessation of the discharge thus suddenly occurs it is most likely a result of the pus having broken into some new and larger channel, as, for instance, into the cranium, and not to a sudden lessening in the quantity of the formation of the pus. Cessation of the aural discharge may be a symptom of meningitis or sinus thrombosis as well as of the disease under consideration.

When a brain abscess develops somewhat rapidly and attains a size sufficient to produce considerable pressure upon the surrounding structure, the patient's mentality may become impaired and cerebration may be exceedingly slow. In this respect this symptom of brain abscess is similar to the later stages of typhoid fever, since in either disease if the individual is asked a question he will hesitate a very long time before giving even the briefest answer; or if requested to protrude the tongue or close the eyes he will delay several seconds before heeding, although his final compliance furnishes certain evidence that he understood perfectly from the first. Drowsiness also accompanies this mental state, and the patient is apparently always asleep and must be aroused on every occasion when food or medicines are administered. In the advanced stages of the disease the patient may fall asleep again after he is awakened and before he can find words to answer a question or before he has swallowed the proffered food or drugs. When not interfered with surgically this stupor gradually deepens into coma and death; or if the abscess ruptures into the ventricles the death may occur more suddenly.

Paralysis, either partial or complete, may occur as the result of a destruction by the abscess of all or some portion of a given motor area; or the palsy may result from the pressure of the abscess; or to the accompanying zone of inflammation surrounding it. Extensive paralysis is not common, since it is observed only in cases where the abscess is very large or when it is located in the motor area (see Fig. 269). The external rectus muscle is sometimes paralyzed, in which case the affected eye looks inward, producing the conditions of a convergent squint. In its worst forms the paralysis may affect the opposite arm and leg, as was observed by the author in one case in which a large temporosphenoidal abscess was accompanied by a complete paralysis of the opposite arm and a paresis of the opposite leg.

An irritable disposition of the individual has also been noted as an early symptom, but little is usually thought of it until graver conditions have fully developed. As an early symptom and especially when taken in connection with those already given, it has some diagnostic value.

Diagnosis.—The positive determination of the presence of a brain abscess is in most instances impossible in the earlier stages, and is nearly always difficult at any period of the disease. The latent or chronic cases of encysted abscess may remain symptomless for months or even years, and the actual condition within the brain during all this time may never be suspected by any one. The author has seen one such case in which a boy ten years old attended school regularly up to within a few weeks of his death, and was undoubtedly a student of more than average ability; nevertheless the autopsy showed a temporosphenoidal abscess of large proportion, the capsule of which was so thick that it must have been many months, if not years, in forming (see Fig. 274). On the other hand, an acute brain abscess of large dimensions may take place within the short period of two weeks, during all of which time symptoms of some grave affection of the head are constantly manifest.

In addition to the symptoms already given, the diagnosis must be made largely upon the physical examination of the ear itself. A discharging ear nearly always precedes and accompanies a brain abscess, except when of traumatic origin. The fact that the patient or his friends may deny the presence of an aural discharge should not deter the diagnostician from making the most exacting examination of the condition of the fundus of the ear, and of ascertaining to an exact certainty the precise state of the middle ear and its connecting air spaces. Every means of examination known to otology that will aid in the accuracy of this examination should be used, to the end that the information thus gained is positive, and, therefore, of definite value when taken in connection with symptoms which are already present in the case or may shortly develop. While there is not likely to be found present in the ear any condition that is pathognomonic of brain abscess, nevertheless, if granulations, polypi, carious bone, or cholesteatoma be found in or adjacent to the middle ear in a patient who has symptoms of an intracranial disease, this fact would have great weight in the final decision as to the character of the ailment.

Since a mastoiditis is also nearly always included in the pathologic chain that ultimately leads to the intracranial disease, the symptoms of this affection may simulate or even completely mask those which arise from the brain abscess. The diagnosis in such cases cannot be certainly made out until the mastoid has been opened and its connecting cavities are freed from their diseased foci. If the previously existing intracranial symptoms are not relieved by the mastoid operation, and if the presence of concomitant general disease can be eliminated from the case, then an exploration of the cranial cavity for diagnostic purposes is a perfectly justifiable measure and should be undertaken. Particularly is an exploration in the vicinity of the mastoid and middle ear indicated if the symptoms all point to a local disease and the patient shows evidence of doing badly under other treatment.

Finally, when in the course of an aural suppuration symptoms develop which lead to the suspicion of an intracranial involvement, it becomes necessary, in order to make an early and correct diagnosis, to place the patient under frequent observation and to make a complete record of every feature of the progress of the disease, embracing especially a record of the pulse, temperature, the presence or absence of rigors, vomiting, and all other symptoms likely to arise during this complication. Such a record, when carefully and competently made, will usually enable the surgeon to arrive at a diagnosis at a much earlier period than would otherwise be possible—an advantage to the patient which should well repay the trouble of its performance.

Prognosis.—The prognosis in brain abscess is unfavorable. When left to nature or treated by drugs, recovery is exceedingly rare. Cases have been observed in which, because of an extensive destruction of the tegmen tympani and tegmen antri, an opening of sufficient dimensions has been provided through the skull to furnish free drainage to the abscess and thus provide the one most essential condition of recovery. Even where good drainage is by this means provided, the abscess cavity in the brain is constantly subjected to the possibilities of reinfection from the nearby suppuration of the mastoid antrum and middle ear with which it is connected, and ultimate extension of the brain affection and death are the final outcome. A natural cure may result from the absorption of a small brain abscess, but this termination must be reckoned among the rarest possibilities. As has been previously stated, when the abscess becomes encapsulated by thick walls, it may remain apparently harmless for months, years, or even until the death of the individual results from other causes. Most usually, however, such an abscess sooner or later ruptures into the ventricles or upon the surface of the brain, and in either instance death speedily follows.

The prognosis following surgical interference is much better than when the case is left to nature or than that following local or medicinal methods. Macewen states that when the abscess is diagnosed early, its position in the brain accurately determined, and surgical measures are promptly adopted, cerebral abscess is one of the most hopeful intracranial affections. It must be remembered that this ideal

condition, as stated by Macewen, is very seldom met with in ac
practise, and that in the past a large majority of all operations
have been undertaken for the relief of brain abscess have been perfor
at a late stage of the disease and as a last resort.   Large statistics
cerning the percentage of recovery in brain abscess after operation
not been published, but from the sources of information availabl
this point it would seem that about 25 per cent. of all operated c
get well.   Of the author's eight cases of operation for cerebral abs
two are living and in good health after a period of four years.
case died from a recurrence of the abscess after a period of sev
months and after recovery had apparently taken place.

INTRACRANIAL COMPLICATIONS (Continued)

THE TREATMENT OF BRAIN ABSCESS

THE treatment of brain abscess is essentially surgical. While a few cases have been known to recover through the unaided efforts of nature, such a result is too rare to be expected and should never be awaited. When, therefore, the diagnosis has with certainty been made, surgical measures offer the only hope of satisfactory results; and even when the diagnosis is not absolutely certain, but when all the symptoms point to intracranial involvement, and the examination of the ear leaves no question as to the possibility of infection from this source, then an exploratory operation is entirely justifiable on the ground that the mastoid infection can thereby be relieved, the adjacent walls of the mastoid cavity can be accurately inspected for sinuses leading into the cranial cavity, and the condition of the floor of the brain above the mastoid antrum and middle ear, together with the groove of the lateral sinus, can be so exposed that a reliable judgment can be formed as to whether or not the infection has extended to the brain surfaces or sigmoid sinus. If still in doubt concerning the matter, no hesitancy should be felt, indeed the surgeon should consider it his positive duty, to uncover the brain above and the sinus posteriorly to an extent in each instance sufficiently to permit the palpation, inspection, and, when necessary, the incision of the dura covering the sinus or that overlying the tegmen. Thus, operative procedures are sometimes indicated for diagnostic purposes for the reason that it is often impossible to tell beforehand with certainty in exactly what portion of the brain the abscess is located; whether it is extradural, subdural, cerebral, or cerebellar; and since when an abscess is present in any of these locations it is amenable only to surgical methods of treatment, it makes little difference whether or not the previous diagnosis is exact in so far as its precise situation in the cranium is concerned, provided the operator is prepared to deal equally with the particular condition when once it is discovered.

In operations for the relief of intracranial disease which has arisen as a result of aural suppuration, it is best to perform the complete tympanomastoid exenteration as a preliminary step (see Fig. 251), first, because in this way only can the original foci of the disease be eliminated;

second, the diagnosis of the exact condition within the cranium can often be made out only after the performance of the radical mastoid operation, and, third, the channel through which the infection traveled to the brain is thus discovered, if present, and hence great advantage will be gained by following this communicating channel of infection in the subsequent steps of the intracranial surgery.

Should the previous symptoms have pointed to a cerebral abscess, the roof of the mastoid antrum—the tegmen antri—should be removed if this has not already been done during a previous exploratory operation, since the site of a cerebral abscess of the temporosphenoidal lobe, when due to aural infection, is nearly always in the immediate vicinity of this portion of the temporal bone. In case a carious opening already exists in the tegmen, this should be followed, but in any case enough of the bone between the antrum and dura should be removed (Fig. 277) to enable the examiner to satisfactorily inspect, palpate, or, if necessary, to incise the dura. Should the subdural space have become infected through the burrowing of pus from the adjacent osseous cavities, an extradural abscess, with or without a collection of pus in the brain itself, will be found.

Surgical Treatment of Extradural Abscess.—When this form of abscess is present pus immediately pours into the mastoid wound as soon as the tegmen antri has been penetrated by the gouge. After the bone has been removed over a sufficiently large area to permit the introduction of the dura mater separator, this instrument should be inserted between the bone and dura and passed in every direction, at the same time lifting the membrane to an extent that will insure the free outflow of any pus from this locality. Care should be taken not to introduce the separator beyond the point where it meets with even slight resistance, for the reason that protective inflammatory adhesions have possibly already taken place between the dura and bone; the extradural abscess is, therefore, a limited one, and any loosening of the adhesions by the separator would permit a spread of the infection, with a rapidly fatal termination from the resulting meningitis.

The extradural pus having been thus evacuated and the exposed dural area dried, a further examination of the dura should be made to determine if subdural abscess is present. Should a cerebral abscess lie near the surface at this point the dura will bulge through the opening as soon as the underlying bone is removed. If the pus is confined under much pressure the membrane will appear injected, dark, or gray, depending upon the stage of the disease, and no pulsation will be felt when the examining finger is placed upon it. If sufficient bone has been removed to permit palpation of the exposed dura, fluctuation may be detected in the protruding part. In case none of these conditions are found present it may be reasonably supposed that the extradural abscess was the sole cause of the previous intracranial symptoms, and the operation may, therefore, be concluded by placing a thin wick of iodoform gauze between the dura and bone, after which the mastoid is dressed in the usual manner. Should, however, the examination of the exposed dura indicate the presence of pus in the brain, this must be at once evacuated.

Treatment of Temporosphenoidal Abscess (Fig. 275).—If the dura mater at the seat of the exposure above the mastoid antrum or of that overlying the attic of the middle ear is black or grayish and bulging, it should be incised in this location even though it is afterward deemed

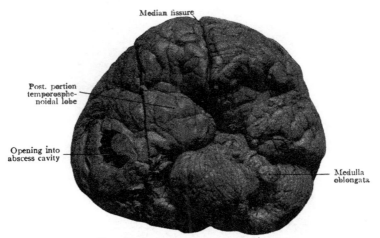

Median fissure

Post. portion temporosphe- noidal lobe

Opening into abscess cavity

Medulla oblongata

FIG. 275.—LARGE TEMPOROSPHENOIDAL ABSCESS.

advisable to trephine the skull at some point above the external auditory meatus, and to connect this latter opening with the mastoid wound below. The author is aware that any method of operating which provides an opening into the abscess so as to connect it with the mastoid wound is open to the criticism that the latter is a septic cavity which remains a constant menace to the subsequent healing of the cerebral abscess. Nevertheless, when the abscess is located over the tegmen antri or teg- men tympani, as above described, the advantage secured by the drain- age of the bottom of the abscess into the mastoid wound is so great that the objection of likelihood of reinfection is of minor importance. Especially is this true when the precaution is taken at the subsequent dressings not to disturb the cerebral wound until the cavity of the mas- toid has first been cleansed and packed with iodoform gauze.

When the abscess cavity is very large or in case it is not thought advisable to open and drain it through the tegmen, the incision through the skin and soft parts is extended as shown in Fig. 276, *C D*. A flap with the pinna at its base is turned downward and forward (Fig. 277) and a trephine with a diameter of ¾ inch is applied to the skull 1¼ inches above Reid's base line at a point perpendicularly above the opening of the external auditory meatus. The button of bone which is removed should be placed in a vessel of warm sterilized normal salt solution for preservation until it is determined whether or not it is advisable to replace the

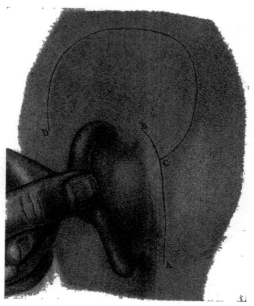

Fig. 276.—Lines of Primary Incision for Opening the Mastoid and Middle Cranial Fossa for the Removal of Diseased Products due to Extension from the Ear.
A B, the line of incision for the preliminary mastoid operation. *CD*, line of extension for making temporal flap.

same in the trephine opening before closing the wound. If upon exposure the dura is found to have a normal color and to pulsate and if no other evidence of an abscess exists, then the button may be replaced either whole or comminuted and the skin flap may be completely sutured over it in its proper place. Should, however, the dura be found to bulge at once through the trephine opening, as shown in Fig. 277, to be free from pulsation, of a dark or gray color, and to give other evidences of the presence of fluid beneath it, an incision should at once be made through the membrane and an exploration of the brain be instituted for the discovery of the abscess. Sometimes thick pus will be found upon the inner surface of the dura, whereas, occasionally when this membrane is incised, the pus escapes at once, there being no other intervening tissue separating the abscess cavity. When the pus is confined under pressure and is thin in consistency, as is frequently the case in acute brain abscesses, it may spurt into the air a foot or more immediately after it is liberated by the incision.

In case the abscess occupies a deeper situation it becomes necessary to incise the dura more extensively, and this is most satisfactorily accom-

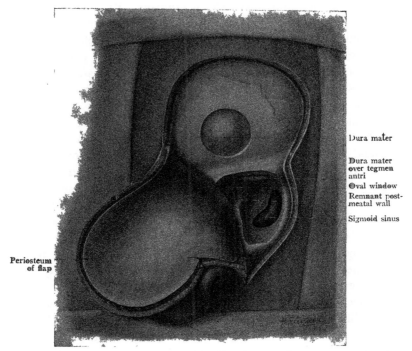

Dura mater

Dura mater over tegmen antri

Oval window

Remnant post-meatal wall

Sigmoid sinus

Periosteum of flap

Fig. 277.—Complete Mastoid Exenteration showing Exposure of the Dura over the Tegmen Antri and over a Portion of the Sigmoid Sinus.

The incision has been extended, following the mastoid operation, along the lines shown in Fig. 276, and a temporal flap including the soft structures of the external auditory meatus and the auricle has been turned down. A button of the squama has been removed with the trephine showing the bulging dura mater of the temporosphenoidal lobe.

plished by cutting a flap from its exposed surface. This flap should have its base at a point in the wound exactly opposite that of the skin flap, namely, at the upper posterior portion of the trephine opening. A small sharp bistoury is used for making this incision, which should follow parallel to the bony margin and $\frac{1}{16}$ inch from it. Sometimes large veins traverse the dura and these should be avoided where possible, since the bleeding which results from their division obscures

29

the field, and it is difficult to arrest blood coming from vessels so difficult to clamp or tie.

After the reflection of the dural flap the operator should note carefully the relation of the exposed portion of brain to the petrous portion of the adjacent temporal bone below, and should recall the most frequent sites in which abscess in this portion of the cerebrum is found. Temporosphenoidal abscesses are near those portions of the petrous which are most frequently carious and which give rise to the brain infection— namely, the tegmen antri and tegmen tympani. By bearing this fact in mind the surgeon will frequently avoid needless wounding of the brain structure in his attempts to locate the seat of the collection of pus. The exploring instrument should, therefore, be first passed in the direction of the tegmen antri, after which, if unsuccessful, it may be directed toward the tegmen tympani, and then again along the adjoining surface of the petrous portion.

The kind of instrument used for this exploration is of importance. Formerly an aspirating needle or a hollow trocar was employed, but was found entirely unsatisfactory. Any hollow needle or canula is apt to become filled with brain tissue, and this class of instrument has, therefore, been known to penetrate the abscess without any pus appearing in the canula to demonstrate that fact. On the other hand, such an instrument may pass entirely through a small abscess and thus deceive the examiner as to the real condition within. Ballance (*Lancet*, May 25, 1901) advocates the use of a sharp-pointed, long and narrow knife as the best exploring instrument, and states that not only is the abscess more certainly discovered by means of such an instrument, but that the clean-cut wound produced by it in the cerebral tissue heals more readily than when produced by other instruments. In very chronic cases of brain abscess, when the pus is contained within a strong capsule, it is possible not to enter the cavity even when a sharp knife is used in exploration.[1]

[1] Ballance reports such a case in which the abscess was missed during explorations at the time of the operation. Post-mortem examination revealed the presence of an abscess containing 4 ounces of pus which was contained in a capsule so dense that the abscess could be hulled out without rupture and rolled about upon the table. The author had a similar experience. A large temporosphenoidal abscess had been evacuated three months previously, and the patient was thereby supposedly cured. A return of the old symptoms resulted in a second operation and evacuation of a secondary abscess. The patient's symptoms did not improve and he was comatose in two weeks from the time of the second operation. At the beginning of the unconscious state a sharp knife was passed into the brain in every direction without discovering further abscess formation. At the autopsy a firmly encapsulated abscess was found which had lain directly in the track of the exploration. So resisting and thick were the walls of this cavity that a sharp thrust of a pointed knife was required to penetrate it.

If the abscess cavity lies in the direction of the tympanic or antral roof and is near the cerebral surface, a counteropening into the mastoid wound is indicated for the purpose of securing the best possible drainage. It sometimes happens that the abscess is located somewhat above, either anteriorly or posteriorly to the center of the trephine opening, and that, therefore, its cavity cannot be satisfactorily explored or subsequently treated through the small and improperly placed trephine opening which has already been made. In this instance the osseous· wound must be enlarged in the direction of the abscess to an extent that the center of the abscess lies approximately under the extended portion of the osseous wound. The removal of any additional portions of the skull for the above or other reasons is best accomplished by means of the Hoffman's or DeVilbiss forceps, with either of which the portion of bone to be removed can be quickly surrounded by the narrow trench which is made through both tables of the skull, and the area thus set free can be lifted out. While the removal of any unnecessary portion of the skull should always be avoided on account of the increased tendency to hernia cerebri or of the subsequent liability to the formation of adhesions between the dura and skin flap, nevertheless when greater advantage can be thereby secured in the way of a better examination and cleansing of the abscess cavity at the time of operation and in the subsequent dressing of the case, the operator should not hesitate to cut away an area of skull sufficient for these purposes. After the evacuation of all pus it may be found that inspissated, cheesy material or brain sloughs yet remain in the abscess cavity which are too thick in consistency to flow out with the other material. These may be cautiously washed away with sterilized normal salt solution, ample provision having first been made for the free return of the· fluid. Or, in case it is deemed more advisable to do so, any remaining sloughs may be removed by the most gentle·use of the curet. When the cavity is thus cleared of septic matter it is advantageous to learn the character of the retaining walls of the abscess. For the purpose of exploration the little finger may be inserted and passed in every direction over the interior surface. Whiting has devised an encephaloscope (Fig. 278), which when inserted into the cavity, the interior of which is subsequently illuminated by reflected light, enables the examiner to actually see the interior surface, to judge the strength of the limiting membrane, and possibly to discover any granulations or fistula that are present. The information thus gained is of great value in the subsequent management of the case. Should it be found that the abscess is a very chronic one and that it is, therefore, completely walled off from the adjoining

brain substance by a thick partition of connective tissue, the subsequent
irrigation or other manipulation necessary for cleansing and drainage
may be accomplished with much less danger than would be the case
if the abscess were acute and no capsule whatever were present.

Although an acute brain abscess may be large, and a large cavity be
present immediately after its evacuation, the elasticity of the surrounding
cerebral tissue has not yet been lost, and there being present no retaining
capsule, the space occupied by the abscess is quickly encroached upon
by adjacent cerebral substance and is soon obliterated.   In this class
of abscess, therefore, it is necessary to cleanse the cavity of all pus and
necrotic brain at the time of the operation if this be possible, and to
make provision for drainage by such means as will not interfere with

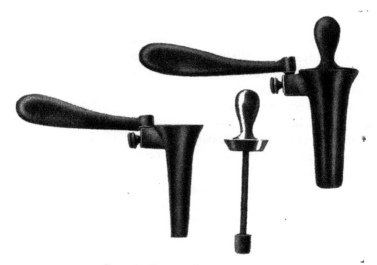

FIG. 278.—WHITING'S ENCEPHALOSCOPES.

the rapid closure of the space by the natural method of brain expansion.
The space resulting from the evacuation of an acute abscess should not,
therefore, be packed with gauze, but if this material is selected as the
method of dressing and drainage, only a thin strip should be inserted
to the bottom, a few folds of which strip should be loosely placed one
over the other and ample space be provided about the point of its
emergence at the dural opening.

When the abscess is chronic and is surrounded by thick walls,
no such expansion of the brain occurs, and the cavity must, therefore,
be ultimately healed by granulation.   The gauze dressing is more
suited in this than in acute cases.   A strip of iodoform gauze $\frac{1}{2}$ inch
wide, with selvage edge, should be seized near one end between the jaws

of a slender dressing-forceps, and the same should be inserted through the encephaloscope, first to the remotest part of the abscess cavity, and then over this coils of the strip are properly placed one upon another. The whole work of packing the abscess must be carried out by means of reflected light, until finally the entire space is snugly but not tightly filled.

In the case of either an acute or chronic abscess if a counteropening has been made through the tegman antri or tympani, the strip of gauze which is inserted through the trephine opening above should be brought out through the lower opening into the mastoid wound, since from this plan the most perfect drainage will be secured.

Instead of the gauze dressing just described, many operators prefer to use a glass or soft-rubber drainage-tube; and when a tube is selected and a counteropening has been provided, one end of the drain should emerge from the upper or trephine opening and the other through that in the tegmen, while the intervening perforated portion passes through the abscess cavity.

In case gauze has been used to fill the cavity and a counteropening has been provided through the tegmen, the gauze should be so arranged in the upper opening that none lies external to the dura. If not too much mutilated or diseased, the flap of dura mater may then be replaced and the skin flap should be stitched into its proper position by means of interrupted catgut sutures. All subsequent dressings are made through the opening in the tegmen. If in any case it is thought necessary to insert a drainage-tube through the upper opening and to bring it out at the lower, it will be advisable to cut a hole through the skin flap large enough to accommodate the upper end of the tube, which is inserted through this hole in the flap, and which latter is then completely sutured in place as before described.

In either instance the mastoid wound is dressed separately from that within the cranial cavity and in the usual way. That portion of the drainage-tube leading from the abscess cavity through the tegmen should not be perforated external to its point of exit through the dura, and this unperforated part should be long enough to pass entirely through the mastoid dressings. The observance of this precaution concerning the preparation of the tube will prevent the leakage of pus from above into the mastoid dressings, and will avoid to some extent, at least, the introduction of sepsis from the mastoid into the abscess cavity above.

Boric acid powder or other antiseptic may be dusted over the line of flap sutures; a large quantity of loose gauze is placed over the end of the drainage-tube to absorb the exuded pus, and the operation is completed by the application of the roller bandage.

The management of the after-treatment is of the greatest importance, for upon the care and intelligence with which this is carried out success or failure will greatly depend. Both pulse and temperature, if previously subnormal, will at once regain the normal and may be slightly elevated. If the patient was comatose, or if paralysis of some portion of the body, or of certain groups of muscles was previously present, but of short duration, and if the nerve center for these had not been destroyed, the function of the parts will be at once restored or at least greatly improved. Consciousness will be regained, sometimes almost as soon as the patient comes from under the anesthetic. Previous pain and tendency to eject all nourishment often disappears at once. The appetite, which had for days been entirely wanting, returns with a most gratifying sharpness. The previously dull mental state is changed to one of acute rational activity, the patient being sometimes unusually talkative and joyous. All former power of cerebration may be again resumed just as though no serious injury to a considerable portion of the brain had ever occurred. Indeed, few diseases present more marked and sudden changes for the better than those which follow the successful evacuation of an uncomplicated cerebral abscess.

The subsequent symptoms will determine the time of changing the first dressing. If the patient's condition remains satisfactory as to temperature, pulse, and freedom from pain, and if the dressings remain dry and sweet smelling the dressing should not be disturbed for four or five days. On account of the very free discharge which follows, particularly in cases of large chronic brain abscesses, the dressings are badly soiled much earlier than this and will need changing. In fact, the amount of subsequent suppuration from a chronic abscess is usually very profuse, and will, therefore, require frequent changes of the gauzes. If at the time of the operation the cavity was filled with gauze it may be found that pressure symptoms rapidly develop, which will require an early investigation of the wound. It may then be found that the gauze has been rapidly saturated with the exudates and that it has hindered rather than facilitated the drainage from the abscess cavity. Should this be found to be the case, a soft-rubber drainage-tube should be immediately substituted for the gauze packing.

Some difference of opinion exists as to whether or not a brain abscess should be cleansed by syringing. It is certain that rude and unskilful methods of syringing in this class of cases would result in harm. In the acute abscess, even the most gentle syringing might wash away portions of the unprotected brain substance; but in chronic cases where a thick-walled capsule exists and no fistulæ are present, this method of cleansing ought to be safe if used with caution, and if ample provision is made for the free escape of the injected fluid. When the interior of such a chronic abscess cavity can be inspected by means of the encephaloscope and reflected light, excessive granulation tissue may be cauterized or even removed. This class of cases heals by granulation and it should be the aim of the operator to secure firm, healthy granulating surfaces in all directions, to the end that the space within is finally obliterated, much after the manner of the closure of a frontal sinus subsequent to an operation and treatment by the open method.

In the after-treatment of the acute case the gauze strip or drainage-tube which was inserted at the time of the operation should at subsequent dressings be gradually withdrawn and cut off as rapidly as the expansion of the brain takes place, to the end that this provision for drainage shall at no time become a hindrance to the closure of the cavity through the natural resumption by the brain of its original dimensions, after once the local pressure of the abscess is removed.

In cases where it was necessary at the time of the operation to remove a considerable portion of the skull in order to reach and thoroughly expose the abscess, a hernia cerebri may subsequently develop. This occurrence may be hastened or even caused by faulty technic at the time of the operation or by the subsequent admission of additional septic material into the wound. Every precaution should, therefore, be taken at all times to avoid infection. Should such a hernia occur, it is best treated by means of sterilized antiseptic dressings, but if it does not subside rapidly from this measure it may be cauterized with silver nitrate or the extruded mass, which consists largely of granulation tissue, may be excised. Proper arrangement of gauze pads over the hernia and the application of slight pressure by the bandages will sometimes satisfactorily relieve this annoying condition.

The convalescence may be interrupted by meningitis or by the formation of a secondary abscess. The appearance of either of these serious complications will be accompanied by the symptoms indicative of the respective disease. Thus, the occurrence of a chill, accompanied by fever, a rapid pulse, and a general headache would indicate that leakage from the abscess had occurred and that a general meningitis had resulted. On the other hand, an abnormal slowing of the pulse, a subnormal temperature, a localized pain over the affected side accompanied by vomiting, would be almost positive evidence that either a new abscess had formed or that the original one is badly drained. Secondary operation is indicated at once when the symptoms of an additional abscess or of the refilling of the former one are well marked.

CHAPTER XXXVI

INTRACRANIAL COMPLICATIONS (Continued)

CEREBELLAR ABSCESS

THE etiology and pathology of this affection have already been discussed in the chapter which dealt in a general way with the intracranial complications (see Chapter XXX.). Moreover, in the several sections of the work relating to the suppurative disease of the temporal bone, it has frequently been pointed out that cerebellar abscess may occur as a complication of any infection existing in the middle ear, mastoid antrum, or mastoid cells.

Symptoms.—The symptoms of a collection of pus in the cerebellum are often vague and misleading. In many instances the symptoms may be such as to lead the examiner to the belief that an intracranial complication exists, but are not indicative of its exact character or location. Some cases are throughout a long period of the existence of the cerebellar abscess entirely symptomless, in so far as suggesting a disease of the cerebellum is concerned. A discharging ear is, of course, always present or there is a history of such a discharge having at one time been present. The discharge may be profuse or scant and is often foul smelling and sanious. The abscess may follow either an acute or chronic aural affection. Many of the symptoms which are present belong to the progress of the original aural disease which has finally led up to the cerebellar abscess. Thus, for many years the carious processes incident to a chronic aural discharge may be going on in some portion of the cellular structure of the temporal bone. During this time more or less pain, deeply seated in the ear, may have been present. The history of one or more attacks of mastoiditis may be given, and headaches, vertigo, and nystagmus may at some time have formed a more or less prominent symptom. The abscess may have been present for a long time, and not having produced symptoms more numerous or severe than the foregoing, the patient continues his usual occupation and perhaps has never regarded his trouble as sufficiently serious to justify him in seeking medical advice. It is only, therefore, when the above symptoms become aggravated and the patient is no longer able to pursue his business that the surgeon is given opportunity to investigate the nature of the affection.

In the most typic cases the pain is located in the occipital region. The pulse and temperature are, in the uncomplicated affection, subnormal, and may, as in the case of a cerebral abscess, be very much reduced. When the abscess is large the respiration is also greatly affected, being slower than normal, and in the worst cases may be both slow and irregular. Optic neuritis occurs in about one-third of the cases, and in some amounts to a complete blindness. In this affection, as in brain abscess, slow cerebration and difficulty on the part of the patient in comprehending what is said are often prominent symptoms.

Objective Symptoms.—The patient may appear robust and healthy unless severe pain, vertigo, and digestive disturbances have been present, in which case a worn and cachectic look may characterize the disease. A physical examination of the ear may furnish evidence indicative of extensive necrosis of the temporal bone. There may be postauricular fistulæ, which indicate in a measure the extent of the osseous necrosis, as well as the continued activity of the suppurative process. Percussion over the occipital region of the affected side frequently gives rise to deep-seated pain.

Diagnosis.—The above symptoms may in any case be sufficiently numerous and so well defined as to point with more or less certainty to the presence of a cerebellar abscess. Early in the disease, however, it is seldom possible to make a positive diagnosis, and hence in any case in which cerebellar complication is strongly suspected it is advantageous to place the patient in charge of a competent nurse with instructions to note and record every symptom as it occurs, for by exercising this precaution a much earlier conclusion as to the nature of the case is often possible.

In many, however, a diagnosis based upon the symptoms alone is not possible. In such instances, if a chronic discharging ear is present, if there is evidence of extensive mastoid necrosis, and if there is a history of pain, vertigo, and perhaps nystagmus, the radical mastoid operation is indicated as a diagnostic measure. During this operation fistulous channels may be found leading through the tegmen tympani or antri and involvement of the middle cerebral fossa may be present, whereas it was supposed, previously to opening the mastoid, that the posterior cranial fossa was involved. The reverse of this statement may likewise be true, and either discovery will justify the exploratory procedure.

Treatment.—The treatment is essentially surgical, and like that for all other intracranial suppurative processes, the operation for the evacuation of the pus should be performed as soon as the diagnosis is made with certainty or as soon as its presence is strongly suspected. Since this class of abscess may be the result of a rupture of pus directly from the mastoid portion of the temporal bone backward into the sigmoid groove (Fig. 267), or may occur as a sequence to the entrance of pyogenic matter into the cerebellar fossa by way of the tympanic cavity and labyrinth, and from thence along the sheath of the auditory nerve to the cerebellar fossa, the surgical technic for the evacuation of the abscess varies, therefore, somewhat accordingly as to whether the collection is located anterior to the sigmoid sinus and in close relation to the adjacent petrous portion of the temporal bone, or as to whether it is posterior to the sinus and in the substance of the adjoining portion of the cerebellum. In either instance if the mastoid operation has not already been performed, this should be done at once, and in addition the bone should be removed posteriorly from the mastoid wound for a distance sufficient to uncover the sigmoid sinus, exactly as has already been advised in operations upon the sinus itself. If pus is found surrounding the sinus, the bone should be removed inward and backward to a sufficient extent to evacuate the same, and to determine whether or not it may have formed a fistulous channel leading to the cerebellum in any direction. A cerebellar abscess and a lateral sinus thrombosis may both exist in the same case, and hence the sinus itself should receive at this time an inspection such as has been previously indicated (see p. 426). Any fistula that is discovered in the bone as the operation progresses must be followed to its source; and if necessary for this purpose additional bone may be removed in the direction taken by the fistulous channel. ·Should the perisinuous pus be found to exude from the anterior and deeper portions of the wound adjacent to the sinus, the fact would indicate the probability of its labyrinthine origin, and the dura should, therefore, be lifted from the cerebellar surface of the petrous portion of the temporal bone, provided the collection of pus is seen to be extradural. The instrument best suited for this extradural exploration is the blunt separator of Horsely. The separator should not be introduced to a depth of more than ¾ inch measured from the anterior lip of the groove for the lateral sinus, for the reason that the facial and auditory nerves may be injured at a greater depth at their point of entrance into the internal auditory meatus. The auditory nerve may be already destroyed by the necrosis, but the function of the facial nerve, if still active, should, if possible, be preserved.

In case the location of the abscess has been previously and definitely determined to be posterior to the sigmoid sinus, much time would be saved by trephining directly into the cerebellar fossa without first performing the mastoid operation and afterward continuing the removal of bone in a backward direction, as above advocated. When this plan is chosen a flap of the skin and soft tissues extending to the bone is turned upward. The center-pin of the trephine is then placed on the bone at a point 1½ inches posterior to the center of the external meatus, and ½ inch below Reid's base line, at which point the anterior edge of the instrument will not injure the descending portion of the sinus. In this position the upper edge of the trephine rests just below Reid's base line, and hence the horizontal portion of the lateral sinus will lie above and well out of harm's way (Fig. 279). A button of

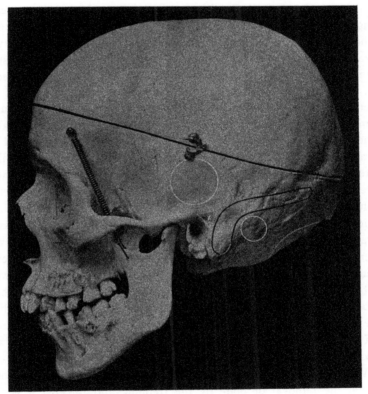

FIG. 279 —POINTS OF ELECTION ON SKULL FOR OPENING THE MIDDLE CEREBRAL AND CEREBELLAR FOSSA. Also the relation of the suprameatal triangle to the floor of the middle fossa, and to the lateral sinus. From the points of election for trephining here shown, the bone may be removed in any necessary direction until the required area of dura mater has been exposed. X, suprameatal triangle.

bone is here removed and the opening may then be enlarged with bone forceps backward and downward as far as necessary, or at least to the extent that 1¼ inches of dura are exposed in a vertical and anteroposterior direction. Enlargement of the trephine opening in an anterior direction is not usually advisable on account of the course of the sinus in front, but if subdural pus is present or if the sinus itself is diseased, the vessel should unquestionably be uncovered and any diseased condition which is found in the vessel should be dealt with in a surgical manner.

The question as to whether or not the mastoid antrum shall be opened prior to and as a part of the operation on the cerebellum, must be decided by the amount of information obtainable concerning the exact condition that is present in the case, and to some extent also by the physical condition of the patient at the time the operation is undertaken. If the surgeon can be reasonably positive that the abscess is situated posterior to the descending portion of the sinus and the patient's strength is so far wasted that prolonged operating would greatly increase the hazard, then there should be no question about the advisability of primarily turning down the flap and trephining as a primary measure. The mastoid operation can be done at some later period if found necessary. In view of the fact, however, that the original source of the infection is in the mastoid, if this be not removed by operative measures, the mastoid suppuration will continue as a menace to subsequent healing of the adjacent wounded structures, and may defeat the purpose of the operation on the abscess, even though the latter appear for a time entirely successful. Moreover, in the extension of the suppurative process backward from the mastoid, the lateral sinus is so frequently involved that it should always be closely scrutinized and sometimes surgically dealt with at the same time that the cerebellar abscess is operated; and this can be best done by first opening and clearing away the mastoid antrum and cells. Finally, diagnostic methods for determining the presence of this class of abscess are by no means always reliable, and what may have previously seemed most certainly to be a cerebellar abscess may prove, at the time of operation, to be nothing more than an extradural collection of pus in the vicinity of the sinus, relief of which through the performance of the mastoid operation and exposure of the sinus is all that is surgically indicated.

When the dura over the site of the abscess is sufficiently exposed through the removal of bone by the trephine and forceps, it is first examined, a flap of the dura raised, and the cerebellum is explored exactly as in case of examination of the temporosphenoidal lobe for a collection of pus. Should, however, the abscess be situated in the anterior and deeper portion of the affected cerebellar hemisphere it is safer not to employ the knife as the exploring instrument, but in its stead the exploring trocar and canula should be used. Ballance (*Lancet*, May, 1901) recommends the use of a canula having exterior rings, so placed that when the abscess has been penetrated and evacuated by the instrument the same may be left *in situ*, serving as a drainage-tube, which may be retained in place by means of sutures passed through the skin and attached to the rings. This author states that cases have been frequently lost because after the abscess has been evacuated the operator fails to reintroduce the tube properly into the abscess. The suggestion as to the method of management given above, he states, would if followed, obviate the possibilities of an error of this kind.

The presence of the abscess within the cerebellum often causes respiratory slowing previously to the operation for relief. During operations upon the cerebellum for the relief of this condition, the difficulties of respiration are sometimes increased and occasionally the breathing is altogether arrested while the heart action continues. The possibility of arrested breathing, therefore, should be borne in mind, the amount of anesthetic given should be as small as possible, and every step of the operation should be as expeditiously executed as is consistent with safety and thorough work. The after-treatment of cerebellar abscess differs in no important particular from that of the cerebral variety, which has already been described (see p. 454).

CHAPTER XXXVII

INTRACRANIAL COMPLICATIONS (Continued)

INFECTIVE MENINGITIS

INFLAMMATION of the brain envelopes, when originating from a suppuration within the temporal bone, is of three varieties—namely, pachymeningitis, leptomeningitis, and serous meningitis. Tubercular meningitis due to an infection which is secondary to tuberculosis of the ear is probably very rare.

Symptoms.—At the onset the symptoms of meningitis are often ill defined and may be identical with those present at the beginning of a brain abscess or a lateral sinus thrombosis; and this similarity should be expected, since these latter diseases are in many instances accompanied by a circumscribed meningitis at the site of the infection.

Either an acute or chronic discharge from the ear is usually present as a symptom. If acute, the discharge is or has been very profuse and the entire aural affection has probably been of unusual severity. Acute mastoiditis frequently accompanies the purulent otitis media and precedes the meningitis. In case the aural suppuration is chronic all the symptoms which accompany this disease (see Chapter XXVII.) may be present at the onset of the meningitis. It should be remembered that in chronic suppurative otitis media the aural discharge is sometimes very scant and may not be sufficient to appear in the external auditory meatus. In such instance the patient may deny the presence of aural suppuration, but this statement should not deter a thorough physical examination of the ears in any case in which the symptoms of meningitis are present.

Headache is the most constant as well as the most prominent symptom. In the developmental stage of the disease when arising from an aural infection, the headache is usually limited to one side of the head and may be designated by the patient as consisting of only a pain in and around the affected ear. This pain, in the majority of cases, however, soon spreads over the whole head and becomes so intense as to cause the patient the greatest agony. The pain is due to the pressure of the inflammatory exudate upon the dura, to an increase of fluid within the ventricles, or to an inflammatory edema of the brain substance. Photophobia develops early, the patient, therefore, turns from the light, avoids conversation, is extremely irritable, desires to be let alone, and lying in a room from which all light is excluded and with the head held between the hands, he moans or cries aloud during the severest moments of his suffering. Delirium is a frequent symptom, especially in children, who then utter a peculiar, piercing cry, a series of cries, or even repeat some short familiar sentence in a high-pitched and most pitiable tone of voice.

Convulsions, or at least convulsive movements, may accompany the delirium. These may amount only to the twitching of certain muscles or groups of muscles or may be of an epileptiform character. Rigidity of the muscles of the posterior part of the neck is characteristic of this disease; the head is drawn backward and any attempt to straighten it causes a decided increase of the pain. In the worst cases, when the disease is well advanced and involves the upper portion of the spinal cord, all the muscles of the back may be involved, and a complete opisthotonos may take place and may recur several times in the twenty-four hours. Spasm of the muscles of the jaw, amounting to a condition of trismus, has also been observed.

At the onset the pulse is slow and the blood-pressure high; but as the inflammation of the meninges spreads, the heart action becomes rapid and the blood-pressure greatly reduced. The temperature varies from 101° to 106° F., and is, therefore, in marked contrast to the temperature of brain abscess, in which disease the temperature is subnormal, normal, or but very slightly elevated. The temperature-curve in meningitis also differs from that of sinus thrombosis, inasmuch as the remissions are not so sudden or marked as is the case in infective thrombosis of one of the large sinuses.

Certain phenomena connected with the nervous system are also observed. Thus, hyperesthesia of the entire integumentary surface may be present to such an extent that the skin reflexes are greatly exaggerated. Vasomotor paresis of the vessels of the skin sometimes takes place, as can be demonstrated by drawing the finger-nail or some blunt instrument firmly across its surface, in which case a persisting white line will mark the site thus disturbed. Among other symptoms of a nervous origin may be mentioned herpes labialis and erythematous eruptions upon the general surface of the body.

The fundus of the eye is frequently involved. The eye-grounds may be only congested or a perineuritis or choked disc may occur. The views of different observers vary greatly concerning the frequency with which changes at the fundus of the eye occur as a symptom of infective meningitis. Zaufal, Kneiss, and Hansen state that these changes are often observed, and they, therefore, consider the presence of an optic neuritis as of great diagnostic value. On the other hand, Pitt and Körner found ocular changes only as a rare objective symptom of this disease, while Gruening states that optic neuritis never occurs as a symptom of meningitis. In 31 cases of meningitis reported by Tenzier (*Annals O. R. and L.*, Vol. XIV., No. 1), 11 or about a third of all reported showed changes at the fundus. The conjunctivæ, especially should the disease approach a fatal termination, become deeply injected, and showing between the widely open lids the eyes present at this time a peculiar bleared appearance.

The pupils of the eye are sometimes unequal, sometimes both are contracted. Paralysis of the motor oculi nerve, when occurring, results in strabismus or other motor changes of the eyeball, and nystagmus is occasionally observed.

Kernig's sign, although demonstrable in most cases, is not conclusive evidence of the presence of a meningitis. The tendon reflexes are all exaggerated.

Vomiting is a symptom which occurs frequently in meningitis, but is an indication of intracranial disease rather than of any particular variety of such disease.

Constipation is the rule in the beginning and throughout the greater part of the course of this as of other forms of meningitis; but toward the end looseness of the bowels and involuntary evacuations sometimes occur.

Diagnosis.—The diagnosis can be made only after a full consideration of all the symptoms of the patient, together with a thorough physical examination of the ear and of the fundus of the eye. Inspection of the ear will show the presence of either an acute or chronic tympanic suppuration. In either instance the pathologic changes that may be present in the auditory canal, drum-head, or middle ear should be determined with a view of tracing the direct progress of the infection from the middle ear to the meninges. Any change of structure that has already been described as a possible outcome of aural suppuration may be found present in the ear during this examination (see p. 321). Lumbar puncture is also a valuable aid to the diagnosis, not only as to the fact of the presence of a meningitis but also as to whether or not it is of the serous or purulent variety. When employed as a diagnostic measure, lumbar puncture is made by the method of Quincke, and 10 or 15 cc. of the spinal fluid are withdrawn for the purpose of inspection, microscopic examination, or chemical test. In meningitis serosa the cerebrospinal fluid thus withdrawn will be clear, whereas in the purulent variety it is clouded. Normal cerebrospinal fluid has a specific gravity of about 1.010 and contains no albumin or at least only traces. When meningitis is present the specific gravity is higher than normal and the amount of albumin is greatly increased. The statement has been made that the presence of more than 1 per cent. of albumin in the spinal fluid is positively indicative of a meningitis; and should the microscopic examination of the fluid in such a case show the presence of pus and an increase of polymorphonuclear cells, the diagnosis of meningitis can be positively made.

DIFFERENTIAL DIAGNOSIS IN UNCOMPLICATED INTRACRANIAL DISEASES OCCURRING AS THE RESULT OF AURAL SUPPURATION

	Meningitis	*Sinus Thrombosis*	*Brain Abscess*
Aural discharge.	Either present now or there are found on physical examination of the ear evidences of former suppuration.	Present or has been present.	Present or has been present.
Temperature.	Sometimes high, usually moderate, and remissions gradual.	Nearly always high with decided remission. Often suddenly rises, then markedly drops. Remissions may occur more than once in twenty-four hours.	May be at first elevated, soon falls to near the normal, normal, or even subnormal. Remains low throughout unless abscess ruptures and meningitis develops as a complication.
Pulse.	Greatly accelerated.	Rapid and often small and weak.	Accelerated at first, is later normal or abnormally slow and full. Becomes weak and rapid if abscess ruptures and death approaches.
Pain.	Always present in form of headache; severest over forehead, but extends to all parts of the head. Pain in the neck, which is stiff and immovable.	Seldom diffused over whole head. Not always present, but when so, is located in ear, over mastoid or along neck of affected side.	Usually present, at first in the ear or over mastoid; later localizes over temporal or frontal region of same side. Usually persistent and severe, and may be remote from seat of abscess.
Chill.	Chilly sensations or a marked chill may occur at onset, but are not frequent or characteristic during later stages.	Chill or chilly sensations frequent throughout disease. Sometimes occur more than once in twenty-four hours. Very severe and characteristic during disintegration of clot.	Not frequent nor characteristic.
Sweating.	Seldom occurs and is not a diagnostic feature.	Occurs frequently; is profuse and exhaustive, and is very characteristic in typic cases.	Seldom present. Not distinctive.
Vomiting.	Nearly always occurs during some stage of the progress of the disease, is of "cerebral" type, and independent of ingestion of food.	Seldom present; not characteristic.	Frequently present, persistent, and "cerebral."
Respiration.	Rapid, and in proportion to the acceleration of pulse and rise in temperature.	Not markedly affected, unless lungs are involved by septic pneumonia.	Slow and full. When pressure of abscess is considerable the breathing may become stertorous.

	Meningitis	Sinus Thrombosis	Brain Abscess
Muscular disturbances.	Stiffening of the muscles of the back of the neck usually occurs. The head is retracted and somewhat fixed. Rigidity of muscles of abdomen and back occur and sometimes general convulsions are present.	Very seldom occur.	Convulsions rarely occur. Stiffness of neck absent.
Mentality.	Unimpaired except by pain. Patient irritable and desires to be let alone. Later stages, mentality may be greatly impaired or lost.	Unimpaired except in prolonged cases and toward a fatal termination.	Sometimes unimpaired even when large abscess is present. More frequently mental processes are slow and typhoid in character.
Eye symptoms.	Perineuritis, congestion, or choked disc present in about one-third of all cases. Contracted or unequal pupils frequent. Photophobia almost constantly present.	Perineuritis, choked disc, etc., occur in about one-fourth of all cases.	Optic neuritis frequent in later stages. Inequality of pupils and photophobia sometimes present.
Kernig's sign.	Demonstrable in 80 to 90 per cent. of cases.	Not present.	Not present.
Paralysis.	Infrequent until late.	Not often present.	Paralysis of ocular muscles frequent. Where abscess is large, arm and leg of opposite side may be involved. If on the left side speech center may be implicated, aphasia resulting.
Course and termination.	Leptomeningitis usually runs a rapid course. The patient at once prostrated and appears seriously ill. Death may occur in three days, but sometimes is delayed two or three weeks.	Usually severe and rapid, with symptoms of extreme exhaustion. Occasionally terminates in resolution and recovery. Death occurs from septic pneumonia or metastatic abscess of brain, lung, liver, or extremities.	May be of short duration if acute. Chronic abscess may be "latent," encapsulated, and continue for months or years. Death occurs from rupture of abscess into brain with resulting meningitis.

Prognosis.—A majority of all cases of circumscribed meningitis recover, provided the radical mastoid operation is performed and the accompanying epidural abscess is evacuated before the infection spreads and results in a general purulent meningitis. This latter disease is almost certainly a fatal one, only a few instances of recovery having as yet been recorded as a result of treatment by lumbar puncture and subdural drainage. Serous meningitis is, however, a much more hopeful affection, and a majority recover following the prompt removal of the septic foci from the temporal bone and the relief of the intracranial pressure by means of lumbar puncture.

Treatment.—The treatment of infective meningitis depends upon the extent and character of the disease. In case the diagnosis of a localized external pachymeningitis is made, the radical mastoid operation should be performed as early as the symptoms of the extension of the septic inflammation to the dura is discovered. Such a circumscribed inflammation of the dura frequently occurs in long-standing cases of aural suppuration over the tegmen antri or tegmen tympani above, or in the region of the sigmoid groove posteriorly, and in either of these situations it is frequently associated with an extradural collection of pus. When the dura is sufficiently laid bare during the mastoid operation by the removal of the underlying bone and free drainage is thereby secured and maintained until the healing takes place, recovery is the rule provided the operation has been done before the pus has burrowed through the dura and set up an internal pachymeningitis or before it has ruptured into the arachnoid space and has resulted in a purulent leptomeningitis. These latter varieties prove fatal almost without exception under any form of treatment. When the meningitis has once spread and has become general, free exposure and incision of the dura is indicated and furnishes the most hopeful means of treatment, but even surgical measures have as yet met with little encouragement in the way of favorable results.

The technic of the operation best suited for all forms of general meningitis consists in turning back a flap of the soft tissues about 1 inch above and behind the affected ear, of trephining the skull at this point, and of enlarging the trephine opening by means of bone forceps. All extradural collections of pus which may be found upon exposing the dura should be washed away by a gentle stream of hot boric acid or normal salt solution, after which a blunt spatula may be used to separate the dura from the adjoining skull and press it away from the inner table; at the same time the patient's head is held in a lowered position in order to favor the outflow of pus or other exudate from every direction in the vicinity of the wound. After thus cleansing as broad an area of the dura as possible, a flap should be cut from the dura, the convolutions of the brain should be gently lifted by the spatula, boric solution may be used for irrigation, and finally a sterile gauze wick or a cigarette drain should be placed through the opening in the dura and brought out at the lower angle of the flap. The skin flap, including all the extra cranial soft tissues, is finally sutured in place, leaving, of course, an opening at its lower angle through which the gauze drain emerges. A large quantity of loose gauze should then be placed over the site of the external wound for the purpose of catching the serum which subsequently exudes, and this should in turn be covered by cotton, rubber protective, and finally by a roller bandage.

The patient should subsequently lie in such a position as to favor the drainage, which in most instances is very profuse. When the dressings become saturated from the discharge a change of the outer portion should be made, but the gauze wick leading through the incision in the dura must be left undisturbed so long as it is thought necessary to continue this mode of treatment. The gauze will, however, be pushed out as rapidly as the wound fills with granulations, provided, of course, subsidence of the inflammation occurs and a subsequent cure takes place.

Lumbar puncture has been tried in leptomeningitis, both by itself and in conjunction with subdural drainage, but aside from its diagnostic assistance this measure has proved of but little permanent benefit. In the treatment of serous meningitis, however, lumbar puncture is of great value, should be early performed, and as much as 25 to 100 cc. of the clear fluid be thus removed. The lumbar puncture and aspiration of fluid may be repeated one or more times, after which, if marked improvement or recovery does not promptly take place, drainage through

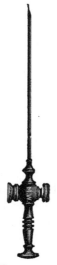

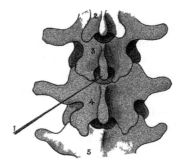

FIG. 280.—NEEDLE FOR WITHDRAWING SPINAL FLUID (KRÖNIG).

FIG. 281.—LUMBAR PUNCTURE (SCHEMATIC). 1, Paracentesis needle; 2 to 5, second to sixth lumbar vertebræ (Brühl-Politzer).

the dura may be established according to the method just described in the treatment of leptomeningitis.

Since lumbar puncture according to the method of Quincke is now frequently employed to secure a specimen of the cerebrospinal fluid for microscopic or chemical examination, as an aid to diagnosis, or as a means of treatment of serous meningitis, Ménière's disease, etc., a brief description of the method of its performance is essential: The puncture is made and withdrawal of the spinal fluid is accomplished by means of a sharp, stout hollow needle (Fig. 280). The point selected for the insertion of the needle is between the third and fourth lumbar vertebra. The skin of the adjacent area having been thoroughly sterilized and the needle freshly boiled and immersed in alcohol, the point of the instrument is entered at a distance of about 1 inch to one or the other side of the spinous process of the third lumbar vertebra, at which point it is thrust in a direction that will insure its entrance into the dural sac under this spine and exactly in the median line (Fig. 281). Lumbar puncture is not a painful operation if skilfully performed and anesthesia of the part is, therefore, usually not necessary. However, in the case of very sensitive individuals a 10 per cent. solution of phenol in glycerin should be applied to the area of skin to be punctured, and this will to some extent render the skin—the most sensitive part— somewhat anesthetic.

CHAPTER XXXVIII

SUPPURATION AND NECROSIS OF THE TEMPORAL BONE AND ITS PRACTICAL RELATION TO LIFE INSURANCE

To the life insurance examining surgeon the vital question concerning the applicant will always be, Is the risk safe? In so far as known to the author, no company of prominence omits in any case to investigate both the present and past condition of the applicant's ears. It must be, therefore, that life insurance companies have recognized the full importance of such investigation, and have accepted as a fact that actual dangers to life lurk in every discharging ear—dangers equally as grave as those which may be found in the urinary, circulatory, or nervous system, or in the faulty habits of the applicant for life insurance.

The insurance company justly expects that the examining surgeon will discover the weakness and dangers, if any exist, of all applicants for life insurance. The deep-seated situation of the ear and consequently the difficulties attendant upon the efforts to obtain accurate knowledge concerning any aural affection, are responsible for frequent errors on the part of the examiner in advising the acceptance of non-insurable applicants; or, on the other hand, in rejecting those in whom it is merely surmised that some serious aural ailment is present, when, in fact, only the most trivial disease exists and when the applicant is undoubtedly a safely insurable one.

The chief points relating to this subject may be briefly stated in answering the three following questions:

1. What symptoms given by the patient and what pathologic conditions found in the diseased ear by the examining surgeon should be regarded as sufficiently dangerous to justify the rejection of the applicant?

The author believes that no just decision can be made as to whether any applicant is or is not insurable, unless the examiner takes into consideration not only the symptoms stated by the patient himself but also the more reliable facts which he is able to obtain from a most thorough, painstaking, and accurate examination of the condition of the middle ear and its accessory cavities. It is the duty of the examining surgeon to make such an examination of every applicant who states

470

that he has once had a discharging ear, for it is a noteworthy fact that most extensive destruction of the soft structures of the ear and of the adjoining osseous structures of the temporal bone may take place during a prolonged suppuration within the tympanic cavity, without the individual ever making any sort of complaint as to pain or other discomfort. Neither is there present in many cases any evidence superficially to indicate the dangerous and hidden process which is going on within. Cases of suppurative middle-ear disease have been reported in which the individuals followed their usual occupation up to the very hour of the rupture of a brain abscess, due to extension of the suppurative process from the ear, and the author has reported a case in which the patient was in school, making his grades, for many months during a time when the right temporosphenoidal lobe of the brain was largely filled by an otitic abscess. It must, therefore, be conceded that there are non-insurable applicants who may present symptomless records with the exception of a discharging ear; and the presence of this symptom is often lightly regarded or even honestly denied by the applicant.

If an applicant with an aural discharge, however slight, or with the history of having had at one time an aural suppuration, should also be found to suffer from headache, occasional and unaccountable fits of irritableness of disposition or of dizziness, such group of symptoms would undoubtedly lessen the degree of safety of the risk. Headache on the same side of the head as the affected ear is an early and most constant symptom of brain extension, and should never fail to be given proper significance. This headache is usually not in the immediate vicinity of the diseased ear and, therefore, unless the examining surgeon is alert to the possible import of this important, early, and almost constant symptom of brain involvement, he may in no way connect the aural suppuration with it. In this class of cases, therefore, the subjective symptoms of aural suppuration are of very greatly less value to the examiner than is the information which may be obtained by the most searching examination of every part of the ear itself and of the open cavities of the temporal bone, provided, of course, that the surgeon skilfully uses every known and modern otologic method in his investigation.

If the middle ear or its accessory cavities, the mastoid antrum or mastoid cells, contain diseased and polypoid mucous membrane; if the mucous membrane is wanting in places, leaving the underlying bone bare; if the bony structures are carious or sequestered, abundant experience has shown that the suppurative process is a progressive one, and that, unless checked by surgical interference, it is apt to result ultimately in some intracranial complication and premature death. In long-standing suppuration, where the perforation of the drum membrane is of considerable size, the epithelium of the skin of the external auditory meatus is apt to grow through the opening and into the attic and antrum, where there is an accumulation of those curious and dangerous masses known as cholesteatoma. In the author's opinion no case of cholesteatomatous ear should ever be considered a safe risk, because both operative interferences for the cure of intracranial complication and post-mortem examination of the cranial contents of those who have died as the result of aural suppuration have shown the presence of cholesteatoma as a causative factor of the death in a large proportion of cases.

If in any case of aural suppuration the external auditory meatus should be occluded to any considerable degree as a result of chronic eczematous thickening of the skin, osteoma of the bony canal, or by the presence of a foreign body, the individual should be considered unfit for insurance. If one or more fistulæ exist in the external auditory canal or over the mastoid surface, the risk should, without question, be regarded an unsafe one, because such fistulæ always lead into the depths of the temporal bone, where there are in progress necrotic processes which are highly dangerous to the life of the individual.

2. In what class of discharging ear, if any, is an individual safely insurable, and what symptoms are indicative of the fact? Also, What pathologic conditions may be present in a discharging ear without serious danger to the life of the applicant?

Without question, there are many suppurating ears which are apt to continue indefinitely without serious risk to the life of the individual; or, at least, the risk is so small that the examining surgeon, could he know the exact pathology, would not hesitate to recommend the acceptance of the case. Unfortunately no intelligent subjective symptom or group of symptoms indicative of either the innocence or danger of the discharge are present in such cases, and, therefore, the deep cavities of the middle ear must be thoroughly inspected and the nature of every condition which is found to be present must be interpreted by an experienced aurist before it should be said that any given case of otorrhea is safely insurable. Briefly stated, if the following conditions exist, the case is one of minimum risk: (a) Cause of discharge primarily due to catarrhal conditions of nose or nasopharynx, and not the result of violent infection from scarlet fever, la grippe, or diphtheria. (b) The character of the discharge mucopurulent and free from blood or odor;

or if pungent odor is present it may be readily checked by antiseptic cleansing. (c) A perforation in the lower half of the drum membrane which is of ·sufficient size to insure efficient drainage. (d) Entire absence of caries, or necrosis of ossicles, or of bone in the middle ear or antrum, and also of exuberant or necrotic granulations. The existence of the above conditions should be ascertained by actual examination, and not by inference or conjecture, before recommendation for acceptance is made.

3. What class of case may be safely insurable after local treatment or after the employment of some surgical procedure instituted for a cure?

In the present highly developed state of the otologic science it may be stated that there are but comparatively few discharging ears that cannot be cured, and the patient, therefore, become an entirely safe risk in so far as the aural disease is concerned. The presence of tubercle, advanced syphilis, or cancer of the ear is here, as elsewhere, often beyond the help of the surgeon, and, therefore, furnishes an exception to the above statement. The well-trained aurist of to-day views a discharging ear from the same standpoint as does the general surgeon any case which is put before him. He asks *why* an ear discharges and has continued to discharge and does not consider himself competent to attempt treatment until he has ascertained the cause. If the "why" is found to be only a lack of aural cleanliness, the cure is easy and the risk safe. If adenoids or nasal obstruction be the cause, the remedy is at hand, is certain of results, and again the risk is good; if a dead ossicle is acting as a foreign body in the ear, setting up granulation, polypi, or bloody discharge, no surgical procedure could be more sensible than its removal, for cure will certainly follow and, therefore, the patient will become safely insurable. Again, if examination has made certain the fact of extensive denudation of bone in the tympanic cavity and consequent caries or necrosis; or, if the formation of cholesteatoma is determined, the radical mastoid operation is of such far-reaching nature that it can be made to include the removal of almost any tissue that is liable to disease from a suppurative process within the temporal bone, and when properly performed and when skilful after-attention is given until the parts are thoroughly healed, the procedure will undoubtedly render the individual safely insurable. It should not, however, be understood that solely because an ear patient has had an ossiculectomy or a radical mastoid operation performed that, therefore, such individual is cured and has become a good risk. The pertinent question in each such case which the examining surgeon should ask himself, and be certain to ascertain, ought to be: "Has the operating surgeon completely removed the diseased tissue

which formerly caused the discharge, has the operative wound satisfactorily healed, and has the aural discharge ceased?" Because in aural
surgery perhaps more than elsewhere the operation which removes all
the diseased parts will usually cure, whereas the operation which fails
in thoroughness fails to cure. In general it may be said, however, that
if after a surgical operation which is instituted for the cure of a discharging ear, that when the ear has remained dry and free from accumulation
for a period of six months preceding the time of the application for
insurance, the risk may be considered safe.

CHAPTER XXXIX

CHRONIC NON-SUPPURATIVE OTITIS MEDIA

Preliminary Statements.—Chronic non-suppurative otitis media is usually described consecutively to the several varieties of acute inflammation of the middle ear. Such an arrangement breaks the continuity in the description of the natural subsequent history of the acute inflammatory diseases of the tympanum, and since this history often begins in a simple catarrhal otitis media, passes through the stages of acute and chronic suppuration, and ends in some complicating aural ailment, as acute or chronic mastoiditis or an intracranial involvement, it has seemed wisest to continue the description of all the suppurative aural diseases to the end without interruption. Should, therefore, this present classification appear to be an unnatural one when viewed from the standpoint of pathology, it is an entirely justifiable one when considered in the interest of the student, who is best served by an unbroken study of all the pyogenic aural affections.

The above title is intended to include the various forms of aural disease which have been described by different writers under the names of "Chronic Middle-ear Catarrh," "Dry Middle-ear Catarrh," "Adhesive Catarrh of the Middle Ear," and "Hyperplastic Middle-ear Catarrh."

The affection usually has its beginning in an acute exudative catarrh of the middle ear which for some reason fails to undergo those processes of resolution necessary for restoration to the normal, and continues into an indefinitely chronic state in which hypertrophy first occurs and, later, true hyperplasia of the structures of the middle ear takes place.

This disease, therefore, when once its natural tendency toward the deposit of new tissue within the cavity of the tympanum has been accomplished, forms one of the most difficult aural problems, in so far as relief or cure of the ailment is concerned. Many patients afflicted with this variety of aural affection represent a condition of neglect on the part of those who had charge of the bringing up of the individual during childhood; for although most of this class of patients are incurable after the disease has persisted into adult life, there *was* a time in the history of most of those who suffer from chronic catarrhal otitis media when

475

treatment, properly directed toward the relief of pathologic conditions existing in the upper air tract of the child, together with proper attention to the Eustachian tube and middle ear, would have either cured or greatly modified the subsequent aural disease. ˙One of the greatest avenues open to the future progress of otology lies in the direction of prevention rather than the cure of this common, but intractable aural disease. One of the unpleasant duties of the aurist is to dismiss daily one or more of these patients after a careful examination has shown the hopeless nature of the case, with an unfavorable prognosis, and the statement that treatment will probably accomplish little or nothing in the way of relief or cure. On such occasions the otologist misses an opportunity for doing future good if he neglects to state to these incurable patients that should they have children or grandchildren who are just beginning to develop an aural ailment they should not be persuaded into the error of letting them "outgrow it."

Pathology.—Chronic catarrhal otitis media is caused by nasopharyngeal diseases, such as hypertrophy, atrophy, hyperplasia of adenoid tissue, and ulcerations. Chronic catarrh of the Eustachian tube may extend to the middle ear, or acute catarrh, after five or six weeks' duration, is called chronic catarrh. Constitutional conditions, anemia, diabetes, and general diseases, such as tuberculosis and syphilis, favor chronic catarrh.

In the middle ear there is the formation of a non-suppurative inflammatory exudate, with deposit of new tissue and consequently resulting in changes in the mucous membrane. The exudate is a mixture of exudate and transudate; the exudate resulting from inflammatory changes, the transudate from the closure of the Eustachian tube, as explained under the chapter on Acute Catarrh of the Middle Ear. From the growth of a new tissue and the collection of exudate plus transudate two forms of catarrh are distinguished: the hypertrophic and the exudative. These two forms cannot be easily separated and blend into each other like colors of the rainbow. The mucous membrane may be very slightly swollen or so much thickened as to completely fill the tympanic cavity. In this latter condition the mucosa resembles the embryonic cushion found in the middle ear of the infant at birth. Instead of affecting all parts of the mucosa equally the swelling may be limited to certain parts; thus, the windows of the labyrinth or only the mucosa around the Eustachian tube may be affected. The exudate is sometimes serous and again of mucoid consistency. The disease may stop in time for reparative processes to take place or it may go on to atrophy of the mucous membrane. Adhesions may have formed and these sometimes cause complete rigidity of the ossicles. Chalky deposits may be found in the mucous membrane, membrana tympani, and tympanic cavity; especially in the membrane of the cochlear window and in the drum membrane.

Causation.—Probably the most frequent cause of this disease is previous and frequently repeated attacks of acute catarrhal otitis media; and it has already been pointed out that the acute affection usually depends in a great measure upon a diseased condition of the nose and nasopharynx, chiefly in the form of adenoids, enlarged faucial tonsils, or a chronic nasopharyngitis. Chronic adhesive middle-ear catarrh may, therefore, be frequently traced to a diseased state of the upper air tract which was allowed to go untreated until late childhood or perhaps was not treated at all, with the result that frequent tubo-tympanic aural congestion occurred, the formation of exudates in the middle ear took place, and ultimately there was a deposit of connective tissue upon the tympanic membrane, about the ossicular articulations, and—most harmful of all—in the pelvis ovalis and upon the foot-plate of the stapes.

Other causes are usually only secondary to the one already mentioned. Thus, heredity is assigned by many as a leading factor in the production of this affection, and without question many instances may be cited of the disease attacking different members of the same family and for several generations.[1]

It is also true that tendencies toward lymphatic enlargement are equally frequent in different members of the same family, and through several generations, and whereas such lymphoid hypertrophy is not always boldly in evidence in every case of chronic catarrhal disease, yet if careful examination of the nasopharynx be made in every instance of chronic catarrhal otitis media, it will be seen that a patch of adenoid tissue exists in the vault of a vast majority of all, and certainly a large enough percentage of cases, to establish the very frequent causative relationship of the one to the other disease.

Patients are, however, seen in whom the most careful examination of the upper air tract will furnish no reasonable explanation for the

---

[1] It is highly probable that many of these cases in which heredity seems to be the chief factor in the causation of this disease, that the ailment is really an otosclerosis and not a dry middle-ear catarrh. Politzer has expressed the opinion that the particular form of progressive deafness which runs its course from its very incipiency without visible evidence of catarrhal symptoms should be regarded as essentially different from aural affections in which the adhesive process is secondary to some catarrhal state. In other words, those cases occurring independently of inflammatory states in the nose, nasopharynx, and Eustachian tube should, more properly, be classed under otosclerosis (see p. 511).

existence of the aural affection. In cases like this, and in those in whose family there is a history of this particular aural disease, the causation may no doubt be justly attributed to heredity.

The exposure to prolonged dampness and cold, which is necessitated by the pursuance of some occupations, is another exciting cause. This, however, is most active in those who are predisposed to frequent cold catching, and, therefore, scarcely applies to those who have healthy throats and strong constitutions. Persons who have nasal or naso-pharyngeal growths or chronic inflammation of the upper air space bear exposure to cold and wet very badly, and it is in this particular class of individuals that connective-tissue deposits are most apt to take place in the tympanic cavity. Certain general diseases, as tuberculosis, syphilis, and anemia, also predispose the individual to this particular aural affection.

Symptoms.—The chief complaints made by the patient are of impairment of hearing and of head noises. Neither of these symptoms are, as a rule, markedly annoying in the early stages of the disease, and the average patient usually ignores both until the aural affection is well advanced, until the function is impaired to an extent that conversation is heard with difficulty, and until such a time as the tinnitus aurium becomes an ever-present and distracting part of the disease. Hence, whereas the patient may honestly state at the time of the first examination that he thinks the disease is of only a few months', or at most only one or two years' duration, yet careful inquiry into the history of the case, together with the evidence secured by a physical inspection of the ear, will prove beyond question that the disease is of many years' standing.

Tinnitus aurium is complained of most bitterly by the patient. In the earlier course of the disease tinnitus is usually present in some degree, but it is commonly intermittent at this period and is seldom of distressing severity except during the acute exacerbation of the ear disease which arises from a head cold or other cause. Gradually, however, in the typic case the head noise becomes louder and the periods of intermission shorter, until in the fully developed case of chronic catarrhal otitis media the tinnitus is constant, usually loud or high pitched, and is always exceedingly distressing to the patient. The character of the sound heard by the patient varies greatly, and seems to be determined, to some degree at least, by the occupation or environment of the individual. Thus the cook may describe the noise as a singing which resembles the steaming teakettle; the engineer will compare it to the high-pressure escaping steam from the locomotive, while those who live in rural districts will often liken it to the noise of insects. Tinnitus aurium is sometimes described as "beating," in which instance it is found to occur synchronously with the pulsation of the heart, and is no doubt due in such case to some disturbance of the arterial circulation within or near the ear. Sometimes it is intermittent and "snapping" in character, and this is due either to the passage of air through the Eustachian tube, which contains thick mucus, or, in rare instances, to the contraction of the tubal muscles which open the orifice—namely, the tensor palati and the levator palati.

The tinnitus is frequently less intense during the early morning hours, while during the day it is to some extent forgotten if the patient is constantly busy and is in the midst of more or less noise, as, for instance, when upon the railway car, in the busy street, the store, or factory. In the evening, however, when all is quiet and the nervous system is somewhat exhausted as a result of the day's exertion, the head-noise is at its height, and in the worst cases the individual is driven by it into a state of semimadness. Such patients are sometimes unable to go to sleep on account of the noise, are sometimes awakened by it in the night, and are compelled to lie awake for hours, only to listen to the incessant confusion of sounds within their own ears. In this state melancholia is common and suicidal tendencies and insanity more rarely occur. *Impairment of function* is always present. The degree of deafness is governed largely by the amount of obstruction in the Eustachian tube, the extent of the deposit of new tissue in the tympanic cavity, and by whether or not the labyrinth is secondarily involved. The deafness, like the tinnitus aurium, is bilateral, although the degree of impairment is usually greatest in one ear. The patient may assert that he hears perfectly in one ear, while the hearing in the other is greatly impaired; but a careful test of the ear which the patient believes is normal by means of the voice, whisper, or other accurate method will often cause the examiner to wonder at the statement, so greatly impaired will the function of this ear be found. The degree of impairment of the function varies greatly in many cases according to the state of the weather, the general health of the individual, and particularly as to the quality of the nerve tone. The hearing will be correspondingly reduced in proportion to the amount of exhaustion from overwork, overanxiety, or from nerve fag due to any cause. Thus, the business man, the student, or the society woman may hear without particular difficulty on arising in the morning, but following a day of strenuous activity along one of these lines the function may be very greatly impaired for all conversational tones. To one who hears badly, the effort put forth to catch every word of the day's conversation that is necessary in the transaction of business or the discharge of social duties is of itself a severe strain upon the nervous system, and one that as a factor in the production of deafness is not always taken into account. These patients often become neurasthenic from a too constant and overanxious effort to understand those with whom business or social affairs may bring them into contact.

A *feeling of fulness in the head* and sometimes of giddiness may accompany the deafness and tinnitus. Rarely faintness and vomiting occur, in which instance the hearing is suddenly and more profoundly impaired and the patient is for a time compelled to remain quiet in bed. These symptoms are occasionally so severe as to simulate Ménière's disease (see p. 529). The occurrence of the latter symptoms indicates increased labyrinthine pressure from hyperemia of the labyrinth vessels or from an actual exudate into the labyrinth.

Pain is a symptom of which complaint is rarely made at any time during the progress of this long-continued affection, and this fact is no doubt chief among the reasons why those afflicted with this form of aural ailment so frequently delay seeking attention until irreparable damage has been done to the ear. The absence of pain is, therefore, an unfortunate circumstance in so far as the results of treatment are concerned, since sufficient suffering does not occur to warn the patient of impending danger and to drive him to seek relief for the aural condition. When pain is at all referred to by the patient it is not usually located in the ear, but more often along the angle of the jaw and over the course of the Eustachian tube; or it may be said to be situated in the throat in the region of the faucial pillars or lingual tonsil. The pain in all these instances is of a neuralgic character and mild type; it is usually produced more by the condition existing in the throat than by the pathologic state within the ear. Occasionally, when there is sudden occlusion of the Eustachian tube, pain of aural origin may occur. The objective symptoms are usually well marked and should be accurately determined in so far as possible at the time of the first examination of the patient, for the reason that the prognosis and treatment will depend in great measure upon the character and amount of the deposit of new tissue that has taken place in the Eustachian tube and drum cavity.

The *appearance of the drum-membrane* varies greatly. It may be thickened or atrophic, translucent or opaque, retracted or normally situated. Chalky deposits are sometimes observed. Adhesions of some portions of the membrana tympani, most frequently at the umbo (see Figs. 286 and 288), are of common occurrence. The drum membrane is also sometimes thickened in one portion, whereas it is atrophic in another.

Opacity and retraction of the membrana tympani constitute the most frequent changes in this structure, and when present in any case which gives a history of long-standing deafness and tinnitus aurium, must be given great diagnostic weight. Opacity of the membrane may exist in the form of a crescent which lies near the annulus tympanicus or it may run parallel to the annulus, but midway between it and the umbo (Fig. 282). Sometimes it consists of an irregular circular, whitish disc of membrane surrounding the umbo. In cases of very long standing the opacity may include all or the greater portion of the membrana vibrans; in this instance the appearance of the entire structure is that of frosted glass or milk-glass, in which can usually be seen the faint outline of the handle of the malleus, leading upward and forward to the short process.

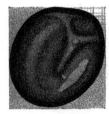
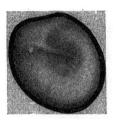

FIG. 282.—CRESCENTIC OPACITY IN POSTERIOR HALF OF MEMBRANA VIBRANS.
Calcareous deposit in anterior half. Shrapnell's membrane greatly depressed.

FIG. 283.—GREAT RETRACTION OF DRUM MEMBRANE AND MALLEUS HANDLE.
Membrane is opaque and milk-white. Landmarks almost obliterated. Case of long standing hyperplastic middle-ear catarrh.

All other landmarks of the drum membrane are obliterated by the hyperplastic process (Fig. 283).[1] Where only partial opacity has taken place, other portions of the same drum membrane may have a nearly normal appearance; or atrophy of some part may have occurred to such an extent that the structures within the middle ear may be clearly visible. Thus, the area lying behind the malleus handle and just below the posterior fold is often so thin that the malleo-incudal articulation can be plainly seen (Fig. 284).

Calcareous deposits constitute one variety of opacity of the drumhead. These may be found single or multiple, may occupy a position before or behind the handle of the malleus, and often lie midway between it and the annulus tympanicus. The lime salts are frequently deposited

[1] The peculiar tendon-white color of the membrana tympani when due to sclerosis is almost unmistakable after it is once recognized. The only other condition for which it might be taken is one of otitis externa, in which necrosis of the dermoid layer of the drum membrane has taken place, is not yet exfoliated, but continues to cover the membrane and gives it a dirty white appearance.

so as to form an opacity of a somewhat semilunar or horseshoe shape (Fig. 285), although it may rarely assume an irregularly circular outline. When viewed by means of reflected light the marked contrast of the dead-whitish, chalky area with the somewhat glistening membranous appearance of opacities of the milky variety will not likely be mistaken for each other.

The extent of retraction that has taken place in the drum membrane varies somewhat with the length of time the disease has progressed. In the earlier stages but little inward displacement may have occurred, but later it may be considerable, and usually forms one of the diagnostic features (see Figs. 286 and 289). The fact that the drum-head occupies an indrawn position is determined largely by the change it causes in the position of the handle of the malleus and light reflex. The malleus handle is usually displaced upward, backward, and inward, but may

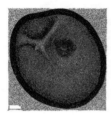

FIG. 284.—PARTIALLY OPAQUE DRUM MEMBRANE WITH SMALL AREA OF ATROPHY OVER MALLEO-IN-CUDAL ARTICULATION.
An outline of this articulation is seen through the atrophic area. The atrophic spot might easily be mistaken for a perforation.

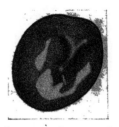

FIG. 285.—CALCAREOUS DEPOSIT IN DRUM MEMBRANE.
Case of long-standing deafness.

rarely be drawn forward by contraction of the newly formed tissue in that direction. When displaced backward the rotation of the malleus upon its axis causes the angular edge of the handle to present toward the examiner, and hence the appearance of the manubrium is narrower and sharper than normal, the umbo occupies a higher plane, and the distance between the umbo and the short process appears very much shortened. The short process appears more prominent and whiter than normal. The light reflex is lengthened and, owing to this fact, seems narrower. It is often broken or multiple (Fig. 286). The posterior fold is exaggerated and sometimes a supernumerary fold extends downward and backward from the short process almost parallel to the handle of the malleus, close to the latter, and is finally lost in the marginal ring.[1] This supernumerary fold (Fig. 287) may be easily mistaken for the

[1] This supernumerary posterior fold has been described by Bing and Pomeroy.

handle of the malleus unless careful examination regarding this point· be made.

When a forward and inward displacement of the handle of the malleus occurs, the latter assumes a more or less perpendicular position, the short process presents directly toward the examiner, and is therefore not so prominent as in the case of posterior indrawing of the membrane. Sometimes, especially during the early history of the affection, posterior rotation of the malleus takes place independent of any retraction of the drum membrane, in which case the manubrium appears abnormally broad (see Fig. 282). But should sinking of the drum membrane occur at the same time as the ossicular rotation, the malleus handle would seem narrowed, as already described (see Fig. 286).

The color of the membrane may remain normal or almost normal during the earlier stages of the disease. Frequently, however, some congestion of Shrapnell's membrane or of the membrana vibrans

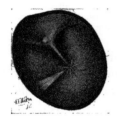

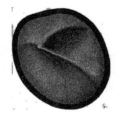

FIG. 286.—GREATLY RETRACTED DRUM MEMBRANE SHOWING SHARP BORDER OF MALLEUS HANDLE, PROMINENT SHORT PROCESS LONG LIGHT REFLEX, AND ADHESIONS AT UMBO.

FIG. 287.—SUPERNUMERARY POSTERIOR FOLD.
Note the position of the handle of the malleus, which appears as a narrow line just in front of this fold. Membrana tensa greatly sunken. Light reflex absent.

along the handle of the malleus occurs. During this period the membrane may at times have a slightly pinkish hue. This is owing to the fact that during the hyperplastic progress of the affection the mucous membrane of the middle ear is greatly congested, and the color of this cavity shows through the semitransparent membrana tympani when illuminated during the examination. The changes in color due to opacities from the deposit of fibrous tissue and calcareous matter have already been described (p. 481). During the earlier or hyperplastic stages of the disease the tympanum may also contain yellowish mucoid exudates which give rise to a yellowish appearance of the drum membrane covering the area below their level in the drum cavity; and the surface level of the exudate is frequently marked by a thin black line (Fig. 137).

Adhesions of the drum membrane may occur between the promontory and umbo (Fig. 288). An adhesion at this point may be suspected when the umbo seems very greatly depressed, even though no other appearance may indicate such an occurrence. Frequently, however, sharply defined bands of fibrous tissue radiate from this point and furnish unmistakable evidence of the fact that the drum membrane and malleus handle are firmly united to the inner tympanic wall at the promontory (see also

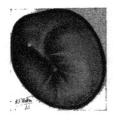

FIG. 288.—ADHESIONS RADIATING FROM THE UMBO AND MANUBRIUM.

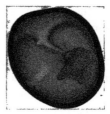

FIG. 289.—SHOWING AN ATROPHIC AREA IN THE MEMBRANE BELOW THE UMBO.
Immediately following the inflation of the tympanum by means of the catheter, this area is seen to bulge outwardly into the external canal like a thin bladder, as shown in Fig. 291.

Fig. 286). Adhesion of Shrapnell's membrane to the neck of the malleus also takes place at times, and this may be recognized by the sunken appearance between the bands of membrane leading to the anterior and posterior spines of the tympanic ring. An adhesion or depression at this point often gives the appearance of a perforation.

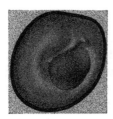

FIG. 290.—ATROPHIC AREA IN ANTERIOR HALF OF DRUM MEMBRANE.
Showing a small point of rupture as the result of tympanic catheter inflation.

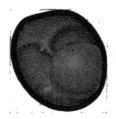

FIG. 291.—BLEB SEEN IN AUDITORY CANAL AFTER CATHETER INFLATION OF TYMPANIC CAVITY IN CASE SHOWN IN FIG. 287.
The atrophic area bulges like an inflated toy balloon.

Atrophic areas in the drum membrane are not uncommon. These are somewhat round or oval, are often surrounded by thickened rims of fibrous tissue, and have very much the appearance of old perforations that have been filled in by the formation of a delicate new membrane. These areas are most frequently found posterior to the manubrium and below the posterior fold (see Fig. 284), or at the umbo (as shown in Figs. 289 to 291). In examining the drum membrane for points of adhesion, for atrophic areas, or for the determination of the condition of the ossicles as to their mobility, the use of Siegle's otoscope (see Fig. 97) is of great assistance. When used for this purpose the attached bulb should first be partially emptied of air, the speculum portion is then inserted into the external auditory meatus so that it fits air-tight, the auricle is retracted in the usual way, and finally, while the fundus of the ear is illuminated, the hand holding the air-bag is relaxed sufficiently to produce suction upon the membrana tympani. If there is no adhesion at any point over the membrana vibrans, and if the ossicles are not ankylosed, the tympanic membrane, together with the handle of the malleus, will be seen to make free and unimpeded outward and inward excursions as the air in the external auditory meatus is alternately rarefied or condensed by the manipulation of the air-bulb. Should some point of adhesion exist, the same may be detected because of its stationary position during the movement of all the adjacent parts. In case there is ankylosis of the whole ossicular chain or of the malleo-incudal articulation, the membrane on either side of and below the handle of the malleus will bulge outward under the influence of the suction exerted by the otoscope, whereas the handle itself will remain stationary.

Atrophic areas in the tympanic membrane may be detected by the same process. Thus, whereas other portions of this structure are displaced only under a rather powerful suction, or perhaps are not at all movable, these thin portions will be disturbed by the very slightest suction from the ball of the otoscope, and if strong suction be made upon them, momentary bleb-like projections will be formed which will mark their size and location with the greatest degree of accuracy.

The *Eustachian tube is more or less stenosed* in the beginning of this affection, and in many cases this condition persists throughout all or a greater portion of the course of the disease. The physical examination must, therefore, include an accurate investigation of this portion of the hearing organ. In this as in every other aural affection the condition of the nose and nasopharynx should also be noted. During the earlier stages of chronic non-suppurative catarrh of the middle ear it will usually be found that adenoids, chronic nasopharyngitis, or nasal disease exists, and even in the more chronic cases of aural disease an inflamed pad of adenoid tissue—the remnants of an adenoid growth in earlier life—may be found. The nasopharyngeal mouth of each Eustachian tube will often be seen in the earlier cases to be thickened, chronically inflamed, and filled with a plug of ropy secretion. As the disease reaches the hyperplastic stage this hypersecretion disappears, the inflammatory redness of the tubal orifice subsides, and the Eustachian mouth frequently appears unduly large and pale.

The patency of the tube can only be accurately determined by the use of the Politzer air douche or, preferably, by means of inflation with the Eustachian catheter. Should the Eustachian tube be greatly narrowed, the sound heard by the examiner through the auscultation tube during the performance of an inflation (see p. 190) will be abnormally high pitched because of the passage of the injected air through an opening which is narrower than normal. If total occlusion of the tube has taken place the inflation sound will be distant and pharyngeal. In many cases of long-standing non-suppurative otitis media the tube is abnormally patent and the air entering through the catheter in great volume is much lower in pitch.

An *accurate functional examination* is essential to correct diagnosis, and, therefore, all the physical tests should be carefully made. The hearing distance for the voice, watch, and whisper will be found reduced in all cases; very much reduced in many, and the various tests are heard with difficulty or not at all in the most advanced forms of this disease. Most patients will hear the whisper test relatively better than the voice. Many who hear quite well if close to a speaker whose words are clearly enunciated, will hear a less carefully trained voice very poorly. Patients will also sometimes hear words distinctly when they are making no particular effort to hear, when, if conscious that tests of the hearing are being made, will entirely fail to distinguish the same words if spoken with equal clearness and intensity.

In uncomplicated cases the hearing for the lower tuning-forks is bad and the lower tone limit is, therefore, said to be raised. Beginning in the series of the Hartmann tuning-forks with C, the examiner may reach C_1 or even C_2 before the patient is able to detect the sound (see Fig. 115). The hearing for high notes is but little or not at all impaired unless labyrinthine complication exists, in which case the high tone limit may be greatly lowered. In uncomplicated cases bone conduction is better than air conduction, and the vibrating C fork when placed on the center of the forehead will be heard better in the worst ear. In making this latter test many patients will declare that they heard the sound better in the good ear, without really thinking in which ear the sound is really louder. They do this largely as a matter of habit and because they think they really ought to hear all sounds better in the good ear. Accurate information can only be obtained, therefore, after repeated trials, and after requesting the patient to observe carefully to which ear the sound seems to go and be heard the louder, before making an answer. In this way the patient will usually detect the error of his former statement at once and will make the proper correction. The examiner should, of course, give no indication as to which ear he thinks the patient will hear the better in.

Prognosis.—The prognosis as to restoration of function and complete relief from the tinnitus aurium is unfavorable in the great majority of cases. During the earliest period of the chronicity of this aural affection and particularly when it has been originally caused by and is yet kept alive because of a coexisting nasal or nasopharyngeal disease, much benefit and sometimes complete cure may be promised as the result of treatment. At a later period, when tissue changes have taken place in the Eustachian tube, and possibly in every part of the tympanic cavity; when these have displaced the various structures comprising the conducting portion of the organ of hearing, and have bound them into an immovable mass, no means of treatment has as yet been devised whereby the new deposits can be absorbed and the contents of the middle ear be thereby restored to a normal condition. Left to nature's course the disease is generally a progressive one, each decade of the patient's life ending with a more greatly impaired function than the preceding one, until, finally, the individual is able to hear only the loudest conversational tones when the speaker is near by. It is a noteworthy fact that the disease when uncomplicated seldom ends in total deafness, this latter condition, as well as the severer forms of defective function, being usually caused by some intercurrent but severe illness in which a labyrinthine complication is developed. Profound deafness may also result from tertiary syphilis should this disease complicate some stage of the adhesive aural catarrh.

The environment and social position of the individual governs to some extent the prognosis; for while the tendency of all cases is to grow gradually worse, there are, nevertheless, conditions of life which cause the progress of the disease to be more rapid than that normally observed. Among these may be enumerated exposure to cold and damp, overwork, either of a mental or physical variety, undue social activity, and constant worry or anxiety. Excessive indulgence in tobacco and liquors have also been enumerated as factors favoring the rapid progress of the disease. Intervals of arrested progress of the disease occur in some individuals; these sometimes last for several months, but finally the disease is resumed with increased severity. Occasionally, however, spontaneous resolution takes place to some degree and the patient finally recovers a serviceable portion of the lost function.

The prospect of material benefit in any case is often a doubtful one. Often those which seem most promising either do not improve at all from treatment or else get worse; on the other hand, material benefit occasionally results from the careful treatment of even the most unpromising aural condition.

Although this class of patients is noteworthy from the fact that for many years perhaps little thought is bestowed by the individual upon the gradual loss of function, nevertheless, when that stage is reached in which conversation is no longer heard with ease and the individual begins to feel that he must soon be ostracised from society, he suddenly becomes highly anxious to secure relief and never fails to solicit a positive statement concerning the prognosis of the case as soon as the first examination is completed. If such an examination has been carefully and intelligently made the examiner should be able to give a statement concerning the probable future of the case that will be almost certainly verified by time. If the disease is not far advanced, if it is yet dependent in a large measure on the presence of nasopharyngeal or nasal disease, and if no labyrinthine complication exists, the patient should be given a prognosis of at least the possibility of arresting the progress of the disease if not of great improvement or cure. Should, however, the drum membrane be adherent to the promontory, the same be thickened and opaque, the ossicles more or less ankylosed, and the Eustachian tube widely open, the prognosis is bad, and slight or no improvement should be promised. Such an unfavorable prognosis is particularly justifiable if, in addition to the above physical conditions, the functional tests should indicate a labyrinthine complication.

The prognosis as to satisfactory relief or cure of the tinnitus aurium is also unfavorable, and particularly so after that period of the disease has been reached in which new deposit of connective tissue has taken place in the tympanic cavity. In the earliest stages, when the tinnitus is partly due to closure of the Eustachian tube by the swollen mucous membrane which lines this channel, or to a congestion of the tympanic mucous membrane with a resulting collection of exudates in the cavity of the middle ear, great relief and frequently cure of the head noises may be promised. When, however, this symptom is due to ankylosis of the foot-plate of the stapes in the oval window and, therefore, occurs as the result of increased labyrinthine pressure from this or other causes, the prognosis should be carefully guarded, because the condition is then not often amenable to successful treatment; and in cases where relief is fortunately experienced the improvement is usually of short duration and the tinnitus quickly returns with its former and sometimes with an increased severity. It is a matter of common observation, however, that in many cases where the disease has been worse in one ear, that after a period of years the perception for the tinnitus seems to be exhausted, and the patient experiences spontaneous relief in that ear. Unfortunately, however, the tinnitus often becomes simultaneously worse in the better ear, in which latter it runs a more violently exasperating course than in the ear first affected.

CHRONIC NON-SUPPURATIVE OTITIS MEDIA (Continued)

TREATMENT

THE treatment consists in efforts to arrest the progress of the disease and to restore as far as possible the affected parts to the normal. More practically speaking, the treatment should aim to restore the impaired hearing and to abolish the intolerable tinnitus.

Should the patient be so fortunate as to consult the aurist early in the course of the disease and, therefore, before sclerotic processes have been established, the first duty should be to restore the diseased nose or nasopharynx as nearly as possible to the normal. It has already been pointed out that hypertrophies or new growths and inflammatory states of the upper air tract are not only the chief causes of the affection in question, but that their continued presence in this location also furnishes the main reason for its continued progress. · All such abnormalities should, therefore, be removed as speedily as possible, since no treatment of the ear alone, however well directed, can prove permanently beneficial so long as a diseased environment of this organ is allowed to remain and to exert a continuously harmful influence upon that organ (see Chapter XIX.).

The character of the treatment of this disease at any stage of its progress should depend entirely upon the pathologic conditions found to be present at the first and subsequent examinations. No set rules of practise can, therefore, be established which would be applicable to every case, for it must be remembered that one patient may be seen by the aurist before the disease is of many months' standing, whereas it may be found that the next patient may have been afflicted for a period of twenty-five years or more. The conditions present in each may, therefore, be vastly different and the methods of treatment must be correspondingly so.

When the Eustachian tube is partly or wholly occluded, the same should, if possible, be restored to its normal degree of patency. The *Eustachian catheter* furnishes the best means of inflating the tympanic cavity, and whereas the patient will receive the benefit of the air which is injected by this method, the operator will also be able to judge, by means of the auscultation tube, the degree of obstruction present. In case the occlusion is due solely to a congestion of the mucous membrane of the tube, as is frequently true in the early stage, and especially when this congestion is due to the presence of nasopharyngeal disease, the repeated inflation of the tympanic cavity will often prove sufficient to relieve the congestion and thereby correct the stenosis of the tube. The free admission of air into the tympanum as a result of the catheter inflation likewise replaces the sunken membrana tympani, empties the engorged venous channels of both the tube and tympanic cavity, and thus this simple measure ultimately restores the lost function and abates the tinnitus. The catheter inflation should not, as a rule, be practised oftener than every second or third day, for the reason that when too frequently performed the aural condition sometimes becomes worse instead of better.

When the inflation of air alone fails to make satisfactory improvement, *medicated vapors* (see foot-note) should be substituted, and the treatment by this means carried out for a period of from four to six weeks. Stimulating vapors may be conveniently substituted for air during catheter inflation by the interposition of a reservoir containing the substance to be vaporized between the cut-off and the catheter. By this means the air current passes over the volatile substance which it is desired to blow into the tympanum before it enters the catheter. Several vaporizing devices are in use. Those of Hartmann and Pynchon are simple, convenient, and efficient. Each consists of a small elliptic shell of glass, metal, or hard rubber, with a fitting at one end for insertion into the mouth of the Eustachian catheter, while in the other end is a receptacle for the nozzle of the air-bag or cut-off. A small amount of cotton is placed in the interior of the vaporizer and on this is dropped a few drops of the stimulating solution which is inserted for the vaporization just before the performance of the inflation.[1]

Dench's vaporizer (Fig. 292) provides an excellent means of inflating the tympanic cavity with medicated vapors. The instrument is so constructed that by merely turning a key in the top of the bottle either air alone or medicated air may be used. This provision is of advantage

---

[1] The substances most frequently employed as stimulating vapors for tympanic inflation are iodin, menthol, camphor, eucalyptol, oil of pine, and chloroform and ether. Iodin is most conveniently used in the form of the official tincture. Combinations of the above drugs are sometimes more efficacious or soothing than one single remedy. The liquid which results from the trituration of equal parts of camphor gum and menthol crystals forms the most convenient method of using these two combined. A few drops of this camphor-menthol solution are dropped on the cotton contained in the vaporizing instrument, and the subsequent inflation of the tympanic cavity is both soothing and stimulating to the auditory tract.

in those cases where there is an oversecretion of mucus, which fills the Eustachian tubal orifice and perhaps extends for some distance inward toward the tympanum. In such instances it is desirable to use air alone until the tube is blown free from mucus, after which the key in the bottle is turned and the tympanic cavity is inflated with the medicated vapor. Should neither of these methods result satisfactorily or should

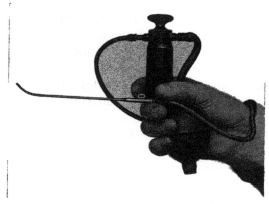

FIG. 292.—DENCH'S VAPORIZER WITH CATHETER ATTACHED READY FOR INSERTION.

it be found that the Eustachian tube is so narrow that but little or on air can be injected through the catheter into the tympanic cavity, the inflation must first be preceded by the passage of the Eustachian bougie (Fig. 293).

The *technic of introducing the Eustachian bougie* should be executed with the greatest precision and gentleness, since otherwise abrasion of

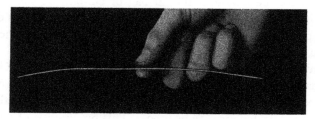

FIG. 293.—EUSTACHIAN BOUGIE.

the mucous membrane of the Eustachian tube may be produced, and subsequently, during the inflation through the tube, a quantity of air may be forced through the rent, under the mucous membrane, and a troublesome or even dangerous emphysema may thus result. All nasal and nasopharyngeal mucus should be first removed by spraying the nose and nasopharynx before the attempt is made to pass the bougie. Particular attention should be given to this latter cavity, especially in the region of the mouth of the Eustachian tube.[1] A Eustachian catheter is selected with a short shank and a beak of long curve (Fig. 106). The caliber of this instrument should be large, in order to permit the passage of the bougie without the necessity of any undue forcing. The bougie is then dipped in vaselin and passed through the catheter until its tip appears at the mouth of the beak, but does not project from it. The catheter thus prepared is next inserted through the nostril in the usual way (see p. 185), and when the beak is known to have entered the pharyngeal mouth of the tube and to fit snugly and deeply into the tubal orifice, the bougie is gently pushed inward through the catheter for a distance not to exceed 1¼ in. (Fig. 294); the distal end of the bougie meanwhile traversing the length of the Eustachian tube. During

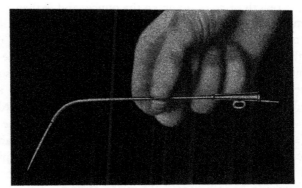

FIG. 294.—BOUGIE AND CATHETER AS SEEN IMMEDIATELY AFTER INSERTION.
The bougie projects from the catheter 1¼ in.

the successful passage of the bougie the patient complains of a slight stinging pain in the ear, neck, or occiput, and sometimes in the teeth, whereas if the bougie has doubled upon itself, as it may sometimes do, and its point has returned into the nasopharynx instead of pursuing the desired course, the patient will complain of the pain in this latter region instead of in the former, as above stated. The chief means of knowing that the bougie has taken the desired course through the Eustachian tube are furnished by the location of the pain during its passage and by the distance of its insertion following the proper introduction of the catheter. In case the posterosuperior quadrant of the membrana tympani is atrophic and semitransparent, an examination of the fundus of the ear while the bougie is in place may

[1] In the very chronic stages of the disease no secretion will likely be present in the neighborhood of the tubal orifices, and the cleansing part of the procedure is, therefore, unnecessary.

reveal the tip of the little instrument in the cavum tympani. When seen under such circumstances the head of the bougie occupies a position slightly below and posterior to the short process of the malleus. Should it be pushed more deeply through the catheter, and consequently further into the Eustachian tube, it would perforate the membrana tympani in this position. When once the bougie has been properly passed through the Eustachian tube it will hold the catheter in place without further assistance from the operator, and in this position it should be allowed to remain for from five to ten minutes in order to secure the full benefit of the dilating force. In cases where the tubal stenosis is due largely to congestion or inflammatory swelling and not to connective tissue or fibrous deposits, better results will be secured from the passage of the bougie if it is first dipped into a solution of silver nitrate of a strength of 30 or 40 gr. to the ounce, and is then passed into the swollen tube and allowed to remain for a few minutes, as stated. In addition to the application of a silver nitrate solution to the whole length of the Eustachian tube, additional good results will be obtained if the same solution be painted over the vault of the nasopharynx, around the lips of the pharyngeal mouth of the tube, and as deeply into the tubal mouth as possible by the use of a cotton-tipped, curved applicator. In making this application the soft palate must be retracted by White's retractor (Fig. 118), and the application is made to the desired areas by means of reflected light and the postrhinoscopic mirror. Iodin and astringent applications may be substituted for the silver if such be thought to be indicated. When the stenosis of the Eustachian tube is of very long standing and is due to the deposit of fibrous tissue, the electric bougie, as advocated by Duel and others, is of greater benefit than the passage of the simple catgut or whalebone instrument.

Whatever may have been the cause of the narrowing or closure of the tube, and whatever may have been the means of relief, recurrence of the trouble is the rule, and it must be expected that the dilation will need repeating after an interval of some weeks or months. Moreover, the same degree of relief is not always obtainable during subsequent treatment that was secured at the first.

In those cases of exudative middle-ear catarrh of the acute variety in which resolution has not taken place and in which the disease has entered the chronic state, this exudate must, if possible, be removed from the tympanic cavity and the attempt be made to prevent its further formation. The methods of dealing with such exudates within the tympanic cavity have already been described in a previous chapter (see p. 247); and the plan of dealing with these products in the chronic form differs in no way from that stated therein, with the exception, of course, that the more chronic the form of the disease the more stimulating must be the treatment and the more persistent the efforts to secure the desired result. The employment of medicated vapors in the middle ear by means of catheter inflation should be, therefore, persistently carried out after the evacuation of the exudate has been accomplished by incision. These vapors prove beneficial through their stimulating action upon the vascular supply to the middle ear. Under their employment an additional inflammatory action is set up in the mucous lining of the cavity, during the subsidence of which absorption of the newly deposited tissue elements takes place. Since these vapors are introduced by means of catheter inflation of the tympanic cavity, much of the benefit arising from this plan of treatment should probably be attributed to the inflation alone.

Dry Middle-ear Catarrh.—After the continuance of the exudative form of the disease for a varying length of time, from one to several years, all catarrhal exudate ceases as a result of glandular destruction and a dense fibrous tissue is formed throughout the middle ear and tube. Owing to the tendency toward the formation of adhesions between adjacent surfaces, the disease is at this period often called adhesive catarrh of the middle ear; and again, because of the absence of secretion, it is designated otitis media catarrhalis sicca, or, as more commonly stated, dry middle-ear catarrh. At this stage all hope of accomplishing a cure must be abandoned and the most that can be expected in any case is to improve the hearing and mitigate the tinnitus; and even this hope is not always realized, for many cases must be dismissed following the first examination with the statement that all treatment would be useless.

The chief methods of dealing with this advanced condition are: Inflation by stimulating vapors, massage of the membrana tympani and of the ossicular chain; general medication, including hygienic measures; and, lastly, surgical procedures directed toward the relief of tension or obstruction due to the advanced adhesive processes.

By the inflation of medicated vapors into the ear it is believed that the adhesive process is often retarded in its progress or is perhaps sometimes arrested and the adventitious products of the disease to a slight extent absorbed. In some instances the hearing is improved by the inflation of these vapors, and the distressing tinnitus is thereby lessened or greatly relieved. On the contrary, however, the opposite effects are sometimes obtained. When improvement is to follow this plan of treatment some increase in the hearing will be noticed by the patient immediately after the first inflation is performed, and some additional gain will probably be observed after each of the next several treatments, following which the gain will become somewhat stationary and will likely remain so during the course of subsequent inflations. Inflation, either of air or medicated vapors, should not be given too frequently or continued for too long a period. The best results will usually be obtained from this method when performed every second or third day. When carried out at these intervals for any greatly prolonged period the patient after a time is apt to grow worse. The term of treatment should, therefore, not usually be longer than six weeks, and often four weeks should be the limit. Certainly if the patient complains of an increase of the tinnitus or of a lessening of the hearing at any time, when improvement had followed the first few treatments, the shorter period above mentioned should be considered the limit. Upon dismissal from such a course the patient should be instructed to continue without further treatment until the hearing is found to be again diminishing, at which time the inflations may be profitably repeated. In any case in which no betterment is secured from the first few treatments, the plan should be abandoned. If made worse by the first inflation this procedure should not be repeated.

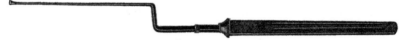

FIG. 295.—LUCAE'S PRESSURE PROBE.
The base of the probe rests upon a spring situated in the handle of the instrument.

Massage of the drum membrane and ossicular chain is best performed in connection with the simultaneous inflation of vapors into the tympanic cavity. Its purpose is to prevent the formation of adhesions between the membrane and inner wall of the middle ear and also to prevent or to break up the ankylosed state of the ossicular chain. The accomplishment of these ends is desirable in all cases and if accomplished even in a small measure, both the hearing and the tinnitus will most usually be benefited. The chief instruments employed for this purpose are some form of Siegle's otoscope (see Fig. 97), Lucae's pressure probe (Fig. 295), and Delstanche's masseur. The first and last-named appliances act upon the drum membrane by means of a rarefaction of the air which their use produces in the external auditory meatus and, as a result of which, the membrane is caused to make outward and inward excursions. Because of the attachment of the ossicular chain to the drum membrane the oscillations produced upon this structure by rarefaction and condensation of the air in the external auditory meatus, also moves the ossicles at the same time. Not every ear in which the adhesive process is present is a proper one for the application of this form of massage treatment, for, as has been already pointed out, the membrana tympani of many of these cases is atrophic in certain areas, whereas the remaining portion may be thickened and adherent to the promontory. The long process of the hammer being thus bound down at its tip, whereas the malleo-incudal joint is firmly fixed by the deposit of fibrous tissue around its articulation, these ossicles are absolutely immovable, and hence any suction exerted upon the membrana by means of any instrument which acts upon the principle of the Siegle's otoscope, will only act upon the atrophic and unattached portions, whereas the hypertrophied areas and the ossicular chain are unaffected by the treatment. Much harm is, therefore, likely to result from the rarefaction of the air in the external auditory meatus, especially if the manipulation be frequently repeated, in all cases where there is either atrophy of the whole or a portion of the membrana tympani. These massage instruments which act through the suction of the rubber hand-ball, as in Siegle's otoscope, or from the exhaust of a small pump propelled by an electric or water motor, are capable, therefore, of doing much harm if indiscriminately employed in this class of disease, for the reason that the suction increases the degree of relaxation in a membrane which is at least in part already too lax. Hence, when conditions of atrophy of the tympanic membrane are present, the use of all instruments of this class is positively contra-indicated.[1] Instruments of this type have been produced in such attractive patterns and alleged utility in the treatment of deafness, that they now form a portion of the armamentarium of many physicians, and the temptation to use them on all cases of deafness, without first having ascertained the exact nature of the disease, and, therefore, without knowing whether or not the particular case is a proper one for suction massage, has been so great that much damage has already been done from this source. The employment of all suction apparatus is positively contra-indicated until, by accurate examination of the membrana tympani, the physician has assured himself that a relaxed drum membrane does not exist.

Lucae's pressure probe acts upon the ossicular chain, and through it upon the membrana tympani. During its use the little cup at the end of the probe is intended to be accurately placed over the short process of the malleus, so that pressure upon the handle of the instrument, exerted by the operator, will move the whole chain of bones. This procedure, even when skilfully executed, is usually quite painful and few patients will tolerate it for any length of time. Lucae

---

[1] Charlatans use the electric suction instrument on every case of deafness regardless of the cause, stage of the disease, or the condition of the membrana tympani.

in his practise wraps a thin layer of cotton over the cup-shaped end and then dips this into ice-water before applying the instrument to the short process. He claims that these precautions very greatly limit the amount of pain produced by the manipulation.

When suction apparatus is employed for the purpose of increasing the mobility of the membrana tympani and ossicular chain, a certain degree of caution must always be exercised by the surgeon in order to avoid actual harm resulting from its ill-advised use or from its overuse. In the first place, no suction apparatus should ever be employed for this purpose unless it is so constructed that the operator is able to actually see the fundus of the ear through the speculum portion, and is thus able to note the effect upon the drum-head of each individual rarefaction that is produced in the external auditory meatus. Siegle's speculum otoscope is, therefore, the best instrument that can be employed for mobilization of these structures, because it is so constructed that the operator can see the exact extent of every movement induced in the whole membrane or in the several segments of the drum-head. By noting precisely the effect of this procedure upon the visible portions of the conducting apparatus the operator may wisely conclude that the membrane is already too much relaxed in whole or in part, that, therefore, massage would be decidedly harmful to the particular case, and that, therefore, this method of treatment should at once be abandoned. It may also be observed through this pneumatic speculum that, whereas the membrana vibrans moves freely under the influence of the suction, the handle of the malleus remains stationary because of adhesions between its tip and the promontory of the middle ear, or because of ankylosis of the malleo-incudal articulation. Persistence in the use of the suction apparatus after this condition is seen to exist will usually result in an increase of damage to the patient's ear. It may also be seen while observing the behavior of the drum-head when influenced by the suction, that whereas both membrana tympani and ossicular chain can be made to move outward and inward at the will of the operator, that a too powerful suction will produce an unnecessarily wide excursion, whereas a weaker suction will produce no excursion at all. The operator will, therefore, be able when using the Siegle pneumatic speculum to accurately judge by actual observation at the instant the drum-head is moved the precise amount of force necessary to produce the desired amount of motion in the membrana and ossicular chain, and by this information will, therefore, be enabled more intelligently to carry out the subsequent treatments. Hence, good result should be expected from the employment of suction massage, only when its use is governed

by the above information concerning the behavior of the drum-head and ossicles when influenced by suction, and as actually witnessed through the pneumatic aural speculum. It is clearly improper, therefore, to use any form of double-suction apparatus which is intended to massage both ears of the patient simultaneously, for the reason that it is impossible for the operator to observe the effect of such treatment upon both ears at the same instant. This topic may be dismissed with the statement that many patients will not be at all affected by suction massage; only a few are improved by its most careful employment and all may be made worse by its indiscriminate and unscientific use.[1]

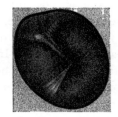

In addition to whatever good effect may result from the massage of the drum mem-
brane by the foregoing method, an increase in the blood supply to the affected parts is induced. Thus, immediately following the manipulations with the otoscope, it will be

FIG. 296.—INDRAWN DRUM-HEAD, SHOWING INJECTED BLOOD-VESSELS ALONG THE HANDLE OF THE MALLEUS AFTER OTOMAS-SAGE BY MEANS OF SIEGLE'S OTOSCOPE.

seen that the blood-vessels along the handle of the malleus become injected and may be traced across the tympanic field, as shown in Fig. 296.

The *internal administration of drugs* is indicated when the patient is anemic, tuberculous, syphilitic, or when the local treatment of the ear has not proved effective for the relief of the tinnitus aurium. Anemia is best combatted by some preparation of iron, taken in conjunction with an outdoor life. The food and exercise of this class of patients should be so regulated as to stimulate the nutritive functions to their fullest physiologic capacity. The tuberculous case which is complicated by this particular class of ear affection must in a general way be treated by the administration of drugs which will improve the nutri-

[1] Another method by which pneumatic massage may be practised upon the drum-head and ossicles has been described by Hommel. This consists of pressing the tragus into the auditory meatus, whereby the air in the auditory canal is condensed, and then quickly relaxing the pressure and allowing the tragus to recover its normal position. The finger of the operator or of the patient is the only instrument necessary for the performance of this method. The movement of quickly forcing the tragus into the meatus and then quickly relaxing the same is repeated one hundred or more times at each daily treatment. If the drum membrane is not greatly thickened or adherent it is stated that some motion can be imparted both to it and to the ossicular chain, and benefit sometimes results from this practise to the extent that the hearing is improved and the tinnitus lessened. Since by it the drum-head is always displaced inward, instead of being lifted outward as is the case when the pneumatic speculum is used, Hommel's method is inferior to the other, and is only suited to home treatment by the patient himself.

tion, and the individual should be encouraged to live as much as possible in the open air and sunshine. If the climate in which he lives is not such as to permit an outdoor life, advantage to the diseased ear, as well as to the tuberculous state will be gained by the removal to a warm, dry, and moderately elevated region. Syphilis affects the ear more frequently than is commonly recognized. In chronic catarrhal otitis media it is most often observed in the tertiary stage of the specific disease and, therefore, the iodids of potassium or sodium are indicated in increasingly large doses and until their effect upon the disease is clearly manifested. If mercury is to be used to improve the luetic aural symptoms it is best employed in the form of an ointment, which should be rubbed into the tissues of the neck once a day for a period of two weeks, then intermitted a week and again repeated, the whole treatment covering a period of six or eight weeks. No doubt much of the good attributed to the mercury when used in this manner is due to the massage of the neck which is necessary in rubbing the ointment through the skin, and, therefore, if the massage be thoughtfully per- formed according to some definite plan the results are apt to be more satisfactory than when the ointment is merely rubbed in.

For the relief of the distressing tinnitus aurium it is often necessary to prescribe some form of internal medication. The drugs most useful for this purpose are the bromids of sodium and potassium and dilute hydrobromic acid. In general, the bromids are more beneficial, because it is frequently the case that the patient who suffers greatly from tinnitus soon becomes highly nervous, sleepless, and often melancholic—condi- tions for which these latter drugs prove especially serviceable. When given for the purpose of relieving head noises the bromids must usually be prescribed in doses of from 15 to 20 gr. one or more times a day. It is found advantageous to give the last dose at least an hour before bedtime and then to repeat the same after retiring if it is found that relief has not been obtained, and that, on account of the continued tinnitus, sleep is impossible. Should the bromids fail to give relief or should relapse occur during their administration, the dilute hydro- bromic acid may be tried in doses of from $\frac{1}{2}$ to 1 dr., freely diluted with water. In the worst cases, when it is found that the preceding remedies are powerless, and the patient is becoming exhausted from worry and the loss of sleep, it is sometimes advisable to try more powerful sedatives or hypnotics, as chloral hydrate or morphin. These latter drugs should, however, be employed only as a matter of urgent necessity and should be withdrawn just as soon as they have produced a temporary rest for the patient. It should be borne in mind that dangerous drug-habits may be easily induced by indiscriminate employment of these powerful remedies for the relief of tinnitus aurium. When medicinal means fail to relieve the tinnitus and the patient's life is made miserable by the continued head noises, surgical interference should be instituted and is under such circumstances entirely justifiable.

In cases where it has been determined by means of a functional examination of the ear that a labyrinthine complication coexists the internal or hypodermic administration of pilocarpin hydrochlorate proves serviceable in some cases, and its use is, therefore, worthy of trial. Of course, the effect is much more certain when given by the hypodermic method, and hence this should be the rule of practise, especially when the patient is too ill to leave the house or if his business will permit him to remain at home and in doors for a few days. The best results will be obtained from this drug when there is present in the labyrinth an increased tension due either to an exudate or to pressure from the footplate of the stapes, as a result of the deposit of new tissue in the pelvis ovalis. The profuse sweating which results from the pilocarpin favors more or less absorption of the intralabyrinthine contents; the pressure irritation upon the perceptive nerve-endings is thereby lessened and the tinnitus and loss of function are in some measure thereby restored. In cases where it is practicable to administer this drug hypodermically this should be done once or twice a day, beginning with the subcutaneous injection of $\frac{1}{10}$, $\frac{1}{8}$, or $\frac{1}{6}$ gr., according to the age and weight of the patient. It is often found necessary to increase the dosage in order to secure the full physiologic effect in the way of profuse sweating. When it is impossible, on account of business or social duties, for the patient to remain constantly indoors during the period of treatment, one hypodermic injection of the pilocarpin may be given at bedtime, and next morning $\frac{1}{6}$ or $\frac{1}{4}$ gr. may be taken by mouth immediately on awakening, so that the period of sweating may be passed before the patient must leave the house. Strychnin sulphate administered by the mouth in doses of $\frac{1}{40}$ gr. three times a day is valuable in those cases which are complicated by labyrinthine disease without evidence of intralabyrinthine pressure. This drug acts as a general tonic as well as a local stimulant to the acoustic nerve and its terminal endings in the organ of Corti. The full effect of this drug upon the ear is often observed only after its administration has been continued uninterruptedly for a period of six or eight weeks. It should then be intermitted for three or four weeks and again repeated as before.

The *influence of climate* upon the adhesive processes of the middle ear after the disease is well advanced is never marked and is usually nil.[1] It is, therefore, seldom wise to recommend a change in this respect unless the disease of the ear is only a complication of some general ailment, as, for example, of pulmonary tuberculosis. In the earlier stages of the aural disease, however, when nasal and nasopharyngeal affections continue to act as exciting causes of the aural affection, a change of residence from a low, damp, and cold region to one which is warmer, dryer, and more elevated, is undoubtedly beneficial. It should be the rule that before such patients are sent to a different climate to remove any adenoid, nasal tumor, or other obstructing growth of the upper air passages, since the climatic effect upon the ear will be much more beneficial if the environment of the ear is free from both obstruction and inflammation.

[1] Black, of Denver, *Trans. Soc. Laryngol. and Otol., A. M. A.,* 1898, states that in his experience non-suppurative inflammation of the middle ear is as liable to progression in Colorado as elsewhere, and that patients have frequently stated that their deafness had markedly progressed since coming to that dry and moderately elevated region.

CHRONIC NON-SUPPURATIVE OTITIS MEDIA (Continued)

TREATMENT BY SURGICAL MEANS

SINCE the pathology of this affection is of such nature that an arrest or cure of the disease through mechanical or medicinal means is seldom or never effected, and since the power of audition finally becomes markedly lessened while at the same time the tinnitus aurium becomes incessant and intolerable, relief from the condition by surgical means has been advocated and practised by many otologists. Unfortunately, the very excellent results that have been reported by Sexton and others have not been secured by other operators, for, with few exceptions, the cases that have been treated by surgical measures have usually resumed their former condition after a short time or have actually grown worse in many instances.

Many of the absolute failures which have followed surgical procedures upon the conducting apparatus have probably been due to the fact that the cases were not properly selected. It is evident that in cases where there is a coexisting labyrinthine affection of marked degree that any operation directed to the removal of obstruction to the sound-waves, which may exist in the conducting mechanism, could not result in benefit to the hearing. On the other hand, if the perceptive portion of the ear remains unimpaired; if the obstruction which exists to the passage of sound-waves can be successfully removed, and the sound impulses be thereby more freely admitted to the perceptive organ, some improvement of hearing and relief from the tinnitus should be anticipated as a result of the removal of such obstruction. It is, therefore, highly essential in all cases where operative measures are contemplated for the relief of deafness due to obstruction in the conducting apparatus to ascertain positively beforehand what damage, if any, has been done by the disease to the inner ear or the perceptive portion of the organ of hearing, and to avoid operations upon the drum membrane or ossicles in the event that perception by bone conductions is found greatly impaired. Chief dependence in ascertaining whether or not nerve deafness is present must be placed upon the results of a carefully conducted functional

503

examination (see p. 193). The various operations that have been advised and practised for the relief of chronic catarrhal otitis media have for their object the relief of tension in the membrana tympani or the ossicular chain, and through these the increased tension within the labyrinth. The operations may be classed as incomplete and complete or radical. Among the former may be placed multiple incision of the drum membrane, division of the anterior ligament of the malleus, incision of the posterior fold, division of the tendon of the tensor tympani muscle, and partial excision of the drum-head. The radical operation consists in the complete removal of the drum-head together with the malleus and incus and of the adventitious tissues that have been deposited in the tympanic cavity during the progress of the chronic catarrh. The more radical operation also frequently includes the incision of the adhesive structures which fill the pelvis ovalis and cover the foot-plate of the stapes, and rarely includes also the removal of this ossicle. Since all of the incomplete operations remedy only a part of the aural defect, and usually not the most essential part, this class of aural surgery is seldom either immediately or ultimately successful. It can be employed, therefore, only in carefully selected cases and is seldom to be advised.

Multiple incisions of the drum membrane have been recommended by Gruber (*Lehrbuch der Ohrenheilkunde*, S. 259) for the purpose of correcting overtension of this structure when the same has been produced by the process of deposit and subsequent organization of connective tissue in the tympanic cavity. This author advocates the incision of the drum-head in four or more places, the direction and location of the cuts being, of course, governed by the position and character of the fibrous bands which are causing the increased tension. Generally, the incisions should radiate from the umbo toward the tympanic ring and, when necessary, other incisions may be made at right angles to the first, and connecting one with another. Sexton states[1] that as many as fifty such incisions may be made in a drum membrane without injury and even to the improvement of function.

The *after-treatment* consists in drying the auditory meatus by, first, the removal of any collection of blood, and of the subsequent insertion down to the fundus of a wick of sterile gauze. Catheter inflation should be performed on the second day and should be repeated every forty-eight hours for a period of ten days or two weeks. The wounds in the membrana tympani quickly heal unless infection occurs, but, unfortunately, whatever improvement may have taken place as a result of the relief of tension usually subsides along with the closure of the

[1] *System of Diseases of Ear, Nose, and Throat*, vol. i., p. 367.

incision. It, therefore, frequently happens that the ultimate result is a worse condition of the ear, both as to function and subjective noises, than existed before the incisions were made.

Partial excision of the drum-head is only one step further toward the radical intratympanic operation, and consists in an effort to secure a permanent perforation through this thickened, calcified, and immovable structure, the object being to provide for the admission of the sound-waves more directly to the perceptive portion of the auditory apparatus. The site chosen for making the window through the drum-head is the postero-inferior quadrant, for the reason that no important structures lie within the cavity of the middle ear at this point. Much difficulty is experienced in permanently maintaining any opening after it is once made, the tendency on the part of nature being to rapidly close the perforation with cicatricial tissue. The opening may be made by turning down and excising a flap of membrane over the area shown in Fig. 297, or the perforation can be established by means of either a corrosive chemical or by the direct application of the electrocautery. When a chemical agent is chosen for this purpose a drop of pure nitric acid is saturated with cocain crystals. A slender aural applicator is selected, its tip is covered by a small pledget of cotton, and this is dipped into the acid-cocain solution. Before it is used this tip is touched to a piece of blotting-paper to absorb any excess of acid and thus to safeguard against spreading of the acid beyond the part to be affected. Under good illumination the acid is carried to the spot on the membrane which it is desired to perforate, and it is pressed firmly upon the same until the acid corrodes the tissue and permits the entrance of the applicator into the

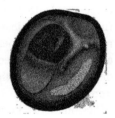

FIG. 297.—EXPLORATORY OPERATION OVER AREA OF INCUDOSTAPEDIAL ARTICULATION.
Showing a flap of the membrana tympani turned down. Same case as shown in Fig. 282.

middle ear. If the electrocautery is chosen the platinum tip of the electrode is inserted against the membrane before the current is turned on. When the tip is in contact the circuit is made, when, if the instrument has been previously tested and the reostat set so that the tip of the electrode will be at cherry-red heat, the opening through the membrane is made almost instantaneously. When using either of the above methods the operator must be cautious not to injure the structures within the tympanic cavity. One chief value of partial excision of the membrana tympani is that through this procedure it is possible to determine the effect upon the hearing that results from the free admission of sound-waves to the foot-plate of the stapes. It may, therefore, be looked upon somewhat as a diagnostic measure and one which is preliminary in suitable cases to the performance of some more radical procedure.

Division of the posterior fold, sometimes called **plicotomy,** is now and then made for the purpose of relieving the subjective noises and improving the hearing. The operation is indicated when the fold is unduly prominent and sharp, forming a sickle-shaped ridge between the short process and the annulus (see Fig. 287), since the condition is found in cases where there is great retraction of the drum membrane with resulting increase of tension. The operation may be performed by means of the paracentesis knife (Fig. 141), the division of the fold being made a short distance posterior to the short process of the malleus. It should be borne in mind that the chorda tympani nerve lies just within this fold (see Fig. 297), and the operator will, therefore, avoid injuring it, if possible, by not cutting more deeply than is necessary. However, it has been elsewhere stated that division of this nerve results in nothing more serious than a temporary loss of taste on that side of the tongue which corresponds to the wounded nerve. No after-treatment is necessary further than the insertion of a sterile gauze wick into the external auditory meatus, and the performance of catheter inflation on alternate days for a period of two weeks. The result of the division of the posterior fold depends upon whether or not the intratympanic structures are or are not immovably fixed. If the ossicular chain is not ankylosed and if no adhesions exist between the drum membrane and the tympanic walls, marked improvement may result. Politzer[1] states that this improvement is not permanent and that after several months have elapsed the former condition of the ear is resumed.

Tenotomy of the tensor tympani muscle was first performed by Weber-Liel in 1868, since which time it has been employed by many otologists. The indication for the division of the tendon of this muscle is based upon the assumption that the cause of the greatly retracted drum membrane, together with the symptoms of deafness and tinnitus aurium, is due largely or wholly to a contracted state of the tensor tympani muscle. Since in chronic non-suppurative catarrh of the middle ear other pathologic conditions, in the form of organized new tissues, are present which bind the ossicular chain and membrana tympani into an immovable mass, it must be clear that a mere division of the tendon of the tensor tympani muscle will not effect a restoration of the structures of the conducting apparatus to either their normal position or to a normal state of mobility. The principle of the operation

[1] *Diseases of the Ear,* p. 306.

is, therefore, based upon a false assumption, and the results of its performance have not been such as to commend it to further use.

Under the section which treats of the pathology of this disease it has been shown that as the affection advances the deposit of new tissues takes place in the tympanic cavity and membrana tympani, and that ultimately the whole conducting apparatus may become so immovably fixed as to provide an actual obstruction rather than an ideal means of conduction to the passage of sound-waves. It is evident, therefore, that none of the foregoing operations which are intended for the correction of only one of the actual conditions present in this conducting apparatus, will prove sufficient to overcome in more than a slight degree the real difficulty. Hence, when surgical intervention is determined to be the proper procedure in this class of cases, it is usually wise to attack the diseased structures in a radical manner and to remove the whole membrana tympani, together with the malleus and incus.

The *technic* of this operation consists in first sterilizing the external auditory meatus and then securing anesthesia either through the administration of a general anesthetic or by the application of cocain directly to the field of operation. The rules governing the employment of the one or the other method of anesthesia are given on p. 245. The following addition should, however, be made to what is there said concerning cocain anesthesia: The membrana tympani, in all cases of dry middle-ear catarrh in which operative measures are indicated, is intact and often greatly thickened. Anesthesia of the operative field by the local application of cocain is, therefore, impossible until an opening of sufficient extent has been made through this membrane to admit the anesthetic solution into the cavum tympani. Aside from the position of the patient, which is erect during the operation under local anesthesia and semireclining under the general anesthetic, the steps of the operation by either method are exactly the same.

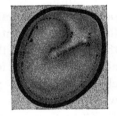

Fig. 298.—Lines of Incision through Membrana Tympani in Ossiculectomy.

With the delicate, sharp-pointed knife (see Fig. 141) an incision is made through the tympanic membrane in the position and to the extent shown by the dark line AB in Fig. 298. A probe-pointed knife (see Fig. 218) is then substituted, and the cut is carried upward to the posterior fold, thence forward along this fold to the short process, thence downward along the manubruim to near the umbo, the whole incision following the course shown by the dotted line in Fig. 298. The flap thus provided is turned down (as shown in Fig. 297) and the site of the incudostapedial articulation is thus exposed.   If care has been exercised when using the sharp-pointed knife for making the initial incision not to insert it too deeply and thereby wound the mucous lining of the middle ear, and if the subsequent course of the probe-pointed knife is not continued too near the annulus tympanicus, but very slight or possibly no bleeding will result from this part of the operation and, consequently, the contents of the exposed portion of the middle ear will be clearly visible.   Division of the stapedius muscles constitutes the next step, which is accomplished by passing the sharp-pointed knife above and posterior to the head of the stapes, pressing it firmly inward against the osseous tympanic wall, and then cutting downward until the tendon is severed.   Immediately following the division of the tendon of the stapedius the head of the stapes should be disarticulated from the long process of the incus, which step is performed by inserting the angular knife between the long processes of the hammer and incus to such a depth that when the handle of the knife is rotated backward the angular blade will fall into a position internal to the long process of the incus, which latter process the blade of the knife should be caused to hug, following it downward as a guide until the joint is reached and severed by the cutting edge.

Following the disarticulation of the stapes and incus the probe-pointed knife is again inserted below X (Fig. 297) and carried around the umbo to the anterior border of this process, and upward as far as the short process of this ossicle.   The knife can then either be continued along the anterior fold, first to the annulus, and following this in the clear membrane to point B, the beginning, or it may be withdrawn when the annulus is reached and reinserted at point B, the reverse course, B, X″ to X, being followed (Fig. 297).   In either case the whole membrana vibrans is thus detached and can be removed.   Should any bleeding occur, pressure upon the bleeding areas may now be made by the insertion into the fundus of a cylinder of cotton saturated with adrenalin chlorid, which is allowed to remain for a moment, or until the hemorrhage is arrested.   The next step consists of the division of the anterior and posterior ligaments of the malleus, which is accomplished by the insertion of the sharp-pointed knife, first, just posterior to the short process of the malleus and then anterior to this process, and in each instance pushing the blade inward to the internal osseous wall, and then depressing the handle to such a degree as to cause the blade to rise sufficiently to completely sever the respective ligaments.   If thought desirable the tendon of the tensor tympani may be next divided, but usually this is unnecessary since this, together with the suspensory, external, and annular ligaments, the only remaining supports of the ossicle, readily yield to the slight force which is subsequently necessary to withdraw the bone by traction. The ossicle is, therefore, at once seized by its neck between the jaws of a strong, though delicate forceps (see Fig. 219), upon which traction is first made in an inward and downward direction until the ossicle is dislocated into the atrium, after which it is withdrawn through the external meatus.

Because of its ligamentous attachment to the incus the removal of the malleus by traction usually dislodges the former ossicle from its normal position, and hence when it is subsequently sought for it is often found to have been dragged downward and backward, and to occupy a position in the postero-inferior quadrant of the tympanic cavity. If any portion of the bone can be seen in either a normal or abnormal position, the same should be seized by the forceps and the ossicle at once be withdrawn. In case the ossicle cannot be seen it becomes necessary to search for it, bring it into view, and then remove it. For the purpose of bringing this ossicle into view when once it has been dislocated and lost, the incus hooks, right and left (see Fig. 220), must be used. One of these, the convexity of whose curved extremity looks backward, is selected and is inserted into the tympanum beyond the tympanic ring and with its convexity lying upon the floor of the middle ear. The instrument is then withdrawn until the outer surface of the angular hook hugs the adjoining portion of the tympanic ring. In this position rotation of the handle of the hook is made, beginning with the concavity of the hook looking upward, and continuing until the hook has made a complete circuit of the tympanic cavity, and, therefore, ends with the concavity of the hook looking downward. Throughout the entire circuit of the hook around the tympanic cavity it should be held so that it constantly hugs the tympanic ring. It will be obvious that when search is made for the incus by using the incus hook after the method just described that it would be impossible to dislodge the ossicle backward into the mouth of the aditus ad antrum, an accident which it is desirable to avoid. However, if the incus is not found by this first hook, the one of opposite curvature should be used to explore the cavity of the middle ear in an exactly opposite direction to that just described. By carefully following these rules for extraction it is scarcely possible not to bring the ossicle into such position that it can be clearly seen and easily removed by the forceps.

After drying away any blood that has again collected in the auditory meatus and middle ear, it is usually possible to see the head and at least

a portion of the crura of the stapes. An examination of this ossicle·
constitutes the next consideration, since it is important to know whether
or not it is movable or is fixed by adhesive bands of connective tissue
running between the crura and adjacent walls of the pelvis ovalis, or possibly by the deposit of fibrous tissue about the foot-plate in the oval
window. These facts may be ascertained by means of a delicate, though
resisting, cotton-tipped applicator, which is pressed firmly against the
head of the bone from all sides, while at the same time it is noted whether
or not any movement of the ossicle results therefrom. Should the ossicle
be found to be immovably bound down and the position of the pelvis
ovalis can be seen with sufficient clearness, the attempt may be made to
mobilize it by severing the adhesive bands which hold it in place. This
may be accomplished by passing the sharp-pointed knife around the
crura of the stapes and to a depth corresponding to the annular ligament
of the foot-plate. The whole ossicle, with the exception of a portion of
the foot-plate, having thus been liberated, a delicate hook is inserted
between the crura by means of which a rocking motion is given to the
ossicle to insure its complete mobilization. It is seldom necessary or
justifiable to remove the stapes, for the reason that if it be properly
mobilized equally good results will follow and labyrinthine suppuration
is a possibility after its extraction.

The *after-treatment* consists in the insertion into the middle ear of
a strip of sterile or borated gauze which should loosely fill the middle ear
and external auditory meatus. Several thick pads of gauze are placed
over the concha and external ear and the dressing is completed by the
application of a roller bandage (Fig. 225). This dressing may be
allowed to remain for one or more days, according to whether or not it
becomes soiled or whether or not pain occurs of sufficient severity to
necessitate an earlier change. If the antiseptic technic at the time of the
operation has been perfect and the subsequent treatment is carried out
with equal care as to cleanliness, suppuration during the process of
epidermization of the exposed drum cavity may be avoided. Since,
however, the continuance of an ideal technic is seldom possible, infection
sometimes takes place, suppuration results, and the treatment should
then be upon the plan of that advised for an acute purulent otitis media
(see Chapter XXIII.).

The *results* of the operation will depend much upon the diagnostic
care with which the cases are selected and upon the skill with which the
obstructive tissues are removed. No improvement will result in any
operated case in which the obstruction to the conducting apparatus is
seriously complicated by labyrinthine affection. In other words, the

more purely the case is one of defect due to hindrance of the passage of sound-waves through the middle ear, the better the results of intratympanic surgery are likely to be. It may be stated that in the main the very favorable results that were obtained by earlier operators[1] are not secured by all those at present engaged in the practise of operative otology. Among the latter it should be stated, however, that Dench has maintained in a commendable way the record established by Sexton and others.[2]

It has usually been found that even those who were most favorably affected immediately after this operation have ultimately resumed their former condition, and in many instances even a worse state than before the ossiculectomy was performed. In all cases there is a tendency toward the re-formation of the drum membrane and in a few months its regeneration is often complete. When this occurs the hearing again becomes worse and it is necessary a second, and even a third time, to excise the regenerated part. Each newly formed membrane is, however, found to be thinner and more insensible than its predecessor and its excision becomes, therefore, a more increasingly trivial matter.

Otosclerosis.—This name has been given to a form of progressive middle-ear deafness which closely simulates that of adhesive catarrhal deafness in every particular except the pathology. In many cases of otosclerosis the tympanic mucous membrane and the membrana tympani are absolutely normal, the sole pathologic change being found in the pelvis ovalis, around the foot-plate of the oval window, and in the labyrinthine capsule. The chief pathologic feature of the disease, therefore, consists in a deposit of osseous tissue on the promontory and walls of the pelvis ovalis, whereby the niche of the oval window is more or less obliterated and in and around the foot-plate of the stapes, with the result that the stapes becomes immovably fixed in the oval window (Figs. 299 and 300).

This osseous deposit may be in sufficient amount to greatly thicken the foot-plate, to obliterate its ligament, and to extend to the adjacent capsule of the labyrinth. In such instance all lines representing the articular boundary of this ossicle in the oval window are obliterated,

---

[1] "The results of the operation have, in the author's experience, been most gratifying. Not only is a stop put to the progress of the disease, but the hearing power usually shows an increase, which, in some instances, is marked indeed. The tinnitus, too, usually disappears altogether."—Samuel Sexton in *Burnett's System Ear, Nose, and Throat*, 1893.

[2] "Of cases where the membrana tympani was intact, including one or two instances in which there had been a suppurative process in childhood, with complete closure of the perforation, 90 have been subjected to operation. Of these there was much improvement in 78 cases, 10 were unimproved, 1 grew worse after operation, and in 1 the result was unknown."—Dench, *Diseases of the Ear*, 1903.

and this portion of the bone is completely amalgamated and buried, so to speak, by the deposit of the adventitious osseous tissue (Fig. 300). The recess of the round window is also sometimes encroached upon,

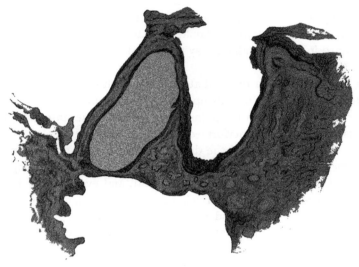

FIG. 299.—DEPOSIT OF OSSEOUS TISSUE UPON THE FOOT-PLATE AND CRUS OF THE STAPES, CAUSING PARTIAL ANKYLOSIS OF THE OSSICLE IN THE OVAL WINDOW. (After Politzer.)

with the result that it becomes greatly narrowed or, perhaps, entirely obliterated.

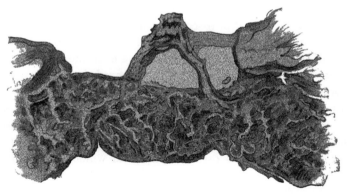

FIG. 300.—SHOWING OBLITERATION OF THE OVAL WINDOW AND PARTIAL FILLING OF THE PELVIS OVALIS BY THE DEPOSIT OF NEW OSSEOUS TISSUE.
The stapes is almost submerged by the deposit and its foot-plate and a portion of the crura are amalgamated with the surrounding structure. (After Politzer.)

The Causation of Otosclerosis.—As factors in the production of this disease hereditary syphilis, faulty states of the blood, and the age of the individual may be mentioned. Many cases develop without any assignable reason. When several members of one family develop a non-suppurative deafness, and when a catarrhal tendency in such individuals can be eliminated, the disease has been found to be one of otosclerosis rather than adhesive middle-ear catarrh. Acquired syphilis is one of the most frequent causes and the disease sometimes follows the hereditary variety. The affection is most frequently found in those past middle life and, according to some observers, occurs oftener in women than in men.

Symptoms and Diagnosis.—The subjective symptoms are much the same as in the adhesive variety of catarrhal deafness just described. A progressive loss of hearing is a most constant symptom, each year the patient becoming more and more hard of hearing until, finally, the speaking voice is heard with difficulty or not at all. While the labyrinth remains unaffected the patient may continue to hear with satisfaction the singing voice or the instrumental musical note long after the speaking voice cannot be heard. In otosclerosis the varying conditions of the weather do not exert as much influence over the failing powers of audition as is the case when a catarrhal process is the chief causative agent of the affection. The individual hears as well, therefore, in winter as in summer and on damp as well as on bright, dry days. The patient often hears better when riding on a railway train or when in some noisy place like a mill than where all is quiet. Such patients may, therefore, be able to carry on a conversation with so much ease under such circumstances that one who is not aware of the deafness might not then suspect it, whereas, when all is quiet the same person is able to hear only the loudest conversational tones.[1]

Tinnitus aurium is probably never absent in otosclerosis and constitutes the symptom of which greatest complaint is usually made. The head noises reach the height of their intensity in this particular disease, and the patient is often driven to the verge of madness by the incessant ringing or buzzing in his ears. Except in their greater intensity, these noises differ in no respect from the tinnitus which accompanies the adhesive catarrhal processes. Pain is an infrequent symptom and is present only in the early stages of the disease and is never severe. Nervousness and neurasthenia finally occur as a result of the tinnitus; and vertigo, due to increased labyrinthine pressure, is sometimes among the symptoms of the fully developed disease.

[1] The ability of partially deaf individuals to hear better in a noise is a symptom which has been described under the name paracusis Willisii. The ability to hear better under these circumstances is usually regarded as a symptom denoting an advanced stage of the aural disease and one not amenable to successful treatment.

33

Objective Symptoms.—The membrana tympani will usually be seen to occupy a normal position and with all its landmarks clearly visible. Sometimes, however, the tympanic membrane is opaque and thickened and calcareous or atrophic areas may be seen upon it. The external auditory meatus is often narrow, collapsed in the aged, and the skin lining this canal is abnormally dry and hard. The nasopharynx, pharynx, and nose are usually free from obstruction or inflammation, but sometimes an atrophic state of the membranous lining is observed and ozena is not infrequently coexistent with the otosclerosis. The nasopharyngeal orifice of the Eustachian tube is seen by postrhinoscopic examination to be widely open and the mucous structures about it to be pale, atrophied, or of fibrous appearance. Upon catheter inflation it is found that the whole Eustachian tube is abnormally patent, and the air enters the tympanic cavity in great volume and without hindrance.

The diagnosis will be based upon the above facts which are obtained from the history of the case, from the physical examination of the external and middle ear, and of the nose, nasopharynx, and Eustachian tube. The main facts upon which reliance in diagnosis can be placed are: The history of a progressive deafness which is accompanied by intolerable tinnitus aurium, in which the deafness is but little or not at all affected by climatic changes; in which heredity and not a previous catarrhal state of the upper air passages seem to form the most rational explanation of the disease; and, finally, the physical examination, which shows the drum membrane to be normal and the Eustachian tube to be abnormally patent. In cases where the drum-head is cloudy and thickened and in which evidences of former inflammatory states of the respiratory mucous membranes still exist, the diagnosis of otosclerosis cannot be made with certainty. Instances of hereditary or acquired syphilis, which are accompanied by all or a majority of the above symptoms, may, with much certainty, be considered as diagnostic of the aural disease in question.

The *prognosis*, in the present imperfect state of our knowledge concerning the treatment of otosclerosis, must be considered most unfavorable. This is not surprising in view of the fact that the pathology of the disease is of such nature and is in such inaccessible situation as to render efficient treatment almost if not quite impossible. Any improvement that may occur as the result of treatment is likely to be of short duration, and the former condition frequently recurs, oftentimes with an increased severity. In a few cases the head noises either exhaust the perceptive centers for their particular tones or else the patient becomes accustomed or resigned to their presence, for in some instances the patient, after a long period of endurance, will cease to complain of this once intolerable and ever-present symptom.

Treatment.—Whereas the past few years have witnessed remarkable advances in both the therapy and surgery of the ear, little has been accomplished toward the cure of otosclerosis, and the otologist is, therefore, just as helpless in the management of this disease to-day as he was a generation ago. Between the years 1885 and 1900, many aural surgeons were busy perfecting operative procedures whereby this disease could be ameliorated or cured. During this time encouraging reports were published concerning the results of these operative measures, and high hopes were expressed to the effect that relief is possible through surgical methods which removed or at least mobilized the stapes, since the accomplishment of this end did away with the hindrance to the passage of the sound-waves through the foot-plate of the stapes. Later reports of these same operators as to the value of otoscleronectomy show, almost without exception, that the improvement which was at first brought about was of a temporary nature and that often the patient was, as a result of the operative measure, made worse both as to the degree of deafness and the intensity of the tinnitus.

In view of the fact, however, that many of these cases when treated only by medicinal or local means other than surgery, progress rapidly to a high degree of deafness, and are annoyed beyond human endurance by the distressing tinnitus from which other means of relief are unavailing, it seems cruel to deny the patient even the temporary relief from those conditions which is sometimes obtained by the removal or mobilization of the stapes (see p. 510). When this operation is undertaken it should be remembered, however, that it is not always possible, because of the welding of the foot-plate into the oval window, which has taken place as the result of the osseous deposit about it (Fig. 300), and the consequent thickening of the bone in this location, to remove the foot-plate without running a risk of great damage to the labyrinth. An infection of the contents of the vestibule, with subsequent suppuration of the labyrinth, occurring as the result of unwise or unskilful attempts to remove the bony deposit in the oval window, would result in vastly more suffering to the patient than would the continuance of the original disease.

The inflation of the Eustachian tube by air, either plain or medicated, or the injection of fluids into the tube, is usually either entirely ineffective or even harmful. Politzer states that pneumomassage of the external auditory meatus, practised in the early stages, is capable of bringing about good results. It must be conceded that any such method when employed after the stapes has become imprisoned in the oval window from the deposit of new osseous tissue will prove e effective and useless.

In the early stages, particularly if a specific origin of the probable, the internal administration of the iodids of sodium sium for a considerable period of time has proved serviceat fixation of the stapes has taken place, however, it is not p affect the course of the disease by any therapeutic measure.

CHAPTER XLII

DISEASES OF THE PERCEPTIVE PORTION OF THE HEARING APPARATUS

General Consideration.—Affections of this portion of the organ of hearing include the vestibule, semicircular canals, cochlea, auditory nerve, and the center in the brain of this special sense. This portion of the ear is commonly known as the labyrinth, and the diseases affecting it are, therefore, properly designated as labyrinthine.

Owing to its protected situation in the depths of the petrous portion of the temporal bone, disease of the inner ear is much less frequently observed than in the tympanic cavity and its accessory air spaces. Primary labyrinthine affections are comparatively rare, but ailments of the perceptive apparatus, occurring secondary to diseases of the middle ear, are more common and constitute a majority of the diseases of the inner ear.

Causation.—Labyrinthine disorders are usually the result of an infection, which may act either through the general circulation or else they are of local origin and extend inward from the cavity of the middle ear by way of the oval or round window; or the extension may be outward from the cranial cavity, the infection finding its way into the labyrinth through the internal auditory meatus, ductus endolymphaticus or aqueductus cochleæ. Infection may also occur as a result of caries or necrosis of some portion of the osseous labyrinth, in which case the pathogenic bacteria, which are present in the suppurating ear, find direct entrance into some portion of the inner ear. As examples of infection and disease of the labyrinth occurring as the result of a general disease, the frequent aural complications of mumps, typhoid fever, diphtheria, etc., may be cited. The auditory nerve is particularly prone to injury as a result of the presence in the circulation of the morbid poisons of the infectious diseases. Extension of the morbid processes of the middle ear due either to suppuration or the deposit of non-suppurative tissues is often observed. It has already been stated (p. 479) that disease of the perceptive mechanism is a common complication of chronic non-suppurative middle-ear catarrh, and especially is this true in those cases in which there is fixation of the foot-plate of the stapes in the oval

517

window as a result of the deposit of connective or osseous tissue in this location.

Certain neuroses are also at times accompanied by deafness, the nature of which is closely associated with diseases of the perceptive mechanism. This condition is most frequently witnessed in individuals whose systems have been weakened by prolonged disease. No visible evidence of any aural affection can be made out in such cases, but the hearing power is nevertheless greatly impaired, the vibrating tuning-fork is heard poorly by bone conduction, and the most reasonable explanation of the trouble lies, therefore, in the assumption that the acoustic nerve or its terminal filaments are, for the time at least, so exhausted that they are no longer capable of normal response to auditory stimuli.

Traumatism is also responsible for some cases of diseases of the internal ear. The labyrinthine affection which follows an injury will usually bear some relation to the force and extent of the injury. Hence, the resulting impairment of hearing with its accompanying tinnitus, and possibly with vertigo and nausea, may be of a mild nature and of short duration, whereas, if fracture of the base of the skull has occurred, and the petrous portion of the temporal is involved, hemorrhage into the the labyrinth, with subsequent infection, may take place; and, should the patient survive long enough, suppuration and complete destruction of the labyrinthine contents may occur. Injury to the labyrinth may also follow the sudden and powerful condensation of air in the external meatus, as, for instance, that which takes place when terrific explosions occur in close proximity to the individual. In such instances the foot-plate of the stapes is driven against the fluid of the vestibule with such suddenness and violence that the entire contents of the laby-rinthine capsule must inevitably suffer as a result. In such cases the middle ear is usually more or less damaged and the drum membrane may be ruptured, particularly if it has already been weakened by previous disease. Another, though infinitely slower, cause of injury by concussion occurs in the presence of continuous and moderately loud noises. From such a cause arises that form of labyrinthine disease commonly known as boilermaker's deafness, although the same affection may be acquired elsewhere than in boiler-shops, as, for instance, in driving railway locomotives.

The cause of many diseases of the perceptive portion of the ear are due to an extension of a previously existing middle-ear disease. Thus, many aural suppurations are at first confined entirely to the tympanic cavity, but in the course of their progress finally implicate the labyrinth-ine structures. The same is true of some cases of the non-suppurative variety of middle-ear catarrh, which disease may for a long time be limited to the conducting portion of the hearing organ, but may ultimately affect the perceptive apparatus because of the injury which results to the foot-plate of the stapes from the deposit of fibrous or osseous tissue upon and around it. In all instances where the labyrinth is secondarily involved as a result of previous diseases in the middle ear, the aecompanying impairment of hearing is designated a *mixed deafness*.

Symptoms.—Since the internal ear is endowed with the function of regulating the static equilibrium as well as of providing the means of sound perception, it follows that deafness is present to a greater or less extent in every case of labyrinthine disease, and disturbance of equilibrium is a symptom in many. When produced by trivial causes, as, for instance, the pressure of hardened ear-wax in the external auditory meatus, the degree of deafness may be slight and will completely disappear upon the removal of the cause and the consequent restoration of the disturbed intralabyrinthine pressure. On the contrary, however, the impairment of the function may be complete and permanent, as happens when there is a total abatement of function of the auditory nerve for any cause. Between these two extremes every degree of impairment of function exists. As a rule affections of the inner ear are progressive, and although the amount of deafness is but trivial in the beginning, in the course of a few months or years the loss of function is sufficient to interfere with hearing the speaking voice and may make it impossible to hear the ordinary voice. Occasionally the progress toward profound deafness is for a time arrested, only to resume at some subsequent period when the individual may, perhaps, be suffering from some general and exhaustive bodily ailment. Some degree of hearing for loud sounds persists so long as the disease is confined exclusively to the labyrinth, and hence complete absence of the perception of sound in any case is certain evidence of the existence of disease of the trunk of the auditory nerve or of the auditory center in the brain.

Certain perversions of hearing sometimes accompany the deafness. Thus, several forms of paracusis have been noted, chief among which may be mentioned diplacusis, paracusis acris, and paracusis loci. The first of these perversions represent a state of auditory perception in which the diseased ear hears a given sound either abnormally high or abnormally low. Hence the individual is capable of recognizing two sounds of different degrees of intensity when only one should be normally heard. Paracusis acris is a term applied to the auditory state in which the individual perceives sounds with a greater acuity than normal. In other words, there is an acoustic hyperesthesia and the sounds are often productive of painful auditory sensations. This auditory phenomenon is usually accompanied by an oversensibility of other special sense organs, and hence, the vision, smell, and taste may be simultaneously acute. These perverted sensibilities are sometimes harbingers of approaching deafness and serious cerebral disorder. In the case of paracusis loci the individual is no longer able to determine in any degree the direction from which any given sound emanates.

Disturbances of equilibrium form one of the most prominent symptoms of many cases of labyrinthine disease. It is a well-known clinical fact that any condition arising in the hearing apparatus, which increases the pressure of the intralabyrinthine fluids, will produce a greater or less degree of giddiness of the individual. Causes acting from without are principally those which act upon the foot-plate of the stapes, drive it inward, and perhaps fix it in an abnormal position through the deposit of connective or osseous tissue in this locality. Hence vertigo is a common symptom of otosclerosis, adhesive middle-ear catarrh, and, less frequently, of chronic suppurative otitis media. It may even result from such simple ailments as closure of the Eustachian tube in tubotympanic catarrh or from the pressure of hardened wax against the tympanic membrane. In all of these instances the vertigo is secondary to influences transmitted from without through the medium of the conducting apparatus.

Within the labyrinth itself vertigo arises from increased pressure and irritation due to a variety of causes, among which may be mentioned hyperemia, primary inflammation with effusion of serum, hemorrhage into any portion of the membranous labyrinth, and infection, either through the general circulation or by the direct introduction into it of pathogenic bacteria from the middle ear or cranial cavity.

Physiologists are practically agreed that the semicircular canals, and especially their ampullæ, have to do with the maintenance of the bodily equilibrium. Hence it should be expected that disease of this portion of the inner ear will give rise to the most severe examples of aural vertigo. Nausea and vomiting at times accompany the dizziness, which in its worst form may be sufficient to compel the individual to remain quiet and in bed. Tinnitus aurium is seldom absent in any case and is due to the same causes which produce the vertigo. Like the latter, these causes are due to disturbance of the normal position of the foot-plate of the stapes in the oval window, or to increased labyrinthine pressure, and irritation of the auditory nerve-endings from other causes. In rare cases the head noises originate external to the ear, as, for instance, in the adjacent blood-vessels, as a result of muscular contraction, or they may be due to hallucination. These latter varieties of tinnitus are seldom due to labyrinthine affection, and usually occur as the result of maladies entirely distinct from the ear, as, for example, in mental diseases or in affections of the carotid artery or jugular vein.

Diagnosis.—The diagnosis will depend much upon the presence of the above symptoms and upon the results of the physical examination. The appearance of the drum membrane and the state of patency of the Eustachian tube are not of so much diagnostic importance in diseases of the perceptive portion of the ear as are the physical changes in these structures in disease of the conducting apparatus. In uncomplicated cases of labyrinthine deafness, particularly when the deafness has been sudden in its onset, the drum membrane will more than likely be normal in appearance and the Eustachian tube will most probably be found normally open. A sudden deafness, therefore, in a case in which the conducting apparatus is found upon inspection to be normal is highly indicative of disease of the perceptive portion of the ear. Progress in the deafness is, on the other hand, very frequently accompanied by marked changes in the structure of both the Eustachian tube and drum membrane, and these changes are clearly demonstrable when examined objectively. In this class of aural affection the labyrinthine disease is secondary to the middle-ear affection, which is a mixed lesion whose exact nature can only be determined by a combination of the results of all the methods of examination, but principally by functional tests by means of tuning-forks.

The functional examination should, therefore, in no case be neglected, especially if the history of the affection points strongly toward disease of the perceptive portion of the ear. Tests by means of the voice, whisper, and acoumeter are essential to a determination of the degree of deafness for these particular sounds, but it is impossible by means of them to ascertain the particular part of the auditory apparatus which is at fault. For this latter purpose the tuning-forks (Fig. 115) are essential. It is a clinical fact that those who suffer from labyrinthine deafness hear the low notes of the tuning-fork relatively well by air conduction, whereas they hear the high notes relatively badly. The reverse of this is true in uncomplicated middle-ear affection. Beginning the functional examination with the lowest fork of the Hartmann set, and running to the highest, if it should be found that C_3 and C_4 are not heard at all, whereas those of the middle scale, C_1 and C_2, are heard quite well, it may be regarded as reasonably certain that the disease is labyrinthine. If in any case where the middle tones only are heard by air conduction it is found that vibrating C or C_1 when placed on the center line of the cranium is heard better in the least affected ear, and if held in firm contact with the mastoid is heard a shorter time than when held in close proximity to the same ear, the conclusion that the disease is labyrinthine will thereby be confirmed. In cases of mixed deafness—*i. e.*, when the deafness is due to disease both of the middle ear and labyrinth—the results of the tuning-fork examination are not always definite. Should bone conduction and air conduction be found equal in an ear that is profoundly affected, this fact would be indicative of a mixed deafness; particularly would such a conclusion be justified if the physical examination revealed a retracted, thickened drum membrane and a disturbed patency of the Eustachian tube.

When a bilateral affection of nearly equal degree exists, the perception of the vibrating fork when placed upon the median line of the cranium will be equal in each ear, whatever the cause of the deafness may be. If, however, the aural defect is in the labyrinth, the perception for the fork during the above test will be greatly shorter than normal. Abnormally short duration for Schwabach's test and a positive Rinné in the same individual are strongly indicative of perceptive deafness.

After it has been definitely decided that the defect lies in the perceptive portion of the hearing apparatus, it yet remains to be determined, if possible, whether the trouble is entirely in the labyrinth or whether it is in some portion of the trunk of the auditory nerve or center of perception in the brain. Localization in this respect is not always easy or possible. It has already been stated that cases of complete deafness occurring suddenly may often be regarded as having an origin either in the nerve trunk or auditory center. Should the latter be the seat of the disease other physical or mental phenomena will likely be present together with the deafness.

The results of treatment upon the hearing have also some diagnostic value, for, whereas in middle-ear affections inflation of the middle ear usually improves the hearing to some extent, such a result is not common in purely labyrinthine deafness. Should benefit result from treatment in any case it is usually slight and transitory. Moreover, the outcome of treatment in this class of aural affection is often quite the opposite to what is desired, the patient growing rapidly worse from the effect of air douches and catheter inflation of the tympanic cavity. Climatic changes do not, as a rule, produce such marked effects upon the hearing in purely labyrinthine as in uncomplicated middle-ear affections. Hence, an uninterrupted course of the disease under all conditions of climate is somewhat diagnostic of labyrinthine affection.

Since nausea and vertigo are symptoms of several other diseases, the particular cause of their occurrence in any case is a matter of no small importance. In a general way it may be stated that these symptoms, when accompanied by deafness and tinnitus aurium and without other assignable reason for their existence, may be attributed to the aural affection. It is now commonly believed that many cases of vertigo which were formerly attributed to stomach derangement were, in fact, the result of internal ear disease. Affections of the middle lobe of the cerebellum are productive of nausea and vomiting and a differential diagnosis is not always easy. Both cerebellar and labyrinthine disturbances may be similarly accompanied by these symptoms in so far as the severity of the actual disturbance in these directions go, but when due to an affection of the central cerebellar lobe the dizziness and nausea are accompanied by others, such as the constant tendency of the patient to fall either forward or backward, nystagmus, difficult speech, strabismus, paroxysms of pain in the occiput, and other more distant reflexes.

Differential Diagnosis Between Middle-ear and Labyrinthine Diseases

	Diseases of the Conducting Apparatus	Diseases of the Perceptive Apparatus
Pain.	Present only in the acute inflammatory affections.	Usually absent.
Deafness.	Present in greater or less degree in all cases. Usually moderate degree of function remains. Deafness never total. Hearing usually better in a noise.	Present in greater or less degree. Often profound and total. Hearing usually worse in a noise.
Tinnitus aurium.	Present in a large majority of cases.	Present in a large majority of cases.
Nausea and vertigo.	Absent in uncomplicated cases.	Present in many cases. Often a most prominent feature of the case.
History of case.	Usually history of injury or inflammation of ear. History of head colds and catarrhal states in early life, with aural discharge in many cases at some time during course of diseases. Frequently follows scarlatina, measles, la grippe, etc.	Often follows general disease, such as cerebrospinal meningitis, typhoid fever, mumps, syphilis, etc. Also scarlatina, measles, and la grippe, but in these latter ailments is secondary to tympanic affection.
Appearance of drum membrane.	Sunken, perforated, granulated, or thickened in the inflammatory variety. Tendon-white, thickened in whole or part, and sometimes contains chalky deposits in non-suppurative variety.	Normal in uncomplicated cases.
Condition of nasopharynx and Eustachian tube.	Adenoids and other nasal obstruction frequently present. Nasopharyngeal inflammation common. Eustachian tube often narrowed.	Adenoids, nasopharyngeal inflammations, and nasal growths absent, or if present no causative relationship to aural affection can be traced. Eustachian tube normal.
Climatic changes.	Conditions of weather affect hearing greatly. Hearing better during bright dry state, worse during damp, cold days.	Have but little or no effect upon hearing or tinnitus.
Effect of catheter inflation.	Usually some improvement in hearing.	No improvement in hearing. Patient often made worse.
Tuning-forks.	Low tones heard relatively bad by air conduction. Vibrating tuning-fork C heard longer by bone than by air conduction. Rinné $\frac{a\,c}{b\,c}$. Vibrating C fork on median line of cranium heard best in worst ear. (Weber test.)	Low notes heard relatively well by air conduction. Vibrating fork C heard longer by air than by bone conduction. $\frac{A\,C}{B\,C}$ Rinné +. Vibrating C fork on median line of cranium heard best in best ear. (Weber test.)

The **prognosis** in disease of the perceptive portion of the auditory apparatus is, in the majority of instances, unfavorable. The nature of the pathology, together with the inaccessible situation of this class of diseases, is largely responsible for the unsatisfactory termination. In some instances, as, for example, in mumps and syphilis, the perceptive mechanism may be hopelessly injured from the first, whereas if the trouble is due only to the irritation of the auditory nerve-endings from an increased pressure of the endolymph, the same may be subsequently absorbed and the perceptive portion of the organ be thereby, at least partially, restored to the normal. When secondary to an injury the damaged labyrinth may also be partially restored and the same may be said of labyrinthine syphilis, provided the true nature of the disease be diagnosed early and an appropriate treatment be at once vigorously instituted.

The *treatment* will be given in connection with the description of the individual diseases comprising this class of aural affections.

DISEASES OF THE LABYRINTH DUE TO CIRCULATORY DISTURBANCES

I. ANEMIA OF THE LABYRINTH

Causation.—Anemia of the labyrinth stands among the mildest of the affections of the internal ear. It is often a mere local expression of a constitutional impoverishment of the blood and, as such, becomes one of the symptoms of general anemia. The cause of this particular affection is, therefore, the same as that which is responsible for the constitutional ailment. Thus, a severe hemorrhage occurring in any part of the body may so deplete the system as to produce immediate disturbance of hearing, vertigo, and nausea. On the other hand, the cause may have come on more slowly and as the result of a prolonged and exhaustive illness, of malnutrition, or perhaps of rapid childbearing. Certain drugs, when administered in excessive amounts or for prolonged periods, are productive of cerebral anemia and, with it, of labyrinthine anemia. Chief among these drugs may be mentioned the bromids of sodium and potassium, hydrobromic acid, and ergot.

Symptoms.—The aural symptoms of this disorder are deafness, tinnitus, and vertigo. The degree of deafness is usually slight and partakes more of the nature of an exhausted perception for sound rather than of an actual defect of hearing. The perceptive mechanism suffers from a similar lack of tone to that which characterizes the mental and physical activities of the individual, all of which are more or less impaired. While the patient seems able to hear almost normally, he is nevertheless conscious that he must constantly put forth an effort to do so and, as a result, it is found tiresome to carry on a prolonged conversation. The tinnitus aurium which accompanies anemia of the labyrinth is to some extent at least produced in the venous circulation of the large cervical veins, and hence it partakes somewhat of the character of the bruit often heard by the examiner during an examination of these vessels in anemic subjects. The noises heard by the patient are, therefore, usually described as more or less continuous and low pitched in character. The vertigo is rather the result than otherwise of the predisposition of the patient toward this affection, which is, of course, greatly increased by the general and labyrinthine anemia. Hence when the individual so affected is quiet, both in mind and body, there may be absolutely no dizziness present; whereas a trivial mental or bodily excitement may give rise to very distressing disturbances of equilibrium, the patient perhaps undergoing a severe faint.

Diagnosis.—The diagnosis of labyrinthine anemia will be justified by the history of a recent hemorrhage or serious illness, by the pallor of the skin and mucous membranes, and by a microscopic blood-count. In addition a physical and functional examination of the ear are essential. The appearance and position of the membrana tympani will usually be normal and the condition of the Eustachian tube will be that of its usual patency. By means of the functional tests it will be ascertained that perception for spoken words is slow, and that the hearing for the higher notes is considerably reduced. The C tuning-fork is heard by bone conduction for a much shorter time than normal.

Prognosis.—The prognosis is good in cases which have resulted from general hemorrhage, and from exhaustive diseases which of themselves, or through judicious treatment, are capable of restoration to the normal. When caused by pernicious anemia or by malignant or incurable disease the aural complication will likely grow worse instead of better, and in some cases the hearing will be lost because of the accompanying degeneration of the auditory nerve.

Treatment.—An effort should be made at the earliest possible moment to correct the cause of the general anemia. Hence if loss of blood continues, as, for example, in bleeding piles, metrorrhagia, or epistaxis, the cause of such waste should at once be remedied. Impoverishment of blood as a consequence of digestive disorder must receive proper medicinal and dietary attention. Regulation of all the habits of the individual, including care as to the amount and quality of the food and the proper amount of exercise and rest, is all that is required to bring about a cure in many cases. The improvement may often be hastened by the administration of drugs. The combination of remedies contained in the elixir of calisaya, iron, and strychnin is valuable in this respect, since the calisaya is an excellent tonic and stomachic, the iron furnishes a needed element in blood making, and the strychnin acts as a stimulant to the sluggish endings of the auditory nerve. Local treatment of the ear is usually not indicated.

II. HYPEREMIA OF THE LABYRINTH

This affection may be of an active or passive nature and may be either primary or secondary. Primary hyperemia of the labyrinth is a rather rare affection, whereas that which is secondary to a similar circulatory disturbance of the meninges or to a congestion or inflammation of the middle ear is of more common occurrence.

Causation.—The primary variety usually results from a general condition of plethora of the individual or from a stasis due to some mechanical interference with the return venous circulation. In the first instance any severe bodily exertion may give rise to the affection and overstimulation of the heart as a result of the use of alcoholics may bring about the same end. Ascent to a great height, as in a balloon or upon a mountain, brings about a labyrinthine hyperemia in conjunction with the general increased flow of blood to the surface of the body. Among other primary causes may be mentioned overeating, gout, rheumatism, and the ingestion of certain drugs. Ether, quinin, or salicin and its compounds, when taken in large and frequently repeated doses, will cause an increased flow of blood to the labyrinth. A more moderate dosage may produce only a physiologic hyperemia, whereas if taken in large quantity, serous effusion into the membranous capsule may result or a hemorrhage into the labyrinth may follow.[1] Passive hyperemia results from any cause which retards the venous return of the labyrinthine circulation. Hence the position of the body, as when the head is hanging down; the thoracic obstruction which occurs during prolonged fits of sneezing, coughing, or from holding the breath while straining, swimming, or diving, are all factors in the production of this particular aural disturbance.

Secondary labyrinthine hyperemia occurs as the result of an extension through the channel of the internal auditory meatus of a similar hyperemia of the meninges; or the disease may enter the labyrinth from without, the affection having first traversed the Eustachian tube and middle ear. Thus, on the one hand, the labyrinthine disease in question may be only a symptom of meningitis, encephalitis, etc., while on the other, it may be a symptom of measles, scarlet fever, la grippe, or other infectious ailment which has a special tendency to involve the middle ear primarily and the inner ear secondarily.

Symptoms.—A feeling of fulness in the head and moderate impairment of hearing may be the only symptoms of the mild and transitory case; such, for instance, as that which results from mountain climbing, sudden, violent exertion, or from hanging the head downward. In cases where the congestion is prolonged or is the result of more serious causes the tinnitus may be violent and may be accompanied by vertigo, disturbed

---

[1] Kirchner, of Wurzburg, administered large doses of quinin to rabbits, which were subsequently killed and the effect upon the ears noted. It was found that congestion and hemorrhage had taken place, both into the labyrinth and middle ear.

equilibrium, and nausea.   A plethoric state of the individual is usually indicated by the tendency toward inflammatory affections and also by the hyperemic state of the capillaries of the skin of the face, particularly of the nose.   In primary congestion the hearing is only moderately affected, whereas when it occurs secondarily to severe inflammatory diseases of the brain or middle ear the loss of function may be very considerable or even complete.

Diagnosis.—In the diagnosis of this affection the history of the mode of onset and progress of the disease, as well as the results of the physical and functional examination of the ear, must be taken into account.   When the labyrinthine hyperemia is primary and due to general plethora the drum membrane will usually show evidences of increased vascularity, just as will the integument of the face and nose. In the secondary variety, particularly when the labyrinthine disorder follows some very active inflammatory state of the drum cavity, the appearance of the drum membrane will be governed by the amount and character of the tissue changes that have taken place in the middle ear, and these will in no way be indicative of the presence of an inner ear complication.   Secondary labyrinthine affections cannot, therefore, be determined by means of the physical appearance of the fundus of the ear.

The severe examples of labyrinthine hyperemia may simulate Ménière's disease.   Indeed, it is probable that such a hyperemia is the immediate precursor of a labyrinthine apoplexy.   Hence it may sometimes be difficult to distinguish the one from the other, except after a lapse of time; for whereas if the case is one of hyperemia only, subsidence of the congestion with recovery will in time probably occur, while if an actual hemorrhage has taken place into the labyrinth such a marked result will scarcely be attained.

Functional tests will show that low notes will usually be heard better than high ones and that bone conduction is better than air conduction.

Prognosis.—Should the affection be recent and due to such causes as overindulgence in food, stimulants, or exercise, improvement or cure may be anticipated.   When occurring as a result of a retarded venous circulation due to the pressure of tumors, when the result of chronic alcoholism, or when secondary to serious inflammatory lesions of the meninges or middle ear, the outlook is not so hopeful and a return to normal is not to be anticipated.   Should hemorrhage into the labyrinth have taken place, a most unfavorable prognosis should be given (see p. 531).

Treatment.—The management of this affection should be determined by its cause in any particular case. Hence, if the result of errors of diet, the excessive use of alcoholics, or of violent and excessive bodily exertion, the individual must be instructed to correct the fault by returning to habits more moderate and normal. Evidences of active labyrinthine hyperemia in plethoric subjects require depletion by purgation, diaphoresis, or the abstraction of blood. In instances where the symptoms are severe and there is great danger of hemorrhage into the labyrinth, 2 or 3 ounces of blood should at once be abstracted from the mastoid region by means of the artificial leech (Fig. 75). If cerebral apoplexy seems threatening, a greater quantity of blood may be more advantageously withdrawn from the arm. In milder cases dependence may be placed upon purgation and sweating. Salines should be given in doses sufficiently large to secure several watery stools. Meanwhile the patient is advised to remain quiet in bed with the head elevated. If satisfactory improvement does not follow the administration of the foregoing measures, pilocarpin should be employed, either in addition or as a substitute. This drug is believed to have an especial value when used in cases where there has been, in addition to the labyrinthine hyperemia, a serous effusion into the membranous capsule. Iodid of potassium is also a remedy of value in case labyrinthine effusion has already occurred, but is of greatest service when employed in those that have not yielded readily to other measures and, therefore, in cases that are subacute or chronic.

III. LABYRINTHINE HEMORRHAGE, MÉNIÈRE'S DISEASE

Causation.—Extravasation of blood into the labyrinth often follows an active hyperemia, particularly when the latter occurs in persons with atheromatous blood-vessels. The hemorrhage may follow a rapidly developed hyperemia of the labyrinth, such, for instance, as accompanies scarlet fever, measles, mumps, variola, and typhoid fever. Postmortem examination of the inner ears of those who have died from suffocation usually reveals ecchymotic areas upon the membrane covering the lamina spiralis, the membrane of the vestibule, and of the ampullæ. The low state of vitality which accompanies pernicious anemia is conducive to the occurrence of small labyrinthine ecchymosis. Those employed in architectural construction requiring several hours each day to be spent in a caisson have been found to suffer from labyrinthine hemorrhages. The chief danger to the labyrinth from this latter cause seems to occur from the too rapid release of the pressure within the vessel in which the workmen are confined.

Labyrinthine hemorrhage may also be of traumatic origin. Severe

34

injuries to the skull, resulting in fracture of the petrous portion of the temporal bone, results in rupture of the blood-vessels of the parts, and the bleeding, therefore, occurs from direct injury. A hemorrhage in this part may, however, take place as a result of concussion of the skull, in which instance the cause acts more or less indirectly. Caries and necrosis of the portion of the temporal bone in which the inner ear is situated is also responsible for some cases of ecchymosis of part of the membranous capsule or of free bleeding into one or more of the labyrinthine spaces. Operative measures in the middle ear, undertaken with a view of removing or mobilizing the stapes, may, if undue force or rudeness is exerted, result in a hemorrhage into the vestibule.

Symptoms.—The symptoms of this affection, which is sometimes called apoplectiform deafness, constitute a complex very commonly known as Ménière's disease. The patient is often suddenly seized with aural vertigo and vomiting of such severity that he falls as from a cerebral apoplexy, and is subsequently unable to sit or stand erect without support, chiefly because of the increased vertigo and nausea. Deafness, which is more or less complete, constantly accompanies the above-marked features of the disease. Complete unconsciousness apparently occurs in the worst cases, although it is characteristic of this disease that the patient is all the time fully aware of his surroundings and can subsequently narrate all that has transpired during the height of the attack. Premonitions of labyrinthine hemorrhage occur in cases of chronic congestion of the middle ear. These take the form of a heaviness about the head, some unsteadiness of gait, and an increase of the previous tinnitus aurium. After the occurrence of the apoplexy the head noises are very much intensified and are often quite intolerable. Genuine cases of Ménière's disease occur most frequently in persons of middle life and of plethoric habit, and in whom the above symptoms take place with a suddenness comparable with that of an individual affected by a severe and genuine cerebral apoplexy. During and immediately subsequent to the labyrinthine hemorrhage the face appears pale and anxious and is covered with a profuse perspiration.

The objective symptoms are either negative or similar to those accompanying labyrinthine hyperemia. If the middle ear is implicated, ecchymotic areas may show in the drum membrane. A careful functional examination shows that both air and bone conduction are greatly lessened or even absent. Perception for the C fork may be equal for both air and bone conduction. It sometimes happens that there is complete loss of hearing for all tones with the exception of that for a small portion of the scale; or gaps in the scale may be found to exist;

that is, in testing all parts of the scale there may be complete deafness for certain tones, then an "island" of perception is discovered, which, being succeeded by an area of deafness, is in turn followed by one capable of perceiving certain sounds. These phenomena of function are explained by the probable fact that the hemorrhage has destroyed certain portions of the basilar membrane in portions of the cochlea, leaving undisturbed only partially destroyed areas between.

The above symptoms usually continue, sometimes to a lessened, but often in a progressively aggravated, degree. Should the immediate apoplectiform symptoms subside sufficiently to permit the patient to be up and around, he usually walks with an unsteady gait, which is made better or worse by every trivial error in diet or exercise. The hearing power often grows progressively worse instead of better and ultimately ends in total deafness. The severity of the tinnitus bears a close relationship to the degree of deafness, but sometimes disappears altogether when the hearing is entirely lost.

Diagnosis.—The diagnosis should usually be made if a majority of the above symptoms are present in a marked degree. Ménière's disease may be mistaken for cerebral apoplexy, but in the latter affection symptoms of paralysis of the tongue, face, or extremities usually quickly shows the cerebral nature of the case, whereas if the inner ear only is involved these paralyses are absent and the other symptoms, together with the functional examination, point strongly to the ear as the seat of the lesion.

Prognosis.—It has already been pointed out in what has been said concerning the causation and diagnosis that the prognosis of this affection is usually unfavorable. In mild cases of recent occurrence partial recovery takes place. The lost hearing can seldom be restored and relapses of the vertigo and tinnitus are the rule.

Treatment.—The same measures that were recommended for the treatment of labyrinthine hyperemia are indicated in case of hemorrhage into this portion of the ear. When the patient is seen during the attack and is plethoric. general blood-letting should be immediately practised. In those only moderately full blooded, natural or artificial leeches may be sufficient. The patient should be put to bed with the head elevated. A hot mustard foot-bath may be administered simultaneously with the employment of other measures intended to relieve the cerebral congestion. Saline purgatives should be given for the double purpose of clearing the digestive tract and of acting as a derivative.

Following the subsidence of the active symptoms, either naturally or as a result of treatment, the diet should be carefully regulated; severe exercise, either mental or bodily, should be prohibited, and the state of the bowels, especially constipation, should be overcome by the use of cascara sagrada and salines. Two drugs are believed to exert an influence in hastening the absorption of effusions of blood or serum into the labyrinth. These are potassium iodid and pilocarpin, the methods of administering which, as well as the resulting action of the same, has been described in another chapter (see p. 529).

IV. EMBOLISM OR THROMBOSIS

These affections of the labyrinth are, no doubt, among the rarest of internal ear disorders. It is possible, however, that, owing to the difficulty with which such occurrences are recognized, the occlusion of the labyrinthine vessels by a blood-clot is not often recognized, a fact which would account for the supposed rarity of the affection.

The cause lies either in the presence of a thrombus in some distant part, from which an embolus, either infected or sterile, is transported to the labyrinth; or the thrombosis of the labyrinthine veins may occur as a result of the direct extension of a thrombus in some of the venous sinuses in the immediate vicinity of the inner ear (see Fig. 274). The thrombus may also extend directly to the labyrinth from the veins of the middle ear during the severe suppurative processes which take place in that cavity during the course of the exanthemata.

Symptoms.—Since the occlusion of the labyrinthine vessel, especially by an embolus, takes place suddenly, it should be expected that the resulting aural symptoms would be correspondingly sudden. The hearing power may or may not be affected, this depending much upon whether or not the vessels supplying the cochlea are occluded or whether the obstruction is in one of the venules of the vestibule or ampullæ of the semicircular canals. If in the former, some degree of deafness will undoubtedly follow, whereas if the latter parts are affected, tinnitus and vertigo will likely be the most prominent symptoms.

Objective symptoms are absent unless the affection is secondary to some variety of otitis media, in which instance the appearances of the fundus of the ear would correspond to that produced by the particular primary disease. The presence of tubal or nasopharyngeal affection is not found except as contributing factors in the production of any accompanying tympanic inflammation or suppuration.

Diagnosis.—The diagnosis is not easy, for the reason that obstruction to the labyrinthine circulation from the above causes gives rise to symptoms very closely resembling several other diseases of the internal ear, especially hyperemia, hemorrhage, and syphilis, in all of which deafness, nausea, vertigo, and impaired bone conduction constitute prominent symptoms. In any case in which vertigo and tinnitus come on suddenly in an otherwise healthy individual and these symptoms are not accompanied by impairment of hearing, it may be assumed, provided no middle-ear disease is present and bone conduction is found greatly diminished, that an embolus or thrombosis of the vestibular veins has occurred. Should more or less deafness accompany the tinnitus and vertigo, it is more probable that the cochlear veins are involved. It must be admitted, however, that a positive diagnosis can seldom be made.

Treatment.—Local treatment is not advisable. If any cause for the affection can be discovered, this should be eliminated, if possible, with a view to preventing a recurrence of the trouble. For the relief of the tinnitus aurium and vertigo, pilocarpin and potassium iodid may be given internally, as described on p. 529. The administration of bromids or of dilute hydrobromic acid are most effectual for the relief of the head noises.

CHAPTER XLIV

INFLAMMATION OF THE LABYRINTH

I. PRIMARY OTITIS INTERNA

BECAUSE of its depth and protected situation, inflammation of the labyrinth, which begins as a primary disease, is among the rarest of aural affections. Voltolini and Politzer have mentioned instances in which labyrinthine inflammation occurred entirely independent of otitis media, meningitis, or other disease of an inflammatory nature. The primary affection occurs in children who are otherwise healthy up to the moment of seizure with deafness, fever, vomiting, delirium, and sometimes unconsciousness and convulsions. All these symptoms subside within a few days, with the exception of the vertigo and deafness, both of which persist for some weeks and may last for an indefinite period. Labyrinthine inflammation may be mistaken for meningitis, which it greatly simulates, and time alone furnishes the best data for a differential diagnosis; for whereas the disease in question may run its course in a few days, the symptoms of meningitis usually persist for many weeks, and the resulting effects of the latter disease upon the auditory apparatus are more marked and lasting.

II. SECONDARY OTITIS INTERNA (ACUTE)

Causation.—While an acute inflammatory involvement of the labyrinth occurs usually as one of the results of scarlet fever, measles, diphtheria, typhus or typhoid fever, it has also been known to complicate an acute otitis media which follows traumatic injury to the drum membrane and middle ear, to follow the accidental entrance of fluids into the Eustachian tube, and to occur subsequent to the infection of the tympanum from pathogenic bacteria during severe attacks of tonsillitis or nasopharyngitis. Age is a predisposing cause of the extension of the inflammation from the middle ear to the labyrinth. Young children are more frequently affected than adults, for the reason that the osseous partition between the several portions of the labyrinth and middle ear is thinner in early than in later life, and for the further reason that nasopharyngeal obstruction is common at this age; and, moreover, the chief cause of acute secondary labyrinthine inflamma-

534

tion—namely, the acute infectious diseases—occur chiefly during child-hood.

In the mildest cases of acute otitis media purulenta the internal ear is probably but seldom involved in a secondary inflammation; in the more severe forms of tympanic suppuration otitis interna more frequently complicates the primary aural affection, whereas in the violently de-structive forms of the otitis media, especially those due to scarlatina, the labyrinth is sometimes exposed by caries or necrosis of the inner tympanic wall, infection of the labyrinthine fluids takes place, and a suppurative otitis interna results. This latter affection, sometimes designated panotitis, deserves a separate discussion.

Symptoms.—The symptoms are those which accompany affections of the labyrinth in general—namely, sudden deafness, tinnitus aurium, vertigo, and vomiting. The onset of the extension of the inflammation to the cavities of the inner ear is very frequently not recognized at the time, either for the reason that the child is too young to enable the examiner to obtain accurate information concerning the nature of the disease or else the accompanying symptoms of the scarlet fever or other causative general ailment which is present are so severe as to overshadow the aural complication, or even to preclude an examination for the purpose of determining its existence. In cases of longer standing there is a history of present or remote middle-ear suppuration, and back of all this is the history of the child having had some general infective disease, as, for example, scarlet fever, typhoid, or typhus fever.

Diagnosis.—In addition to the history of the case, which includes a recital of the above symptoms, the physical examination will show more or less damage to the drum membrane and middle ear. Indeed, any one or more of the many pathologic conditions of the membrana tympani and tympanic cavity which have been described in the chapter devoted to Acute Otitis Media Purulenta may be found present in this disease. The functional examination is here, as in all affections of the labyrinth, an absolute essential to correct diagnosis. If, in a suspected case of secondary otitis interna, it is found that the tuning-forks C_2, C_3, and C_4 are heard badly or are not heard at all by air conduction; if it is found that Rinné is positive, and that the C fork by Weber's test is heard best in the *good* ear, it may be safely stated that the perceptive portion of the ear is involved. It must be remembered in all cases of secondary labyrinthinitis that a mixed deafness is present; that is, a deafness which is due both to a hindrance of the passage of the sound-waves through the conducting apparatus and to an impairment of the perception of the same.

It should, therefore, be expected that the functional tests will give results which differ from those found when the disease is either purely labyrinthine or purely tympanic. Thus, the tests may indicate a normal relationship as to the duration of perception for a given sound by both air and bone conduction, but the actual duration of the hearing for each test will be greatly reduced. In very young children, and even in older ones who are yet too young to give intelligent information concerning the functional tests, an exact diagnosis is impossible; but, during the progress of an acute exanthema, the labyrinthine complication may always be strongly suspected if, in addition to a middle-ear suppuration, there is suddenly added profound deafness, annoying tinnitus, vertigo, and vomiting.

Prognosis.—The prognosis as to recovery of the hearing is not good, yet undoubtedly there are many cases in which recovery takes place and the function is restored to a useful degree. The tinnitus aurium usually subsides as the hearing improves and it may also disappear entirely in case the function is entirely destroyed. Likewise the vertigo and nausea, when present at first, may gradually improve and finally subside altogether, even in cases where the labyrinth is entirely destroyed by the severity of the inflammation.

Treatment.—The plan of treatment must be decided by the nature and extent of the pathologic conditions present in the ear and by the length of time that has elapsed since the beginning of the disease. Prophylaxis should, when opportunity offers, play an important part in the management of these cases. During an attack of the exanthemata or of the acute infectious disease the liability of the general affection to this aural complication should not be forgotten. Middle-ear abscess should be given early and free drainage by a free incision of the drum-head just so soon as the collection of pus or other fluid is discovered in the tympanic cavity. Under such circumstances it is unwise to permit nature to take its course, to await a rupture through the drum membrane, and the subsequent establishment of imperfect tympanic drainage. Provision for a free outflow of intratympanic fluids in these cases will undoubtedly prevent extension to the labyrinth in a large proportion of those so affected. If a rupture of the membrana tympani has already occurred the ear should be managed as outlined in the chapter on Acute Otitis Media Purulenta, great care being exerted to prevent mixed infection, and to secure a free outflow of all the necrotic inflammatory products until healing has taken place. As a matter of course, such general medication should be given as may be indicated by the nature of the particular general ailment, of which the aural disease is only a part.

When seen after the general disease has subsided and while the middle-ear affection is yet subacute, the internal remedies in which most reliance can be placed are potassium iodid and pilocarpin, the proper mode of administering which is stated on p. 529. It must be anticipated that the worst cases will not be improved greatly, in so far as the perceptive portion of the organ of hearing is concerned, by any method of treatment yet devised.

CHRONIC OTITIS INTERNA

Causation.—Mention has already been made of the fact that during the progress of a chronic adhesive inflammation of the middle ear or of a chronic suppurative otitis media a secondary involvement of the labyrinth may take place. The chronic secondary inflammatory state of the internal ear occurs, therefore, as a result of an extension of the middle-ear disease to the capsule of the labyrinth or to the membranous structures in which the acoustic nerve filaments terminate. Not every case of chronic dry middle-ear catarrh or of suppurative otitis media is complicated by an affection of the internal ear, but an extension to the perceptive apparatus, of some degree of severity, probably occurs in the course of these affections much oftener than is commonly recognized.

Symptoms.—The symptoms of chronic secondary inflammation of the labyrinth are those of mixed deafness and have, to some extent, been described in other chapters. The disease is distinguished from most other internal ear affections by its mode of onset, which is in most instances mild in the beginning, but progressive throughout its course. When resulting either from dry middle-ear catarrh or from suppurating otitis media the labyrinthinitis may not develop for several months or even years after the inception of the tympanic disease. Hence, the individual may state that whereas he has had a running ear for several years, that he had only recently become seriously deaf and greatly disturbed by the incessant head noises. It is in this particular form of deafness that the tinnitus aurium is often most intolerable. The character of these noises varies greatly in different persons and at different stages of the disease in the same person. The particular quality or quantity of the sound which is perceived by the patient depends, to some extent at least, upon the portion of the labyrinth most involved. Thus, when the cristæ and acusticæ are principally implicated, the tinnitus may be described as a rumbling, roaring, or booming noise. If the lower turn of the cochlea is the chief seat of the inflammation the noises are most likely to be high pitched and constant. The tinnitus may at first be limited to one ear and long periods of complete cessation of the head noises may occur.   As the disease progresses, however, the noises become continuous and only cease when the acoustic nerve-endings in the labyrinth have become destroyed or are, at least, insensible ,to sound perception.   It frequently happens that as soon as the tinnitus begins to abate in the ear first affected the opposite ear becomes involved, and rapidly assumes a condition, both as to the amount of deafness and the severity of the tinnitus, which is worse than that in the original ear.   In the worst cases the. patient, having no respite from the harassing and everpresent tinnitus, becomes finally despondent, neurasthenic, and sometimes suicidal.

Vertigo and nausea are frequently observed, but do not, as a rule, occur so suddenly as in other labyrinthine affections.   These symptoms are rarely of such severity as to interfere seriously with the individual's locomotion.   In this, as in other labyrinthine affections, a disturbance of the equilibrium is usually regarded as an indication of an implication of the semicircular canals, and may be due solely to an increased tension of the intralabyrinthine fluids, the restoration of which to the normal restores the patient to his usual static control.

Diagnosis.—The chief reliance must here, as in all labyrinthine affections, depend upon the results of an accurate functional examination. The result obtained by functional tests differs so little in this and the labyrinthine inflammation which is secondary to acute middle-ear suppuration that there is no occasion to repeat here what was said concerning the same matter under that heading.   There is this difference, however: In the chronic affection the patients are usually adults and there is no severe general illness at the time of the examination to obtund the intelligence and thus to interfere with the accuracy of the tests. More accurate results should, therefore, be obtained in this instance as a consequence of the employment of these tests.

Physical examination of the drum membrane and middle ear shows a variety of conditions dependent upon the cause of the tympanic affection which has been responsible for the spread of the disease to the inner ear.   In case the primary trouble was a chronic suppurative otitis media a great number of pathologic changes may be discovered, among which may be mentioned the presence of foul-smelling pus, granulations or polypi, perforation or destruction of the membrana tympani, complete absence or partial necrosis of one or more ossicles, and necrosis of the mucous membrane of the tympanic cavity with exposure and caries of some portion of the osseous walls of the middle ear.

Should the labyrinthine involvement be secondary to an adhesive middle-ear catarrh the drum membrane may appear normal in every particular or it may be alternately thickened and atrophic over different areas. Retraction of the drum-head, with ossicular displacement, adhesion, and ankylosis of the ossicular chain are commonly observed. The membrana tympani is at times thickened, opaque, and milk white in appearance; the landmarks are more or less obliterated and both ossicular chain and membrane are absolutely immovable to the suction of Siegle's otoscope.

Prognosis.—When labyrinthine inflammation is secondary to a suppurative otitis media the prognosis is, as a rule, more favorable than when it occurs subsequently to a hyperplastic otitis media. In other instances the involvement of the perceptive portion of the ear may be arrested, to some extent at least, provided the opportunity to treat the disease is given sufficiently early. When observed in connection with any variety of middle-ear disease which has been of long standing, and especially if there has been considerable necrosis of the soft or osseous structures, or if there has been much deposit of new connective tissue in the middle ear, a correspondingly great change in the labyrinth may be inferred, and the prognosis may, therefore, be regarded as very unfavorable. In those instances in which new tissue has been deposited in the capsule and the spaces of the labyrinth have thereby been narrowed or obliterated, the acoustic nerve-endings are destroyed and any favorable termination is therefore impossible. The prognosis, in cases where one ear is seriously involved and the other not at all or but slightly, is usually unfavorable for both the better as well as the bad ear, because the history of such cases shows that the better ear is sooner or later attacked and is often more rapidly impaired than was the first. In such instances the prognosis may be more favorable if the case is seen early and a proper line of treatment is promptly instituted.

Treatment.—Since no known treatment is capable of bringing about satisfactory results after once the disease is very chronic and extensive tissue changes have taken place both in the middle ear and labyrinth, it should, therefore, be borne in mind that all suppurative or hyperplastic processes of the tympanum should receive appropriate attention at the earliest possible time. Purulent otitis media, together with all its evil consequences—necrosis of soft and osseous structures, granulations, polypi, etc.—should be managed in its incipiency according to plans of treatment already given for these conditions (see Chapter XXVIII.). Likewise, the first stages of the adhesive catarrhal processes in the tympanic cavity should be treated so soon as discovered. Prophylaxis, therefore, should be regarded as the best possible treatment for this as for many other aural affections, and every child or young adult who has nasal or nasopharyngeal growths that interfere with free respiration and invite frequent inflammation must be regarded as an individual who is very likely to develop middle-ear disease, with possibly a subsequent labyrinthine inflammation. Attention to the diseases of the upper air tract in early life would undoubtedly eliminate many of the possibilities of later aural affection, and early rhinologic treatment, when necessary, is of greater value to the child than any attention, however skilfully applied, which may be instituted after the organ of hearing is chronically diseased or perhaps hopelessly destroyed.

CHAPTER XLV

LABYRINTHINE SYPHILIS

SPECIFIC involvement of some portion of the labyrinth or of the nervous mechanism supplying it constitutes one of the most frequent forms of primary disease of the perceptive apparatus, and may result either from hereditary or acquired syphilis. Packard (*Jour. Amer. Med. Assoc.*, June 15, 1901) found 4 cases of this affection in a total of 2500 consecutive cases of ear disease.

Symptoms.—These have many points in common with those occurring from other diseases of the labyrinth, among which are sudden and often complete deafness in one or both ears, vertigo, tinnitus aurium, and sometimes nausea. No symptom is, therefore, pathognomonic of the specific complication of the ear. In the hereditary form of the disease the deafness comes on more slowly and is frequently accompanied by inflammatory and ulcerative inflammations of the eye, which latter are also of syphilitic origin.

Diagnosis.—The diagnosis is seldom made except as a result of the more rigid physical examination of the body in general, and of the nose

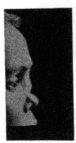

FIG. 301.—PARENT.

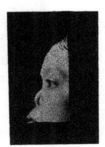

FIG. 302.—CHILD FIVE YEARS OLD.

and throat and eye and ear in particular (Figs. 301 and 302). Since the affection comes on either during the secondary or tertiary stages of the syphilis it is usually possible to discover some evidences of a specific nature upon the skin, upon the mucous membrane of the upper air tract, or in the structure of the eye. In the case of any individual, therefore, who is suddenly attacked by severe labyrinthine symptoms the skin should be inspected for the purpose of determining the presence of syphilis. Mucous patches may be found in the mouth, over the soft palate, or upon the tonsils if there is present a syphilis in the secondary stage, whereas if it has progressed to the tertiary stage, any portion of the hard or soft palate, the tonsils, or the postpharyngeal wall may be found swollen and red from the presence of a gumma; or the gumma may have already broken down, after which deep ulceration or even perforation of the hard or soft palate may be seen as a result. The author has observed one case of labyrinthine deafness due to syphilis, the sole objective evidence of which was found in an ulcerated condition of the epiglottis. The nose likewise furnishes frequent evidence of tertiary syphilis when no other part of the body suggests its presence. Thus, the nasal septum may be found swollen from a gumma or it may be widely perforated or even completely destroyed by the disease. The external deformity known as "saddle-back" nose is most

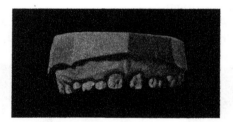

FIG. 303.—HUTCHINSON TEETH OF CHILD.
Note irregular setting and indentations of each tooth.

often due to syphilis. In addition to the above physical evidences of specific infection, the presence of enlarged lymphatics in the cervical, axillary, or inguinal regions may furnish helpful diagnostic information.

Children who suffer from labyrinthine deafness as a consequence of hereditary syphilis are not suddenly seized by the aural symptoms, as is the case in adults when following the acquired variety. The diagnosis of the nature of the labyrinthine affection in this class will usually be based upon the syphilitic history of the parent and upon the evidences of the syphilis itself as exhibited by corneal opacities or active ulceration of the cornea, and upon the presence of the peculiar arrangement and shape of the teeth, generally spoken of as the Hutchinson teeth (Fig. 303).

Since suppurative otitis media sometimes coexists with the syphilitic affection of the labyrinth, the symptoms due to the latter may be attributed entirely to the middle-ear disease unless a differentiation is made by means of functional tests with the tuning-forks. It should be remembered that in case of specific diseases of the labyrinth, as in all other ailments involving the perceptive apparatus, that air conduction for the vibrating C fork will probably be better in the worse ear than bone conduction (Rinné—); that when the vibrating fork is placed upon the center line of the skull it is usually heard longest in the better ear, and that the high tones, especially those above C_3, are often not heard at all.

Examination of the fundus of the ear in most cases of labyrinthine disease due to syphilis shows a healthy drum membrane, and unless a nasopharyngitis is present the Eustachian tube will be found patent when catheter inflation is practised.

Politzer (*Diseases of the Ear*) states that labyrinthine syphilis may occur without the presence of any other symptom of a general infection being discoverable at the time. However, a thorough examination of the skin, the upper respiratory tract, and the eyes of any suspected case will usually enable the diagnostician to find sufficient evidence of syphilis to justify a diagnosis of specific labyrinthinitis in any case where this disease has been the primary cause of the internal ear affection.

Prognosis.—Should the labyrinthine affection be of acquired variety and of only short duration, the prognosis is somewhat favorable, at least in so far as improvement of the deafness, tinnitus, and vertigo is concerned. Cases of long standing, which have progressed unhindered by proper treatment, particularly if in persons of debilitated habit or of advanced age, are likely to grow worse despite any form of treatment. The prognosis is also bad should there have previously existed an adhesive catarrhal otitis media or a suppurative otitis. Inherited labyrinthine syphilis is more unfavorable in its prognosis than is the acquired variety, the disease being often of a progressive nature and continuing until total deafness results.

Treatment.—Specific labyrinthine deafness should be treated at the earliest possible moment by the administration of those drugs most suited to the particular stage of the syphilis in which the labyrinthine disturbance occurs. Should the deafness and dizziness appear during the secondary stage both mercury and the iodids are indicated, the former being given until its full physiologic effect is produced, whereas the latter may be administered in moderate doses. On the other hand, when labyrinthine symptoms rapidly develop during the tertiary period, the iodids accomplish a better purpose than the mercury, and hence should be pushed even to the administration of 3 or 4 dr. of the drug in the twenty-four hours. In this stage mercury is secondary in value to the iodids, but may be given in the form of an iodid or bichlorid, especially if for any reason the iodids of potassium or sodium are badly borne. Mercurial inunctions also provide a good means of giving mercurials and have the decided advantage of saving the stomach for the administration of the more important iodids of potassium or sodium.

Specific medication is not so effective in the treatment of hereditary syphilis and consequently not of the labyrinth complication. Syphilitic children do better when care is given to secure their best nourishment and to insure for them a maximum of time to be spent in the open air and sunshine. Ferruginous tonics and cod-liver oil are helpful in the badly nourished cases.

Local treatment of the ears in any variety of syphilitic inflammation, except in those suffering from a coexisting middle-ear disease, is useless and probably harmful.

CHAPTER XLVI

LABYRINTHINE DISEASES DEPENDENT UPON GENERAL AFFECTIONS

REFERENCE has many times been made in the several chapters of this work to the effect upon the hearing produced by certain constitutional diseases, chiefly those of an infectious character. Among the general diseases that are most likely to be accompanied or followed by an aural complication are the exanthemata, especially scarlatina and measles, epidemic cerebrospinal meningitis, meningitis, typhus and typhoid fever, mumps, syphilis, and influenza. All these affections may seriously impair or even completely destroy the function of the labyrinth. They may attack the labyrinth in the following ways: (a) The systemic infection, of whatever nature it may be, may act directly upon the labyrinthine structures solely through the blood supply to this portion of the ear; (b) pathogenic material may be transported from an infective or suppurative disease of the cerebrum or cerebellum to the labyrinth, through the intercommunicating blood and lymph canals, or the infection may take place more directly through either the vestibular or cochlear aqueducts; (c) the labyrinthine implication may be secondary to a tympanic suppuration, in which case the infection usually finds its way inward into the labyrinth, through the common blood supply of these two divisions of the hearing apparatus. On the other hand, the pus may enter the vestibule or cochlea directly from the middle ear through a perforation in the inner tympanic wall, which has resulted from an osseous necrosis.

Chief among the general diseases which affect the labyrinth through an extension of some infection from the brain coverings, the several forms of meningitis, including epidemic cerebrospinal meningitis, should be mentioned. The labyrinth is perhaps most commonly infected through the medium of the blood-current in typhoid and typhus fever, mumps, and syphilis. Labyrinthine complications when secondary to middle-ear suppuration may follow a number of diseases, chief among which are scarlet fever, measles, la grippe, infective tonsillitis, and diphtheria.

35   545

Epidemic cerebrospinal meningitis is frequently followed by disease of the labyrinth and consequently by an impairment of function which sometimes amounts to total deafness. Beginning at about the end of the second week of the disease the infective inflammation of the meninges, which characterizes the primary disease, may extend into the internal auditory meatus, along the sheaths of the facial and auditory nerves, and finally implicate the various structures comprising the internal ear. Instead of inflammation traveling from the meninges to the labyrinth by this route, actual pus from the meninges may take its way along the same path into the labyrinth. Likewise an inflammation or the actual products of suppuration may enter the labyrinth through one of the aqueducts.

The *symptoms* of the labyrinthine complication, when arising during the process of the cerebrospinal meningitis, are in the beginning the sudden onset of more or less deafness, accompanied by pain in the ear and tinnitus aurium. These symptoms may rapidly increase in severity until a high degree of deafness or even total deafness results. Should the patient be unconscious or even much stupid at the time the labyrinth is so involved, the presence of the above symptoms will not be known until sufficient mentality has been restored to the patient to enable him to recognize the defect.

The deafness due to this cause is usually bilateral and, in case recovery from the meningitis results, is accompanied by intense tinnitus aurium and disturbed equilibrium, the latter sometimes being present to the extent that walking is impossible. When the degree of deafness is total the head noises usually subside and the unsteadiness of gait in time improves and finally disappears. The facial nerve is sometimes injured by the disease during its passage through the internal auditory meatus, and as a result facial paralysis is added to the patient's list of misfortunes, which may also include blindness and the arrest of development or total suspension of mentality. In young individuals deaf-mutism is a common sequence, even in cases in which the cerebrospinal meningitis was not severe.

The *prognosis* in deafness due to this disease is unfavorable for the reason that the damage wrought to the labyrinthine structures is of such nature that restoration is impossible. The outlook for improvement in the hearing is regarded as better in those cases in which the disease is accompanied by tinnitus aurium, for, so long as the head noises are perceived, this fact furnishes evidence that at least some portion of the organ of Corti is still intact.

Treatment of this form of deafness is usually of little consequence.

If the labyrinthine involvement is recognized at the moment of its onset during the progress of the meningitis, the aural ice-bag should be applied to one or both mastoid processes and kept on for two or three days without intermission, while at the same time all other symptoms of the meningitis are met by means most appropriate to the individual case. During convalescence an effort should be made to absorb the exudates that have presumably been left in the labyrinth, and this can best be done by the administration, first, of pilocarpin and, later, of the iodids of sodium and potassium. If a child, and the resulting deafness is too great to permit hearing for the speaking voice, the patient should be sent to an institution for the education of the deaf so soon as the proper age is attained.

Constitutional Diseases which May Implicate the Labyrinth Chiefly through an Infection by the Blood Supply to the Inner Ear.—The diseases included in this classification may also rarely cause middle-ear suppuration, the particular pathogenic bacteria of the disease finding their way into the middle ear through the Eustachian tube (see Chapter on Bacteriology).

Typhus and Typhoid Fever.—During the progress of these diseases it is frequently observed that deafness in some degree—often very severe—has occurred. This may sometimes be attributed to the impaired and often almost completely suspended mentality of the patient which is present as a result of the direct action upon the cerebrum of the specific poison of the typhoid or typhus state. When the deafness is due to this cause, improvement in the hearing takes place subsequently and coincident with the convalescence from the primary disease. Instances are, however, met with in which marked deafness and tinnitus persist indefinitely after recovery from the specific fever, and the functional tests in such cases point unmistakably to an involvement of the labyrinth. In nearly all such cases an objective examination of the drum membrane and middle ear shows nothing abnormal.

The *prognosis* is unfavorable. Local treatment is usually without effect upon the hearing and the internal administration of strychnin and other nerve stimulants offers the best chance of improvement, which, under all circumstances, is likely to be but slight.

Mumps.—The tendency of mumps toward a metastatic involvement of the testes, ovaries, and breasts is well known, and an explanation of the occurrence of deafness during an attack of parotitis has been made upon similar grounds. Whatever the nature of the virus of mumps may be, in the purely labyrinthine cases of deafness which result from its deposit in the inner ear, the effect seems most often to be upon the auditory nerve itself, and to finally cause more or less complete atrophy of its trunk.

The *symptoms* are the onset, during the first week of the mumps, of deafness which is more or less profound, together with the occurrence of tinnitus aurium and sometimes a staggering gait. Both ears are affected in about one-half of all cases. Adults are as frequently affected as children. Pain in the ear is uncommon and usually little or no fever is present, except the same be due to the mumps itself. Sometimes the deafness precedes the swelling of the parotid glands. The labyrinthine complication of mumps is much more frequent in some epidemics than in others.

The *diagnosis* can be made from the known tendency of mumps to affect the perceptive portion of the ear and by means of the tuning-forks, which will show that, whereas the hearing is greatly impaired, bone conduction will be very poor, and in the worst cases the vibration will not be heard at all through the bone. Upon otoscopic examination it will usually be seen that the drum membrane is normal in every re-. spect, and by catheter inflation it may be demonstrated that the normal patency of the Eustachian tube has in nowise been disturbed.

The *prognosis* in this, as in most other affections of the labyrinth, is not very hopeful. Except in the early stages of the complication and in the mildest cases treatment has little effect in restoring the hearing. The best results are obtained by tonic and restorative methods. If increased labyrinthine pressure is indicated by the presence of severe tinnitus and disturbed equilibrium and the patient is plethoric, the administration of saline purgatives and pilocarpin will prove most effective in the absorption of the excessive labyrinthine exudates and consequently in the restoration of function.

Syphilis.—The affect of this disease upon the labyrinth has already been considered (see Chapter XLV.).

General Diseases which Secondarily Affect the Labyrinth through First Establishing a Suppurative Otitis Media.—To this class belong the exanthameta, especially scarlet fever and measles; certain infective general diseases, as diphtheria and la grippe; certain throat inflammations and infections, as the different forms of tonsillitis. The pathogenic bacteria which are present in the pharynx and nasopharynx during the progress of these several affections find entrance through the Eustachian tube into the middle ear, where a violent inflammation and speedy suppuration is at once set up. In a considerable percentage of these cases of otitis media suppurativa the septic products find their way into the labyrinth either through an opening the result of a previous necrosis of the intervening osseous structures or by transportation of the pathogenic bacteria through the blood or lymph channels. In either case extensive damage is done to the perceptive portion of the ear and total deafness may be the consequence (see Chapter XLVIII.). Since the various diseases named under this head act first and chiefly upon the tympanic structures, a more complete consideration of their relation to aural diseases is given in another section of the work (see Chapter XXIV.).

CHAPTER XLVII

LABYRINTH SUPPURATION WITH CARIES AND NE-CROSIS OF THE PETROUS PORTION OF THE TEM-PORAL BONE

INFECTION and subsequent suppuration within the several channels and cavities comprising the labyrinth is now known to occur with considerable frequency. Greater attention to diagnostic methods in the examination of the middle ear, together with more frequent and extensive operations upon the temporal bone for the cure of suppurative

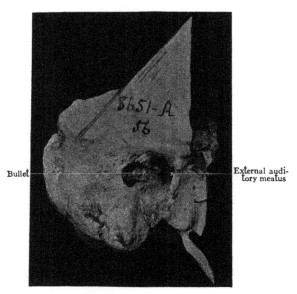

FIG. 304.—COMPOUND FRACTURE OF PETROUS PORTION OF THE TEMPORAL BY LEAD BULLET.
(Warren Museum, Harvard Medical School. J. Orne Green Collection.)

diseases within, have not only demonstrated the frequency of internal ear suppuration but have also stimulated operators to greater activity in determining the correct methods of cure. Indeed the successful invasion of the labyrinth by surgical means may be classed among the greatest of the many recent achievements of operative otology. The cause of such suppuration may be a previously existing middle-ear

550

discharge, or it may result from severe injuries which cause fracture of the temporal bone, as in Figs. 304 and 305.

Symptoms.—The subjective symptoms of an infection and subse_ quent suppuration of the labyrinth are of themselves but little or not at all different from those occurring when the middle and inner ear are involved from other causes. The patient complains of deafness, aural discharge, dizziness, some degree of tinnitus, pain, and frequently of facial paralysis. The deafness may appear suddenly in the course of what is believed to be an ordinary case of suppurative otitis media and may vary in degree from a moderate impairment to a total inability to hear. The affection is usually uni- lateral. Head noises are, as a rule, less troublesome in this disease than in other affections of the inner ear, possibly for the reason that the auditory nerve terminals were in the beginning of the disease de- stroyed. When the semicircular canals are involved the amount of vertigo may be so great as to compel the patient to remain for a consid- erable time in a recumbent position.

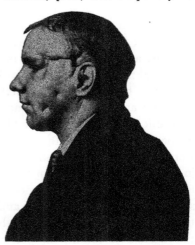

FIG. 305.—CASE OF TRAUMATIC MASTOIDITIS, LABYRINTHINE SUPPURATION, TOTAL DEAFNESS IN INJURED EAR, AND FACIAL PARALYSIS ON AF- FECTED SIDE.

Pain is present on the affected side when the labyrinthine suppura- tion has been of such severe character as to cause caries or necrosis of some part of the petrous portion of the temporal bone. When a seques- trum is forming and during the process of its separation and expulsion there is of necessity much irritation or actual injury to the sensory nerves supplying the parts, and as an inevitable result more or less pain is present, and severe hemorrhage. The pressure resulting from the excessive growth of granulation tissue or polypi from the environment of the sequestra is also responsible for the pain in many cases.

Facial paralysis is a symptom of nearly all cases of labyrinth infec- tion in which there is subsequent suppuration and necrosis. The location of the facial nerve in its tortuous course through the petrous bone would render its injury an almost certainty in every case of exten- sive necrosis and sequestra of the labyrinth. Of 35 cases of labyrinth suppuration and necrosis reported by Bezold, there was only partial facial paralysis in 6; whereas in the remainder there was a very decided paralysis. Should the necrosis of the petrous portion occur at the internal meatus both the facial and auditory nerves, because of their intimate relation at this point, are almost certain to be destroyed, in which instance total deafness and complete facial paralysis will simultaneously result.

Diagnosis.—*Physical Examination.*—Because of the long-continued suppuration the patient is sometimes septic, and this, together with the pain and loss of sleep, may give the individual a worn and haggard look. When absorption of pathogenic products has taken place or when there has been an extension of the disease to the meninges, both the pulse and temperature may be increased. Inspection of the auditory canal and middle ear will detect the aural discharge. The drum membrane will be perforated and perhaps largely destroyed. Granulations or polypi are frequently present, sometimes to the extent of filling the tympanic cavity and external auditory meatus. All the physical changes in the tympanic cavity that were described in the chapters on Chronic Purulent Otitis Media and Chronic Mastoiditis may be found present in this disease. In fact, mastoiditis and suppuration and necrosis of the labyrinth are so often associated in the same case that every effort should be made during the examination of any case of discharge from the middle ear to determine if the suppurative path has been toward the mastoid or toward the petrous portion of the temporal bone; and when the intratympanic exploration has been thorough, it is sometimes found that both portions of the temporal bone have been involved.

The methods of making this examination have already been described and need not be repeated here (see Chapter XXVI.). Should exfoliation of some portion or the whole of the labyrinth already have occurred, the sequestrum may be discovered by the probe as a loose mass of bone embedded in the surrounding granulations. The sequestra thus thrown off may vary in size from that representing the whole labyrinth to that which includes only the cochlea or one semicircular canal. In the former instance the separated mass would be too large to find its way outward through the external auditory meatus; whereas if only the cochlea or one of the semicircular canals is thrown off, the same may be found lying loosely in the tympanic cavity or even in the external auditory meatus, from which it is ultimately discharged or extracted.

Prognosis.—Considering the fact that the labyrinth is surrounded on two sides by dura mater and that the carotid artery and petrosal sinuses pass respectively through the petrous portion of the bone and lie in immediate contact with it, it seems rather remarkable that suppuration and necrosis within the labyrinth is not followed by a greater fatality than is indicated by statistics. In the cases reported by Bezold death occurred in about 20 per cent., the cause of death being due usually to an extension of the infection to the meninges. In those in which spontaneous recovery took place there was an exfoliation of the whole or some portion of the labyrinth, with subsequent discharge of the sequestrum through the external auditory meatus, and in one case through the Eustachian tube into the nasopharynx. In several of the cases cure followed some form of mastoid operation which provided a channel sufficiently wide to permit the extraction of the exfoliated labyrinth. Following a complete exfoliation of the labyrinth healing of the resulting cavity takes place either by means of the cavity filling with granulation and osseous tissue or by an extension into it of the epidermis from the external auditory meatus, by which the space is ultimately lined by a dermoid layer and finally becomes dry.

The prognosis as to function is bad, since if the cochlea is necrosed and exfoliated the auditory nerve terminals are completely and permanently destroyed. In case only the semicircular canals are thrown off and the labyrinth is left, a considerable degree of hearing may remain. The facial nerve possesses remarkable power of regeneration and hence, if the trunk has only been injured through pressure or but a short portion of its course is destroyed, it is probable that more or less complete restoration will take place, and motion will be again possible in the paralyzed facial muscles. Should, however, a considerable portion of the Fallopian canal be swept away, and with it the contained portion of the trunk of the facial nerve, it is entirely improbable that the nerve will be regenerated or that the facial paralysis will ever be improved (see Chapter XXX.).

Treatment.—The treatment of this disease is wholly surgical. In the earlier stages, when the diagnosis remains doubtful, the method of treatment advocated for suppurative otitis media should be employed. When seen at a later period, and the external auditory meatus is found filled with granulations or polypi, it may be necessary to remove these by means of a snare or curet before it is possible to determine the presence of a labyrinthine suppuration or necrosis, and, therefore, before a plan of operative treatment can be outlined. Since the surgery of the labyrinth is always best performed in connection with the radical mastoid operation, the reader is referred to the chapter which deals with this latter procedure (see Chapter XXX.).

CHAPTER XLVIII

DEAF-MUTISM

Definition.—This term is applied to individuals who, because of an early inability to hear spoken language, are both deaf and dumb. Deaf-mutism may be either congenital or acquired. In case of acquired deaf-mutism the child may have lost the hearing before the age when speech is normally learned; or in older children some degree of child language may have been acquired before the damage to the ears has occurred, but this is afterward lost because it can be no longer heard or practised. In the case of children who have lost the hearing power as late as the age of eight or ten, it is probable that ability to speak such language as has already been learned will to some extent be indefinitely retained. In such instances, however, the patient, no longer hearing the sound of the words, ultimately forgets both their combination of tone and accent and is, therefore, no longer able to pronounce them with distinctness; in many instances the speech of such individuals is harsh, irritating to the healthy ear, the words are badly enunciated and hence are difficult, for those unaccustomed to the peculiarities of the vocabulary and accent, to understand.

Pathology.—Some of the pathologic findings in deaf-mutes are as follows: The nerve-fibers in the modiolus are lessened in number. Ganglionic cells in the spiral canal may be few in number. There may be new formation of bone in the scala tympani and the lamina spiralis may be entirely wanting. The vestibular and cochlear windows may be filled with newly formed bone; ganglionic cells may fail or, having once formed, may later atrophy or degenerate. In the aqueductus cochlæ new growths composed of bone, connective tissue, or nerve tissue may take place. Failure of development of some of the essential parts may occur and the lamina spiralis membranacea may be wanting; again, there may be no organ of Corti or spiral ligament with its stria vascularis. The organ of Corti may be stunted (flat) or the hair-cells lacking. There may be a displacement of Reisner's membrane.

Causation.—Congenital deaf-mutism is, in the great majority of cases, the result of heredity or of the intermarriage of those closely related, as, for example, of first cousins. Mr. Graham Bell, in a study of 2262 congenital deaf-mutes, states that there were deaf-mutes in the immediate families of more than one-half of the near relatives, or of 1232. Nevertheless, direct transmission of this defect is not so common, for in Hartmann's statistics it is shown that of 276 couples, of whom one, either the father or mother was a deaf-mute, there were born only 11 children who were congenitally deaf, of a total number of 419 children. When both parents are deaf-mutes, Bell states that about one-third of all the children are born deaf.

Marriage of those of close blood relationship is, therefore, a frequent cause of congenital deaf-mutism. The immediate offspring resulting from such marriage may be deaf or the defect may not occur until the second or third generation. Statistics relative to deaf-mutism as a result of close intermarriage vary, according to different writers, from 6 to 25 per cent. of all children born to such parents. The number of deaf-mutes in proportion to a stated population found in different countries varies very greatly. Thus, in Switzerland the number of deaf-mutes to each 100,000 population has been as high as 245, whereas in Holland, the number per 100,000 has been as low as 43. In certain countries the proportion is, as stated by Wilde, as high as 1 to every 206 of the population. The high rate in Switzerland is accounted for on the ground that in this country the intermarriage of those closely related is a common custom. Opposed to the theory that consanguineous marriage is responsible for the large number of deaf-mutes in Switzerland, Wishard, who lived for eleven years in Persia, where he practised medicine, states that he never saw a case of deaf-mutism there which was due to this cause, although consanguineous marriages are very common.

Acquired deaf-mutism is more frequent than the congenital variety. While statistics on this point vary somewhat, the most reliable information seems to indicate that about twice as many cases are acquired as are congenital. However, Hartmann states that of 8404 cases of deaf-mutism, 66 per cent. were congenital. Between the years of 1844 and 1900, 2227 deaf-mutes were admitted to the Indiana Institution for the Education of the Deaf. Only 754 of this number, or less than 34 per cent., according to the records, were congenitally deaf. The records of deaf and dumb institutions are not entirely reliable concerning this point, for the reason that the statements of the parents concerning the cause of the deafness are relied upon, whereas a most careful physical examination of the ear is necessary to determine whether or not there has been a middle-ear disease present which has been a cause of the impaired perception subsequent to the birth of the child.

Acquired deaf-mutism is the result (a) of primary affections of the ear due to injuries or to suppurative otitis media; (b) of general diseases, the exanthemata, la grippe, typhoid fever, mumps, whooping-cough, and congenital syphilis; (c) of inflammatory affection of the meninges, as cerebrospinal meningitis and simple meningitis. Following any of the above-named general or local diseases the deafness is caused by an extension of the inflammatory or suppurative process into the labyrinth, either from the meninges, in case of meningitis, or from the tympanic cavity when the middle ear is the seat of a violent inflammation.

Diagnosis.—Infants exhibit no evidence of the perception of sounds before the age of four months, and hence it is impossible prior to this period to determine the presence of deafness. Practically speaking, the behavior of the child seldom arouses the suspicion of congenital deafness before it arrives at the age when it should begin to speak articulate words. Hovell says that the ability of a child to repeat the words "papa" and "mamma" is no evidence that it has ever heard these words, for he believes even very young children learn to read the lips of parents who frequently repeat these words while the infant is watching the necessary mouth movements. Even when the child has passed the age when it should be able to begin speaking, many parents are apt to assign some reason other than deafness as a cause of the backwardness in this respect. The opinion that the child has no defect of audition is many times firmly fixed in the minds of the parents of the congenitally deaf, for the reason that they think the infant perceives such noises as are produced by walking across the floor, slamming a door, the falling of a weight, or the passing of heavy wagons in the street. The totally deaf soon acquire a most acute general sensibility, and the above instances of supposed hearing, as stated, are really instances of feeling, the jar of the noise-producing body causing some behavior on the part of the child which is interpreted as effected by hearing. The slamming of a door awakens the child from its sleep or the footsteps of the mother on the floor attract the child to turn around, but not because it hears the sound of either. The statements of the parents regarding the hearing of suspected deaf children are, therefore, misleading, and hence some means of examination of function must be chosen which the child can neither see nor feel. A fairly satisfactory functional test may be conducted as follows: While the child sits upon the floor or in the lap of an attendant it should be completely entertained in some way. The examiner stands behind the child and should not be seen by it. A series of gongs or tuning-forks may be used for making the test.   It is essential to ascertain first whether or not there is total absence of perception for moderately loud noises.   For this purpose the series of Japanese gongs are convenient.   Each bell of the series may be struck with a mallet, while at the same time some competent witness is noting the effect, if any, upon the infant's facial expression. Should the child hear any of the sounds thus produced a pleased and intelligent expression of the face is noted, while at the same time it will turn toward the source of sound.   Should it be determined with certainty that some degree of hearing is present, the Hartmann set of tuning-forks may then be used and the effect, if any, of the same upon the child's face, at the same time be carefully noted.   If these experiments are conducted in such manner as to eliminate the possibility of impressions reaching the child through either sight or jar, and the child shows no change of countenance during the time, it may be reasonably certain that a high degree of deafness is present.   Physical evidence of congenital deaf-mutism may be present in the form of atresia of the external auditory canals, but this is rare as a bilateral defect.

The diagnosis of acquired deafness may be made by the above methods, especially in cases where the aural disease which destroyed the hearing occurs at an age prior to that at which speech has been acquired.   In cases occurring at an age after some degree of speech had already been acquired, but was subsequently lost, the history of the case will be helpful, and a physical examination of the middle ear, in connection with a functional examination by means of tuning-forks, will leave no doubt concerning the nature of the defect.   It should never be understood that total deafness is an essential to deaf-mutism, for such is certainly not the case, since in any individual who in early life hears the human voice only when spoken loudly and near by deaf-mutism is certain to develop.   A large percentage of the inmates of institutions for the education of the deaf are able to hear loud noises, and sometimes to distinguish words or sentences when spoken in a loud voice and close to the ear.   Bezold found among 276 deaf-mutes only 79 who were absolutely deaf.

Prognosis.—The prognosis as to restoration of hearing and the acquirement of speech is extremely unfavorable. Politzer and Hartmann state that cases of congenital deafness sometimes improve, and the former author says that the prognosis is much better in the congenital than in the acquired variety. Occurring as the result ·of measles, scarlet fever, diphtheria, or cerebrospinal meningitis the prognosis is always bad, no case of recovery having as yet been recorded.

Treatment.—When directed toward the cure of the deafness, treatment of the aural condition is usually hopeless. On the other hand, when the treatment is given with a view to the improvement of the child's health and to the proper development of its mental faculties, much good can often be accomplished. If the defect of speech and hearing has resulted from some disease which has left a chronic discharging ear, this should be treated according to the principles stated in the chapter on Chronic Otitis Media Purulenta. Much discussion has arisen of late concerning the causative relation of enlarged tonsils and adenoids to deaf-mutism, and as to the effect upon the deaf-mutism resulting from their complete removal. There can be no question concerning the evil results of these growths when considered in the rôle of predisposing factors in the causation of aural suppuration; and especially is this true when these pharyngeal and nasopharyngeal obstructions are present during attacks of the exanthemata, to which all children are liable. However influential may have been the original causative relation between adenoids and deaf-mutism, when the latter is once established as a result of the more or less complete destruction of the perceptive portion of the organ of hearing, it is extremely doubtful if the subsequent removal of the tonsils and adenoids has ever improved the deaf-mutism materially in any case. As a prophylactic measure and as a means of improving the physical and mental condition of the child, these growths should in every case be thoroughly removed.

In children who have suffered severe damage to both ears as a result of scarlatina or other like disease, but who nevertheless retain enough hearing to distinguish words spoken in a loud voice, it is highly essential that care be taken to give frequent opportunity to such children to hear spoken words and sentences, since otherwise deaf-mutism will be rapidly acquired, when it should have been in some measure at least prevented. Children too deaf to be effectually educated in the ordinary way in the public schools must be sent, at the age of seven or eight, to institutions especially provided for this unfortunate class.

Institutions for the education of the deaf give instruction by three principal methods: (1) Entirely by means of sign language; (2) by the purely oral method, and (3) by the combination of the sign and oral methods. Each of these plans has its advantages and advocates. The sign method is easiest to learn, but the deaf-mute is subsequently at the disadvantage of being unable to converse with the outside world and is put to the constant necessity of communicating with those about him by means of writing. When educated by the oral method the individual is able to converse with those about him provided the mouth of the person with whom he talks is visible and the articulation is proper. Efficient training by this method requires a period of six or eight years in most children. The combination of sign and oral methods gives the obvious advantage of being able to converse by either, but it is asserted that the child will usually neglect the oral for the use of the manual, until finally he is unable to use but the one method efficiently.

INDEX

Peterson *and* Haines' Legal Medicine & Toxicology

A Text-Book of Legal Medicine and Toxicology. Edited by FREDERICK PETERSON, M. D., Professor of Psychiatry in the College of Physicians and Surgeons, New York; and WALTER S. HAINES, M. D., Professor of Chemistry, Pharmacy, and Toxicology, Rush Medical College, in affiliation with the University of Chicago. Two imperial octavo volumes of about 750 pages each, fully illustrated. Per volume: Cloth, $5.00 net; Sheep or Half Morocco, $6.50 net. *Sold by Subscription.*

IN TWO VOLUMES—BOTH VOLUMES NOW READY

The object of the present work is to give to the medical and legal professions a comprehensive survey of forensic medicine and toxicology in moderate compass. This, it is believed, has not been done in any other recent work in English. Under "Expert Evidence" not only is advice given to medical experts, but suggestions are also made to attorneys as to the best methods of obtaining the desired information from the witness. An interesting and important chapter is that on "The Destruction and Attempted Destruction of the Human Body by Fire and Chemicals." A chapter not usually found in works on legal medicine is that on "The Medicolegal Relations of the X-Rays." This section will be found of unusual importance. The responsibility of pharmacists in the compounding of prescriptions, in the selling of poisons, in substituting drugs other than those prescribed, etc., furnishes a chapter of the greatest interest to every one concerned with questions of medical jurisprudence. Also included in the work is the enumeration of the laws of the various states relating to the commitment and retention of the insane.

OPINIONS OF THE MEDICAL PRESS

Medical News, New York

"It not only fills a need from the standpoint of timeliness, but it also sets a standard of what a text-book on Legal Medicine and Toxicology should be."

Columbia Law Review

"For practitioners in criminal law and for those in medicine who are called upon to give court testimony in all its various forms . . . it is extremely valuable."

Pennsylvania Medical Journal

"If the excellence of this volume is equaled by the second, the work will easily take rank as the standard text-book on Legal Medicine and Toxicology."

Church and Peterson's
Nervous *and* Mental Diseases

Nervous and Mental Diseases. By Archibald Church, M. D., Professor of Nervous and Mental Diseases and Medical Jurisprudence, Northwestern University Medical School, Chicago; and Frederick Peterson, M. D., President New York State Commission on Lunacy; Professor of Psychiatry at the College of Physicians and Surgeons, N. Y. Handsome octavo, 937 pages; 341 illustrations. Cloth, $5.00 net; Sheep or Half Morocco, $6.50 net.

JUST ISSUED—NEW (5th) EDITION

This work has met with a most favorable reception from the profession at large. It fills a distinct want in medical literature, and is unique in that it furnishes in one volume practical treatises on the two great subjects of neurology and psychiatry. In preparing this edition Dr. Church has carefully revised his entire section, placing it in accord with the most recent psychiatric advances. In Dr. Peterson's section — Mental Diseases — the Kræpelin classification of insanity has been added to the chapter on classifications for purposes of reference, and new chapters on Manio-Depressive Insanity and on Dementia Præcox included. While the changes throughout have been many, they have been so made as but slightly to increase the size of the work.

OPINIONS OF THE MEDICAL PRESS

American Journal of the Medical Sciences

" This edition has been revised, new illustrations added, and some new matter, and really is two books. . . . The descriptions of disease are clear, directions as to treatment definite, and disputed matters and theories are omitted. Altogether it is a most useful text-book."

Journal of Nervous and Mental Diseases

" The best text-book exposition of this subject of our day for the busy practitioner· · · · The chapter on idiocy and imbecility is undoubtedly the best that has been given us in any work of recent date upon mental diseases. The photographic illustrations of this part of Dr. Peterson's work leave nothing to be desired."

New York Medical Journal

· To be clear, brief, and thorough, and at the same time authoritative, are merits that ensure popularity. The medical student and practitioner will find in this volume a ready and reliable resource."

Frühwald and Westcott's
Diseases of Children

Diseases of Children. A Practical Reference Book for Students and Practitioners. By PROFESSOR DR. FERDINAND FRÜHWALD, of Vienna. Edited, with additions, by THOMPSON S. WESTCOTT, M. D., Associate in Diseases of Children, University of Pennsylvania. Octavo volume of 533 pages, containing 176 illustrations. Cloth, $4.50 net.

RECENTLY ISSUED

This work represents the author's twenty years' experience, and is intended as a practical reference work for the student and practitioner. With this reference feature in view, the individual diseases have been arranged alphabetically. The prophylactic, therapeutic, and dietetic treatments are elaborately discussed. The practical value of the book has been considerably enhanced by the many excellent illustrations.

E. H. Bartley, M. D.,

Professor of Pediatrics, Chemistry, and Toxicology, Long Island College Hospital, New York.
"It is a new idea, which ought to become popular because of the alphabetic arrangement. Its title expresses just what it is—a ready reference hand-book."

Ruhräh's
Diseases of Children

A Manual of Diseases of Children. By JOHN RUHRÄH, M. D., Clinical Professor of Diseases of Children, College of Physicians and Surgeons, Baltimore. 12mo of 404 pages, fully illustrated. Flexible leather, $2.00 net.

RECENTLY ISSUED

In writing this manual Dr. Ruhräh's aim was to present a work that would be of the greatest value to students. All the important facts are given concisely and explicitly, the therapeutics of infancy and childhood being outlined very carefully and clearly. There are also directions for dosage and prescribing, and a number of useful prescriptions are included. The feeding of infants is given in detail, and the entire work is amply illustrated with practical illustrations. A valuable aid consists in the many references to pediatric literature, so selected as to be easily accessible by the student.

Brower and Bannister on Insanity

A Practical Manual of Insanity. For the Student and General Practitioner. By DANIEL R. BROWER, A. M., M. D., LL. D., Professor of Nervous and Mental Diseases in Rush Medical College, in affiliation with the University of Chicago ; and HENRY M. BANNISTER, A. M., M. D., formerly Senior Assistant Physician, Illinois Eastern Hospital for the Insane. Handsome octavo of 426 pages, with a number of full-page inserts. Cloth, $3.00 net.

FOR STUDENT AND PRACTITIONER

This work, intended for the student and general practitioner, is an intelligible, up-to-date exposition of the leading facts of psychiatry, and will be found of invaluable service, especially to the busy practitioner unable to yield the time for a more exhaustive study. The work has been rendered more practical by omitting elaborate case records and pathologic details, as well as discussions of speculative and controversial questions.

American Medicine

" Commends itself for lucid expression in clear-cut English, so essential to the student in any department of medicine. . . . Treatment is one of the best features of the book, and for this aspect is especially commended to general practitioners."

Bergey's Hygiene

The Principles of Hygiene: A Practical Manual for Students, Physicians, and Health Officers. By D. H. BERGEY, A. M., M. D., Assistant Professor of Bacteriology in the University of Pennsylvania. Octavo volume of 536 pages, illustrated. Cloth, $3.00 net.

RECENTLY ISSUED—SECOND REVISED EDITION

This book is intended to meet the needs of students of medicine in the acquirement of a knowledge of those principles upon which modern hygienic practises are based, and to aid physicians and health officers in familiarizing themselves with the advances made in hygiene and sanitation in recent years. This new second edition has been very carefully revised, and much new matter added, so as to include the most recent advancements.

Buffalo Medical Journal

" It will be found of value to the practitioner of medicine and the practical sanitarian ; and students of architecture, who need to consider problems of heating, lighting, ventilation, water supply, and sewage disposal, may consult it with profit."

Kerr's Diagnostics *of* Diseases *of* Children

Diagnostics of the Diseases of Children. By LeGrand Kerr, M. D., Professor of Diseases of Children, Brooklyn Postgraduate Medical School, Brooklyn. Octavo of 550 pages, fully illustrated. Cloth, $5.00 net ; Half Morocco, $6.50 net.

JUST READY—FOR THE PRACTITIONER

Dr. Kerr's work differs from all others on the diagnosis of diseases of children in that the *objective symptoms* are particularly emphasized. The author believes that as the objective symptoms are the main sources of information in diagnosing children's diseases, the subject should be discussed with these symptoms as the foundation. The constant aim throughout has been to render a correct diagnosis as early in the course of the disease as possible, and for this reason differential diagnosis is presented from the very earliest symptoms. The sequelæ of the various diseases have been considered only to the extent that they may be of value in anticipating them and thus aiding in their early diagnosis. The physician will find the many original illustrations a source of much information and help.

Kerley's Treatment *of* Diseases *of* Children

Treatment of the Diseases of Children. By Charles Gilmore Kerley, M. D., Professor of Diseases of Children, New York Polyclinic School and Hospital. Octavo of 550 pages, illustrated.

JUST ISSUED

This work has been prepared for the physician engaged in general practice. The author *presents all the modern methods of management and treatment in greater detail than any other work on the subject* heretofore published. The methods suggested are the results of actual personal experience, extending over a number of years of hospital and private practice. Every method, therefore, has been thoroughly tried and its value as a therapeutic measure proved. Special endeavor has been taken to have the illustrations of a practical nature.

Draper's Legal Medicine

A Text-Book of Legal Medicine. By FRANK WINTHROP DRAPER, A. M., M. D., Professor of Legal Medicine in Harvard University, Boston ; Medical Examiner of the County of Suffolk, Massachusetts, etc. Handsome octavo volume of 573 pages, fully illus.　Cloth, $4.00 net.

A NEW WORK—RECENTLY ISSUED

The subject of Legal Medicine is one of great importance, especially to the general practitioner, for it is to him that calls to attend cases which may prove to be medicolegal in character most frequently come. The medicolegal field includes not only deaths of a homicidal nature, but also suits at law—the fatal railway accident, machinery casualties, and the like, to which the neighboring physician may be called, and later, perhaps, summoned to court. It is evident, therefore, that every practitioner should be thoroughly versed in all branches of medicolegal science. This volume, although prepared as a help to medical students, will be found no less valuable and instructive to practitioners. The author has had twenty-six years' experience as Medical Examiner for the city of Boston, his investigations comprising nearly eight thousand deaths under a suspicion of violence.

Hon. Olin Bryan, LL. B.
Professor of Medical Jurisprudence, Baltimore Medical College
" A careful reading of Draper's Legal Medicine convinces me of the excellent character of the work. It is comprehensive, thorough, and must, of a necessity, prove a splendid acquisition to the libraries of those who are interested in medical jurisprudence."

Jakob *and* Fisher's Nervous System and its Diseases

Atlas and Epitome of the Nervous System and Its Diseases. By PROFESSOR DR. CHR. JAKOB, of Erlangen. *From the Second Revised German Edition.* Edited, with additions, by EDWARD D. FISHER, M. D., Professor of Diseases of the Nervous System, University and Bellevue Hospital Medical College, New York. With 83 plates and copious text. Cloth, $3.50 net. *In Saunders' Hand-Atlas Series.*

The matter is divided into Anatomy, Pathology, and Description of Diseases of the Nervous System. The plates illustrate these divisions most completely ; especially is this so in regard to pathology. The exact site and character of the lesion are portrayed in such a way that they cannot fail to impress themselves on the memory of the reader.

Philadelphia Medical Journal
" We know of no one work of anything like equal size which covers this important and complicated field with the clearness and scientific fidelity of this hand-atlas.'

De Lee's Obstetrics for Nurses

Obstetrics for Nurses. By JOSEPH B. DE LEE, M.D., Professor of Obstetrics in the Northwestern University Medical School; Lecturer in the Nurses' Training Schools of Mercy, Wesley, Provident, Cook County, and Chicago Lying-In Hospitals. 12mo volume of 460 pages, fully illustrated. Cloth, $2.50 net.

JUST ISSUED—NEW(2nd)EDITION

The illustrations in Dr. De Lee's work are nearly all original, and represent photographs taken from actual scenes. The text is the result of the author's eight years' experience in lecturing to the nurses of five different training schools.

J. Clifton Edgar, M. D.,
Professor of Obstetrics and Clinical Midwifery, Cornell Medical School, N. Y.
" It is far-and-away the best that has come to my notice, and I shall take great pleasure in recommending it to my nurses, and students as well."

Davis' Obstetric and Gynecologic Nursing

Obstetric and Gynecologic Nursing. By EDWARD P. DAVIS, A.M., M. D., Professor of Obstetrics, Jefferson Medical College and Philadelphia Polyclinic. 12mo of 400 pages, illustrated. Buckram, $1.75 net.

RECENTLY ISSUED—SECOND REVISED EDITION

The Lancet, London
" Not only nurses, but even newly qualified medical men, would learn a great deal by a perusal of this book. It is written in a clear and pleasant style, and is a work we can recommend."

Reference Handbook for Nurses

A Reference Handbook for Nurses. By AMANDA K. BECK, of Chicago, Ill. 32mo of 177 pages. Flexible leather, $1.25 net.

RECENTLY ISSUED

This little book contains information upon every question that comes to a nurse in her daily work, and embraces all the information that she requires to carry out any directions given by the physician.

Boston Medical and Surgical Journal
"Must be regarded as an extremely useful book, not only for nurses, but for physicians."

Hofmann and Peterson's Legal Medicine

Atlas of Legal Medicine. By Dr. E. von Hofmann, of Vienna, Edited by Frederick Peterson, M. D., Professor of Psychiatry in the College of Physicians and Surgeons, New York. With 120 colored figures on 56 plates and 193 half-tone illustrations. Cloth, $3.50 net. *In Saunders' Hand-Atlas Series.*

By reason of the wealth of illustrations and the fidelity of the colored plates, the book supplements all the text-books on the subject. Moreover, it furnishes to every physician, student, and lawyer a veritable treasure-house of information.

The Practitioner, London

" The illustrations appear to be the best that have ever been published in connection with this department of medicine, and they cannot fail to be useful alike to the medical jurist and to the student of forensic medicine."

Chapman's Medical Jurisprudence

Medical Jurisprudence, Insanity, and Toxicology. By Henry C. Chapman, M. D., Professor of Institutes of Medicine and Medical Jurisprudence in Jefferson Medical College, Philadelphia. Handsome 12mo of 329 pages, fully illustrated. Cloth, $1.75 net.

RECENTLY ISSUED—THIRD REVISED EDITION, ENLARGED

This work is based on the author's practical experience as coroner's physician of the city of Philadelphia for a period of six years. Dr. Chapman's book, therefore, is of unusual value.

This third edition has been thoroughly revised and greatly enlarged, so as to bring it absolutely in accord with the very latest advances in this important branch of medical science. There is no doubt it will meet with as great favor as the previous editions.

Medical Record, New York

" The manual is essentially practical, and is a useful guide for the general practitioner, besides possessing literary merit."

Golebiewski *and* Bailey's Accident Diseases

Atlas and Epitome of Diseases Caused by Accidents. By DR. ED. GOLEBIEWSKI, of Berlin. Edited, with additions, by PEARCE BAILEY, M.D., Consulting Neurologist to St. Luke's Hospital, New York. With 71 colored illustrations on 40 plates, 143 text-illustrations, and 549 pages of text. Cloth, $4.00 net. *In Saunders' Hand-Atlas Series.*

This work contains a full and scientific treatment of the subject of accident injury ; the functional disability caused thereby ; the medicolegal questions involved, and the amount of indemnity justified in given cases. The work is indispensable to every physician who sees cases of injury due to accidents, to advanced students, to surgeons, and, on account of its illustrations and statistical data, it is none the less useful to accident-insurance organizations.

The Medical Record, New York
" This volume is upon an important and only recently systematized subject, which is growing in extent all the time. The pictorial part of the book is very satisfactory."

Stoney's Materia Medica for Nurses

Practical Materia Medica for Nurses, with an Appendix containing Poisons and their Antidotes, with Poison-Emergencies ; Mineral Waters ; Weights and Measures ; Dose-List, and a Glossary of the Terms used in Materia Medica and Therapeutics. By EMILY M. A. STONEY, of the Carney Hospital, South Boston. 12mo of 300 pages. Cloth, $1.50 net.

RECENTLY ISSUED—NEW (3rd) EDITION

In making the revision for this new third edition, all the newer drugs have been introduced and fully discussed. The consideration of the drugs includes their sources and composition, their various preparations, physiologic actions, directions for administering, and the symptoms and treatment of poisoning.

Journal of the American Medical Association
" So far as we can see, it contains everything that a nurse ought to know in regard to drugs. As a reference-book for nurses it will without question be very useful."

Stoney's Nursing

Practical Points in Nursing: for Nurses in Private Practice. By EMILY M. A. STONEY, Superintendent of the Training School for Nurses at the Carney Hospital, South Boston, Mass. 466 pages, fully illustrated. Cloth, $1.75 net.

THIRD EDITION, THOROUGHLY REVISED—RECENTLY ISSUED

In this volume the author explains the entire range of *private* nursing as distinguished from *hospital* nursing, and the nurse is instructed how best to meet the various emergencies of medical and surgical cases when distant from medical or surgical aid or when thrown on her own resources. An especially valuable feature will be found in the directions how to *improvise* everything ordinarily needed in the sick-room.

The Lancet, London

"A very complete exposition of practical nursing in its various branches, including obstetric and gynecologic nursing. The instructions given are full of useful detail."

Stoney's Technic for Nurses

Bacteriology and Surgical Technic for Nurses. By EMILY M. A. STONEY, Superintendent at Carney Hospital, South Boston. Revised by FREDERIC R. GRIFFITH, M. D., Surgeon, of New York. 12mo, 278 pages, illustrated. Cloth, $1.50 net.

RECENTLY ISSUED—NEW (2d) EDITION

Trained Nurse and Hospital Review

"These subjects are treated most accurately and up to date, without the superfluous reading which is so often employed. . . . Nurses will find this book of the greatest value both during their hospital course and in private practice."

Spratling on Epilepsy

Epilepsy and Its Treatment. By WILLIAM P. SPRATLING, M. D., Medical Superintendent of the Craig Colony for Epileptics, Sonyea, New York. Octavo of 522 pages, fully illustrated. Cloth, $4.00 net.

The Lancet, London

"Dr. Spratling's work is written throughout in a clear and readable style. . . . The work is a mine of information on the whole subject of epilepsy and its treatment."

Griffith's Care of the Baby

The Care of the Baby. By J. P. CROZER GRIFFITH, M. D., Clinical Professor of Diseases of Children, University of Penn.; Physician to the Children's Hospital, Phila. 12mo, 455 pp. Illustrated. Cloth, $1.50 net.

JUST ISSUED—THE NEW (4th) EDITION

The author has endeavored to furnish a reliable guide for mothers. He has made his statements plain and easily understood, in the hope that the volume may be of service not only to mothers and nurses, but also to students and practitioners whose opportunities for observing children have been limited.

New York Medical Journal.
"We are confident if this little work could find its way into the hands of every trained nurse and of every mother, infant mortality would be lessened by at least fifty per cent."

Crothers' Morphinism

Morphinism and Narcomania from Opium, Cocain, Ether, Chloral, Chloroform, and other Narcotic Drugs; also the Etiology, Treatment, and Medicolegal Relations. By T. D. CROTHERS, M. D., Superintendent of Walnut Lodge Hospital, Hartford, Conn. .Handsome 12mo of 351 pages. Cloth, $2.00 net.

The Lancet, London
"An excellent account of the various causes, symptoms, and stages of morphinism, the discussion being throughout illuminated by an abundance of facts of clinical, psychological, and social interest."

Abbott's Transmissible Diseases

The Hygiene of Transmissible Diseases: Their Causation, Modes of Dissemination, and Methods of Prevention. By A. C. ABBOTT, M. D., Professor of Hygiene and Bacteriology, University of Pennsylvania. Octavo, 351 pages, with numerous illustrations. Cloth, $2.50 net.

SECOND REVISED EDITION

During the interval that has elapsed since the appearance of the first edition investigations upon the modes of dissemination of certain of the specific infections have been very active. The sections on Malaria, Yellow Fever, Plague, Filariasis, Dysentery, and Tuberculosis have been both revised and enlarged.

The Lancet, London
"We heartily commend the book as a concise and trustworthy guide in the subject with which it deals, and we sincerely congratulate Professor Abbott."

Register's Fever Nursing Just Issued

A TEXT-BOOK ON PRACTICAL FEVER NURSING. By EDWARD C. REGISTER, M.D., Professor of the Practice of Medicine in the North Carolina Medical College. Octavo of 350 pages.

The work completely covers the field of practical fever nursing. Just sufficient of pathology, symptoms, and treatment is given to enable the nurse to care for the patient intelligently. The work is thoroughly practical and nurses will find it most valuable. The illustrations show the nurse how to perform those measures that come within her province; such as bathing, hypodermoclysis, pulse and temperature taking, etc.

Hecker, Trumpp, and Abt on Children Just Ready

ATLAS AND EPITOME OF DISEASES OF CHILDREN. By Dr. R. HECKER and Dr. J. TRUMPP, of Munich. Edited, with additions, by ISAAC A. ABT, M.D., Assistant Professor of Diseases of Children, Rush Medical College, Chicago. With 48 colored plates, 144 text-cuts, and 453 pages of text. Cloth, $5.00 net.

The many excellent lithographic plates represent cases seen in the authors' clinics, and have been selected with great care, keeping constantly in mind the practical needs of the general practitioner. These beautiful pictures are so true to nature that their study is equivalent to actual clinical observation. The editor, Dr. Isaac A. Abt, has added all new methods of treatment.

Lewis' Anatomy and Physiology Recently Issued

ANATOMY AND PHYSIOLOGY FOR NURSES. By LEROY LEWIS, M.D., Surgeon to and Lecturer on Anatomy and Physiology for Nurses at the Lewis Hospital, Bay City, Michigan. 12mo of 317 pages, with 146 illustrations. Cloth, $1.75 net.

A demand for such a work as this, *treating the subjects from the nurses' point of view*, has long existed. Dr. Lewis has based the plan and scope of this work on the methods employed by him in teaching these branches, making the text unusually simple and clear.

The Nurses Journal of the Pacific Coast

"It is not in any sense rudimentary, but comprehensive in its treatment of the subjects in hand. The application of the knowledge of anatomy in the care of the patient is emphasized."

Friedenwald and Ruhräh's Dietetics Recently Issued

DIETETICS FOR NURSES. By JULIUS FRIEDENWALD, M.D., Clinical Professor of Diseases of the Stomach, and JOHN RUHRÄH, M.D., Clinical Professor of Diseases of Children, College of Physicians and Surgeons, Baltimore. 12mo volume of 365 pages. Cloth, $1.50 net.

This work has been prepared to meet the needs of the nurse, both in the training school and after graduation. It aims to give the essentials of dietetics, considering briefly the physiology of digestion and the various classes of foods and the part they play in nutrition.

American Journal of Nursing

"It is exactly the book for which nurses and others have long and vainly sought. A simple manual of dietetics, which does not turn into a cook-book at the end of the first or second chapter.

Paul's Fever Nursing Recently Issued

NURSING IN THE ACUTE INFECTIOUS FEVERS. By GEORGE P. PAUL, M.D., Assistant Visiting Physician to the Samaritan Hospital, Troy, N. Y. 12mo of 200 pages. Cloth, $1.00 net.

Dr. Paul has taken great pains in the presentation of the care and management of each fever. The book treats of fevers in general, then each fever is discussed individually, and the latter part of the book deals with practical procedures and valuable information.

The London Lancet

"The book is an excellent one and will be of value to those for whom it is intended. It is well arranged, the text is clear and full, and the illustrations are good."

Paul's Materia Medica for Nurses Just Issued

MATERIA MEDICA FOR NURSES. By GEORGE P. PAUL, M.D., Assistant Visiting Physician to the Samaritan Hospital, Troy. 12mo of 240 pages. Cloth, $1.50 net.

Dr. Paul arranges the physiologic actions of the drugs according to the action of the drug and not the organ acted upon. An important section is that on pretoxic signs, giving the warnings of the full action or the beginning toxic effects of the drug, which, if heeded, may prevent many cases of drug poisoning. The nurse should know these signs.

Pyle's Personal Hygiene Just Issued
The New (3d) Edition

A MANUAL OF PERSONAL HYGIENE: Proper Living upon a Physiologic Basis. By Eminent Specialists. Edited by WALTER L. PYLE, A. M., M.D., Assistant Surgeon to Wills Eye Hospital, Philadelphia. Octavo volume of 451 pages, fully illustrated. Cloth, $1.50 net.

To this new edition there have been added, and fully illustrated, chapters on Domestic Hygiene and Home Gymnastics, besides an appendix containing methods of Hydrotherapy, Mechanotherapy, and First Aid Measures. There is also a Glossary of the medical terms used.

Boston Medical and Surgical Journal

"The work has been excellently done, there is no undue repetition, and the writers have succeeded unusually well in presenting facts of practical significance based on sound knowledge."

Galbraith's Four Epochs of Woman's Life Recently Issued
Second Edition

THE FOUR EPOCHS OF WOMAN'S LIFE. By ANNA M. GALBRAITH, M.D. With an Introductory Note by JOHN H. MUSSER, M.D., University of Pennsylvania. 12mo of 247 pages. Cloth, $1.50 net.

Birmingham Medical Review

"We do not as a rule care for medical books written for the instruction of the public; but we must admit that the advice in Dr. Galbraith's work is in the main wise and wholesome."

Starr on Children Second Edition

AMERICAN TEXT-BOOK OF DISEASES OF CHILDREN. Edited by LOUIS STARR, M.D., assisted by THOMPSON S. WESTCOTT, M.D. Octavo, 1244 pages, illustrated. Cloth, $7.00 net; Half Morocco, $8.50 net.

American Pocket Dictionary

AMERICAN POCKET MEDICAL DICTIONARY. Edited by W. A. NEW-MAN DORLAND, M. D., Assistant Obstetrician to the Hospital of the University of Pennsylvania. Containing the pronunciation and definition of the principal words used in medicine and kindred sciences, with 64 extensive tables. Handsomely bound in flexible leather, with gold edges, $1.00 net; with patent thumb index, $1.25 net.

" I can recommend it to our students without reserve."—J. H. HOLLAND, M. D., *Dean of the Jefferson Medical College*, Philadelphia.

Morrow's Immediate Care of Injured

IMMEDIATE CARE OF THE INJURED. By ALBERT S. MORROW, M. D., Attending Surgeon to the New York City Hospital for the Aged and Infirm. Octavo of 340 pages, with 238 illustrations. Cloth, $2.50 net.

Dr. Morrow's book on emergency procedures is written in a definite and decisive style, the reader being told just what to do in every emergency. It is a practical book for every day use, and the large number of excellent illustrat'ons can not but make the treatment to be pursued in any case clear and intelligible. Physicians and nurses will find it indispensible.

Powell's Diseases of Children

ESSENTIALS OF THE DISEASES OF CHILDREN. By WILLIAM M. POWELL, M. D. Revised by ALFRED HAND, Jr., A. B., M. D., Dispensary Physician and Pathologist to the Children's Hospital, Philadelphia. 12mo volume of 259 pages. Cloth, $1.00 net. *In Saunders' Question-Compend Series.*

Shaw on Nervous Diseases and Insanity

ESSENTIALS OF NERVOUS DISEASES AND INSANITY: Their Symptoms and Treatment. A Manual for Students and Practitioners. By the late JOHN C. SHAW, M. D., Clinical Professor of Diseases of the Mind and Nervous System, Long Island College Hospital, New York. 12mo of 204 pages, illustrated. Cloth, $1.00 net. *In Saunders' Question-Compend Series.*

" Clearly and intelligently written; we have noted few inaccuracies and several suggestive points. Some affections unmentioned in many of the large text-books are noted."—*Boston Medical and Surgical Journal.*

Starr's Diets for Infants and Children

DIETS FOR INFANTS AND CHILDREN IN HEALTH AND IN DISEASE. By LOUIS STARR, M. D., Consulting Pediatrist to the Maternity Hospital, Philadelphia. 230 blanks (pocket-book size). Bound in flexible leather, $1.25 net.

Grafstrom's Mechano-Therapy

A TEXT-BOOK OF MECHANO-THERAPY (Massage and Medical Gymnastics). By AXEL V. GRAFSTROM, B. Sc., M. D., Attending Physician to the Gustavus Adolphus Orphange, Jamestown, New York. 12mo, 200 pages, illustrated. Cloth, $1.25 net.